Network Approaches to Diseases of the Brain

Edited by

Matt T. Bianchi

Sleep Division
Neurology Department
55 Fruit Street, Wang 7
Massachusetts General Hospital
Boston, MA 02114,
USA

Verne S. Caviness and Sydney S. Cash

Neurology Department
55 Fruit Street, Wang 7
Massachusetts General Hospital
Boston
MA, 02114
USA

CONTENTS

FOREWORD

Is it possible to make a walk crossing each of the seven bridges of the Pregal River in Konigsberg only once? This does not sound very much like the question modern neurologists are likely to ask when dealing with their patients and the complexities of neurological disease. Surprisingly, however, this book by Drs. Bianchi, Caviness, and Cash will show how this type of question has recently become very relevant for understanding how complex brain networks develop and function, and how this enchanted loom breaks down in neuropsychiatric disease. The famous problem of the seven bridges of Konigsberg was solved by the brilliant mathematician Leonhard Euler. To do this he had to invent a completely new branch of mathematics: graph theory. Graph theory deals with complex networks by reducing them to their bare essentials: collections of network nodes or 'vertices' and their interconnections called 'edges'. How could this esoteric piece of mathematics teach us something useful about the brain and its disorders?

The Hungarian writer Frigyes Karinthi may have been one of the first to hit upon some unexpected properties of large-scale networks. In a short story called *Chains*, one of the characters wonders whether every human being might be connected by at most six intermediate persons. This phenomenon is the basis of popular games such as the Kevin Bacon game, where one has to connect an arbitrarily chosen actor to Bacon by a series of movies in which the two actors played together. Another variant of the game is the Erdos number: this indicates how close you are to the famous and eccentric mathematician using a chain of co-authorships. The first to study this phenomenon of small distances in social networks more scientifically was a psychologist from Harvard: Stanley Milgram. With his famous letter experiment he showed that indeed distances between arbitrary persons in social networks are surprisingly small, on average close to six intermediate persons. This gave a scientific basis to the notion of six degrees of separation, but it was completely unclear how such a property of social networks could arise. We should not forget an average person has only about 150 acquaintances (Dunbar's number), and there are close to billion people in the world.

The problem was solved by Duncan Watts and Steve Strogatz in a brilliant Letter to Nature published in 1998. Using graph theory they proposed a network model that could span the whole range from fully ordered networks (each node connected to a fixed number of neighbors) to completely random networks. Networks in the intermediate regime, so-called 'small-world' networks, were characterized by high clustering as well as short distances between any pair of nodes. The discovery of the 'small-world' model, and the 'scale-free' networks by Barabasi and Albert one year later, revolutionized the study of complex networks. It has now been shown that high clustering, short path lengths, and scale-free properties are the typical properties of a wide range of complex networks found in nature, ranging from metabolic and gene networks to transportation systems and social networks, providing a scientific basis for Karinthi's intuition and Milgram's observations.

What about the brain? Neuroscientist have seized upon the new possibilities offered by modern network science to study the anatomical and functional organization of the brain, ranging form *C. elegans* to cats, macaques and humans. We now know that brains of all sizes and at various levels show the typical signature of small-world networks: they are highly clustered, and have very short path lengths. In addition, they are characterized by highly connected nodes called hubs, which hang together in the form of a 'connectivity backbone'. Furthermore, complex brain networks have a delicate hierarchical structure, with modules and sub-modules. These topological features are closely related to brain function. For instance, very recently it has been shown that the path length of anatomical and functional brain networks, that is, the number of steps it takes to travel from one region of the brain to any other region, is closely related to intelligence. How our brains are wired up is strongly predictive of how smart we are.

If modern network theory is so promising for gaining a better understanding of the structure and function of complex brain networks, what does this imply for neurology and psychiatry? Can we understand neural diseases in terms of various scenarios for network breakdown? An increasing number of studies have addressed this question in recent years. Although it is too soon to make up the balance, some interesting patterns can be seen to emerge. Many degenerative disorders are characterized by a breakdown of the normal, optimal small-world structure, resulting in a more random topology of brain networks. In Alzheimer's disease, there are indications that the disease process specifically targets the hubs of the network, which are also associated with the highest levels of amyloid deposition.

In epilepsy, there is increasing evidence that certain network topologies might underlie abnormal low thresholds for network synchronization and seizure spread.

Drs. Bianchi, Caviness, and Cash have attempted to give an overview of this exciting field of network studies in neurology and psychiatry. For anyone who is not familiar with graph theory, the basic concepts are explained in various chapters, avoiding the mathematical details that would distract from the overall understanding. This e-Book gives and excellent overview of the state of the art of network theory and oscillatory synchronization, both in relation to normal brain development, sleep and cognition, as well as with respect to a range of neurological disorders, ranging from degenerative disease to epilepsy. This e-Book is a 'must' for any scientist and clinician involved with network studies. Neurologists, neurosurgeons, psychiatrists, psychologists and neuroscientists who are not familiar with these new developments will find that this e-Book is an exciting as well as accessible introduction. Hopefully, many will get 'hooked up', and turn their attention to a complex network perspective of the brain.

The Harvard psychologist Stanley Milgram was one of the pioneers of the 'small-world' idea. Now, this e-Book edited by neurologists and neuroscientists of Harvard and Massachusetts General Hospital continues this Boston tradition by pointing out the importance of the 'small-world' in our brains. Hopefully, one day, we will be able to prove network theorems about the brain, as Euler did for the seven bridges of Konigsberg.

Cornelis J. Stam
Bussum

PREFACE

This endeavor grew out of a reading group of neurology residents begun several years ago and based on the foundational work of Buzsaki's *Rhythms of the Brain* as the centerpiece. Although many of us found the language of networks and oscillations to be somewhat unfamiliar to the parlance of our clinical training in the traditional connectionist approach to diseases of the brain, with each chapter we collectively felt the importance of these unique perspectives to understanding brain disorders. These monthly meetings brought neuro-minded individuals together for discussion, and we are deeply indebted to this group for sharing in our continued learning process across these fascinating fields. In particular, we extend our thanks and appreciation to Drs. Ali Atri, Justin Baker, James Bartscher, Adam Cohen, David Kaplan, Joshua Klein, Atul Maheshwari, Kazuma Nakagawa, Jay Pathmanathan, David Stark, Vivek Unni, Brian Wainger, Zelime Ward, Brandon Westover, and Timothy Yu. In particular we would like to thank the late Dr. Edward Bromfield for valuable discussions in the early phases of our writing.

Certainly our own conceptual framework has drawn profoundly from the growing literature spanning basic and clinical neurosciences. While the translation of these techniques and perspectives into clinically relevant diagnostic, prognostic, and treatment strategies are in their infancy, the trajectory of the learning curve appears already quite steep. Adding these facets to the clinician's conceptual armamentarium promises to rapidly narrow the gap between the theoretical and the practical implications for individual patient care.

The text is not meant to be a specialized compendium reference, nor a highly technical niche review, but rather a linking "edge" between the nodes of basic and clinical researchers and practitioners - and with any such attempts, sharing a common language is a crucial first step. We hope that these chapters will shed light bi-directionally, as the basic scientists and clinicians who study and treat disorders of the brain have much to learn from one another.

Whether one cares about the brain from the perspective of neurology, psychiatry, or philosophy, there is a certain shared sense of awe inspired, perhaps equally, by the careful observation of normal and pathological brain function. It is therefore with humble appreciation that we thank those who contributed to the current collection. On behalf of all of the authors, we hope that our attempt to capture the excitement of this field will inspire further collaborations and development of novel approaches, with a keen eye towards the clinical relevance of these exciting endeavors.

Matt T. Bianchi

Sleep Division
Neurology Department
55 Fruit Street, Wang 7
Massachusetts General Hospital
Boston, MA 02114,
USA

Verne S. Caviness and Sydney S. Cash

Neurology Department
55 Fruit Street, Wang 7
Massachusetts General Hospital
Boston
MA, 02114
USA

List of Contributors

Bassett, Danielle S.
Brain Mapping Unit, Department of Psychiatry, University of Cambridge, UK; Biological and Soft Systems, Department of Physics, University of Cambridge, UK

Bianchi, Matt T.
Sleep Division, Neurology Department, 55 Fruit Street, Wang 7, Massachusetts General Hospital, Boston, MA 02114, USA

Bullmore, Edward T.
Brain Mapping Unit, Department of Psychiatry, University of Cambridge, UK

Cash, Sydney S.
Neurology Department, 55 Fruit Street, Wang 7, Massachusetts General Hospital, Boston, MA, 02114, USA

Caviness, Verne S.
Neurology Department, 55 Fruit Street, Wang 7, Massachusetts General Hospital, Boston, MA, 02114, USA

Chu-Shore , Catherine J.
Divisions of Pediatric Neurology and Neurophysiology, Department of Neurology, Massachusetts General Hospital, 175 Cambridge Street, Suite 340, Boston, MA 02114

Klein, Joshua P.
Neurology Department, Brigham and Women's Hospital, 75 Francis Street, Boston, MA 02115, USA

Kramer, Mark A.
Department of Mathematics and Statistics, Boston University, 111 Cummington St, Boston, MA, 02215, USA

Laufs, Helmut
Department of Neurology and Brain Imaging Center, Goethe-University Frankfurt am Main, Theodor-Stern-Kai 2-16, 60590 Frankfurt am Main, Germany

Pascual-Leone, Alvaro
Department of Neurology, Berenson-Allen Center for Noninvasive Brain Stimulation Beth Israel Deaconess Medical Center Harvard Medical School, 330 Brookline Ave, KS 454 Boston, MA 02215, USA

Phillips, Andrew J.
Division of Sleep Medicine, Brigham & Women's Hospital, Harvard Medical School, 221 Longwood Avenue, Boston, MA 02115, USA

Shafi, Moushin
Neurology Department, 55 Fruit Street, Wang 8, Massachusetts General Hospital, Boston, MA 02114, USA

Singer, Wolf
Department of Neurophysiology, Max Planck Institute for Brain Research, Deutschordenstrasse 46, Frankfurt am Main, 60528, Germany, Frankfurt Institute for Advanced Studies, Johann Wolfgang Goethe University, Max-von-Laue-Strasse 1, Frankfurt am Main, 60438, Germany

Uhlhaas, Peter J.
Frankfurt am Main, Department of Neurophysiology, Max Planck Institute for Brain Research, Deutschordenstrasse 46, 60528, Germany, Laboratory for Neurophysiology and Neuroimaging, Department of Psychiatry, Johann Wolfgang Goethe University, Heinrich-Hoffmann-Strasse 10
Frankfurt am Main, 60528, Germany

CHAPTER 1

Synchronizing Bench and Bedside: A Clinical Overview of Networks and Oscillations

Matt T. Bianchi[1,*], Joshua P. Klein[2], Verne S. Caviness[3] and Sydney S. Cash[3]

[1]*Sleep Division 55 Fruit Street, Wang 7, Massachusetts General Hospital, Boston, MA, 02114, USA;* [2]*Neurology Department, Brigham and Women's Hospital, 75 Francis Street, Boston, MA 02115, USA and* [3]*Neurology Department, 55 Fruit Street, Wang 7, Massachusetts General Hospital, Boston, MA, 02114, USA*

Abstract: Technological and computational advances offer increasing capacity to quantify what neurologists have long appreciated as the complexity of the brain. The information-rich techniques of electro- and magneto-encephalography, as well as structural and functional MRI, are increasingly being examined through the lenses of network theory and oscillations to capture complex brain dynamics. Although still in the early stages of clinical application, these "network" approaches have the potential to shed new light on the diagnosis, prognosis, and treatment of neurological diseases. We review the basic principles of network theory and oscillation dynamics, including the recently discovered "small-world network" concept, and provide and introduction to how these techniques are being applied to routinely available clinical data (such as MRI, EEG, and MEG). Specific clinical applications span normal brain functions (cognition and sleep) and disorders of the brain such as epilepsy, dementia, movement disorders, pain, autism, and schizophrenia. These interrelated approaches respect the fundamentals of anatomically-driven diagnosis while providing a theoretical and practical armamentarium to investigate aspects of neurological disease that may challenge the scope of traditional clinical tools.

Keyword: Network, small world, oscillation, clinical applications, pathophysiology.

INTRODUCTION

The clinical practice of neurology is heavily influenced by a classical approach emphasizing gross anatomical localization in the context of a connectionist view that the brain is comprised of connected but discreetly localized functional domains. This approach not only informs the neurological examination and clinical decision making, but also provides insight into the anatomical division of labor of various nervous system functions. This is perhaps most famously manifested in the diagnosis of ischemic stroke, with its protean clinical presentations yielding clues to lesion localization. However, the relationship between pathophysiology and clinical presentation is not always straightforward in stroke and other settings. Similar strokes might recover differently, similar patients may respond differently to psychotropic medications, and similar degrees of white matter abnormalities may have disparate clinical consequences. Moreover, many central nervous system conditions do not conform to a specific lesion-based (connectionist) model *per se*, in that multiple pathological mechanisms influencing multiple brain circuits may be involved.

The respect neurologists develop for the nuance of clinical presentations across individual patients is not matched by a diagnostic framework for systematically understanding what makes one patient classic and another atypical. The interrelated ideas of networks and oscillations may contribute to such a framework for clinical neurology. We review the principles of networks and oscillations that are beginning to find application in the challenges presented by disease categories that may be less amenable to traditional localization strategies, such as epilepsy, neurodegeneration, pain, sleep, movement and psychiatric disorders. Two fundamental clinical challenges may benefit most from ongoing developments in these techniques: 1) non-invasive diagnostics for brain diseases with minimal or nonspecific structural abnormalities evident on routine MRI, and 2) prognosis and treatment monitoring for neurological disorders, including those with traditionally localizable damage.

*Address correspondence to Matt T. Bianchi: Sleep Division, Neurology Department, 55 Fruit Street, Wang 7, Massachusetts General Hospital, Boston, MA, 02114, USA; E-mail: mtbianchi@partners.org

The Network Approach: Anatomy and Physiology

It seems intuitive that brain function depends on the interplay of its components at multiple levels (molecular, cellular, circuit, etc.). So-called network approaches may provide insight into clinically relevant questions of diagnosis, prognosis, and treatment by extracting information from available non-invasive diagnostic tools that may not be readily apparent through routine (mainly visual) interpretation [1-2]. These tools include structural (MRI, diffusion tensor imaging (DTI) and diffusion spectrum imaging (DSI)) and functional interrogations (EEG, MEG, and functional MRI (fMRI)), each with distinct advantages and limitations (Table **1.1**). Advanced approaches to analyze these metrics may capture not only the anatomical complexity of brain circuits, but also their rich temporal dynamics. Note that the term "network" in this sense need not refer to the microscopic connections among neurons, but is rather more general and can be applied to larger scale connections (or more precisely, interactions) inferred by the non-invasive techniques outlined here. Computational tools applied to these datasets may prove to have pertinent clinical parallels: performance efficiency in a network may correspond to cognitive function clinically, and robustness in the face of damage may correspond to clinical symptoms and functional recovery in a patient suffering from a brain lesion [3]. Understanding the basics of networks and oscillations as biomarkers of brain function provides a foundation for future clinical application of these concepts.

Table 1.1. Clinical Tools Used in Network and Oscillation Analysis, Along with a Summary of the Type of Data Measured by Each Technique and the Type of Information Provided

Technique	What it Measures	Network-Related Information Provided
EEG	Cortical oscillations 0.01-200 Hz	-Task-specific activation -Default Networks - Coupling between network nodes (electrodes) -Small world network metrics[1]
MEG	Cortical oscillations Subcortical oscillations 0.01-200 Hz	-Task-specific activation -Default Networks - Coupling between network nodes (electrodes) - Small world network metrics[1]
Functional MRI	Cortical oscillations Subcortical oscillations 0.01-0.1 Hz (limited time domain)	-Task-specific activation -Default Networks -Coupling between network nodes (voxels) - Small world network metrics[1]
Diffusion-based tractography (DSI and DTI)	Water diffusion in axon bundles of white matter tracts	-Gross anatomy of white matter connectivity -Combines with MRI/fMRI analysis

[1]such as path length and cluster coefficient (see glossary)

Networks

Integrating the anatomically distinct functions attributed to different lobes, tracts, and nuclei is necessary to overcome biological constraints in available space (anatomic distances, intracranial volume) and bandwidth (conduction velocities, synaptic delays). These boundaries may be overcome in part through a pattern of connectivity resembling what has become known as a "small-world" network [4]. This powerful concept has been explored in physical, metabolic, informational, and perhaps most famously, social systems. Small-world architecture, considered from a social network standpoint, means that not only are one's friends more likely to be friends with each other (local clustering or cliques), but also that clusters are sparsely interconnected with each other (a few friends in each cluster interact with members of other clusters). From the perspective of neuroanatomy, cerebral small-world organization is suggested by abundant local connections (for example, within particular regions of cortex) and relatively sparse long-range connections (for example, those conducted by white matter axon bundles) [5] (Fig. **1.1**). Considering networks from the perspective of graph theory is explained further in Chapter 2, and the evidence for small world networks in the brain is explored in Chapter 4.

These abstractions can be quantified using metrics derived from the field of graph theory, such as the clustering coefficient and path length of a network (GLOSSARY). Graph theory refers to the quantitative analysis of node connectivity patterns, and the general framework has been applied to many systems outside of neuroscience that involve multiple interacting components (social sciences, the World Wide Web, intracellular signaling, etc). In the case of a small world neuronal network, the presence of relatively few long-range connections markedly reduces the mean path length connecting any two neurons, enabling rapid communication (coupling) between anatomically and functionally segregated regions, each of which has high local connectivity (clustering). The balanced advantages of processing efficiency and resilience to damage has been shown in computational studies [3]. Neuroanatomical data from nematodes to humans demonstrate that this features of small-world organization can be found across species [4, 6]. Diffusion tensor imaging of white matter tracts is consistent with a small-world architecture of connections among regions of the human cortex [7-9]. Dynamic functional techniques (EEG, MEG, fMRI) can be translated into a "graphical" substrate, to allow similar network analyses. This is typically accomplished by inferring connectivity between regions of interest by virtue of functional coupling between spatially separated signal fluctuations (see next section) [10]. In fact, brain network architecture derived from structural measurements (DSI and DTI of white matter axon bundles) correlates well with that derived from functional (fMRI) measurements [11-13].

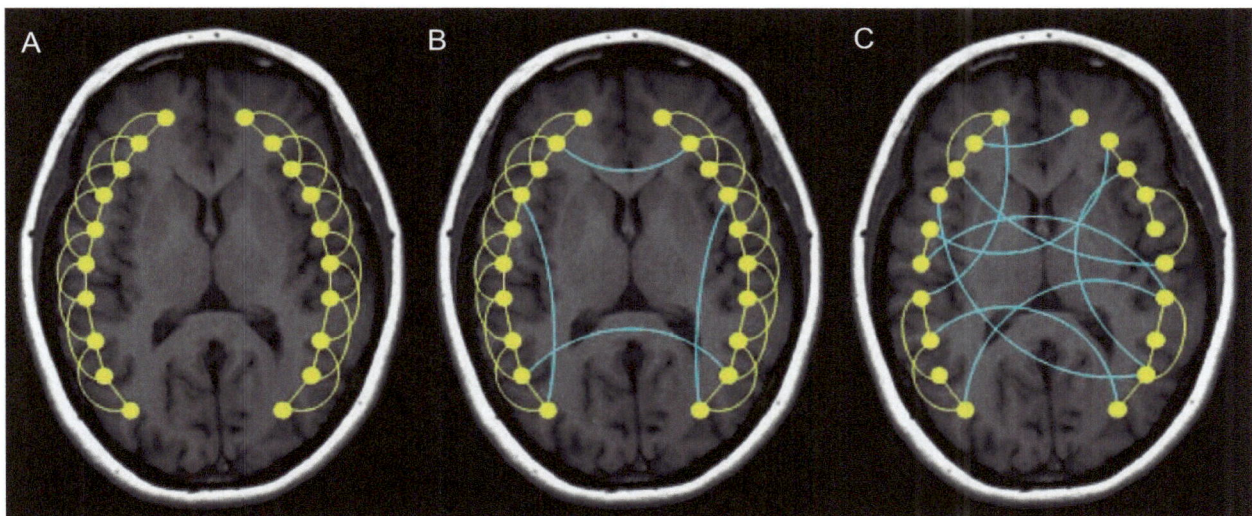

Fig. (1.1). A cartoon version of the graph theory approach to networks overlaid upon axial T1 weighted MRI of a normal adult. Regular (or local) connections are schematized in panel A, random connections are shown in panel C, and the intermediate, or small world pattern is shown in panel B.

Oscillations

The signal oscillations of EEG, MEG and fMRI provide a window into the dynamic function of neuroanatomical circuits involved in normal and pathological brain function [14]. Although the exact physiological meaning of any given oscillation remains actively debated [15], they can be viewed as potential biomarkers of circuit processing, and thus hold promise in combination with network approaches for application to disorders of brain function.

Although certain oscillations may be visually evident (such as occipital alpha waves with eye closure, or sleep spindles in non-rapid eye movement sleep), available automated signal processing techniques can illuminate a rich variety of "hidden" patterns that further capture oscillatory dynamics. These time-domain signals can be mapped to the spatial domain to facilitate network analysis, by inferring functional connections between signals detected by individual EEG and MEG sensors *via* temporal coupling (such as coherence or correlation of signal fluctuations). Such coupling implies a functional relationship (direct or indirect), between regions producing the signal, which may reflect the summed activity of a large population of individual neurons. For example, signal fluctuations at individual electrodes of an EEG or MEG dataset can be compared over time and space (without making assumptions about specific anatomical connectivity). Each electrode can be considered as representing a node in a network, connected to other nodes by virtue of coupled activity (through any number of statistical methods quantifying coherence, correlation, or covariance). The resulting spatial-domain data, consisting of nodes and their connections, is thus amenable to graph theoretic network analysis, as described above. This represents an important technique for linking structural and functional/oscillatory datasets by virtue of a common analytical toolkit.

Overview of Clinical Applications

The toolkit encompassing anatomical and functional connectivity (networks) and dynamics (oscillations) - and the ability to map information from one to the other – is gaining momentum towards clinical translation because of several practical advantages: these techniques are 1) non-invasive; 2) scalable to different numbers of sensors/detectors; and 3) applicable to multiple physiological signal modalities. The common availability of EEG, for example, facilitates testing in virtually any patient or setting. Scalability and versatility means that similar analytical approaches can be applied across data acquisition modalities (EEG, MEG, fMRI, tractography), spanning electrical, magnetic, metabolic, and anatomical information. Although much less common, more invasive techniques (electrocorticography and depth electrodes) can expand on these approaches and even better elucidate the neurophysiologic mechanisms underlying these signals [11, 16-17].

The combination of network and oscillation approaches has the intuitive appeal of respecting traditional localization principles that guide neurological practice, while providing a conceptual and analytical basis for evaluating more complex or dynamic features of disease processes (Fig. **1.2**). As these network approaches become increasingly available to routine clinical use, they may eventually prove to be as fundamental to the clinical practice of neurology as traditional anatomical localization and molecular pathology [18]. Several themes have become apparent, with multiple neurological disorders showing more widespread disturbances in network architecture and/or oscillation dynamics than may otherwise have been suspected. The fields of epilepsy (Chapter) and neuropsychiatry (Chapter 7) have enjoyed particular emphasis in this regard.

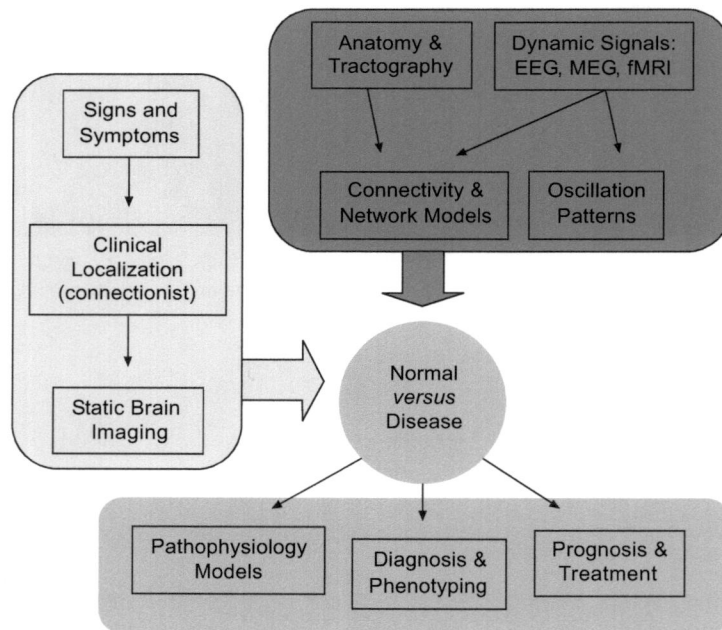

Fig. (1.2). A schematic of the complementary roles of classical and more recent computational approaches, converging on the common goal of characterizing brain function in health and disease, with the final goal of improving patient care endpoints.

Normal Brain Function

Waking oscillations have been extensively probed as markers of cognitive processing. In animals (and humans undergoing invasive monitoring), theta oscillations have been correlated with learning and memory, while human studies using EEG and MEG have linked gamma oscillations with cognitive performance [19]. The recent discovery of a resting or "default" network of brain activity, consisting mainly of posterior cingulate, medial prefrontal, and medial temporal regions, holds particular clinical promise as a readily measured biomarker of brain function that requires no task performance (in contrast to routine fMRI studies) [20]. Default network abnormalities using a spectrum of measurement techniques have been demonstrated in aging, Alzheimer's disease, multiple sclerosis, chronic pain, attention deficit disorder, depression, autism, schizophrenia [21-22]. This work raises the intriguing possibility of implementing a non-invasive task-free imaging assay as a probe of cognitive dysfunction across a variety of disease states [21, 23].

Sleep

Despite abundant interactions between sleep and various disease states, clinical sleep disorder assessments focus mainly upon abnormal breathing, insomnia, and circadian rhythms. The neurological examination may not provide the rich localization opportunity for sleep disorders which are heavily dependent on clinical history and polysomnography. More sophisticated assays of sleep oscillations and network dynamics during sleep, such as small-world features, may improve classification of sleep disorders characterized by insomnia or hypersomnia. Early work suggested that small world EEG patterns are increased in sleep compared to wake in healthy subjects [24]. Similar analyses may prove relevant for linking sleep quality or dysfunction to neurological and psychiatric disease states and symptoms. A related demonstration of how clinically useful information can be extracted from analysis of dynamic biological signals is provided by time series analysis of electrocardiogram fluctuations during sleep. Analysis of cardio-pulmonary coupling has provided a novel metric of sleep "stability" with clinical utility in the evaluation of sleep disordered breathing [25]. Complex physiological patterns such as heart rate variability have long been recognized to contain clinically relevant information not apparent through visual inspection [26]. The application of computational methods to sleep physiology is further discussed in Chapter 5.

Epilepsy

Perhaps the most obvious disease in which oscillatory behavior and network analysis intersect is epilepsy. Epilepsy is classically considered to result from an imbalance between excitation and inhibition caused by any of a wide variety of underlying mechanisms. Efforts to understand the pathophysiology of epileptogenesis, seizure initiation, propagation, termination, and response to treatment are increasingly informed by studies of network connectivity and electrical oscillations [27]. For example, computational models have demonstrated how altered functional connectivity (changes in the architecture or synaptic strengths) may influence epileptiform activity [28]. Approaches mapping temporal signals to the spatial domain by considering electrodes as nodes, and signal coherence between electrodes as connections (see "Oscillations" above), have been applied to EEG signals from epilepsy patients. Characterization of network activity across different stages of seizures revealed an increase in network order as seizures progress [29]. Others have found increased or decreased synchrony of faster EEG frequencies immediately before and during seizures in humans [30]. Particular interest has focused on very high frequency oscillations, 80-300 Hz, or "ripples", as a possible hallmark of epileptogenic cortex [31-32].

The emerging evidence for dynamic network connectivity in epileptogenesis raises questions of what is meant by a seizure focus and whether seizures are always hyper-synchronous. Network and oscillation analysis suggests that epileptogenesis likely involves interactions among multiple structures, and therefore it may prove useful to consider the "seizure-focus" as part of a circuit of abnormally connected cortical and subcortical structures [29, 33-35]. This framework may lead to novel methods for quantitative analysis of EEG, MEG, structural (e.g. DTI) or functional imaging (e.g. fMRI) in pursuit of improved diagnostic and prognostic techniques [32]. For example, network analysis may inform the risk of future development of epilepsy after first seizure [36]. Further details of these applications are discussed in Chapter.

Aging and Dementia

The dementing and other neurodegenerative disorders may also involve abnormal networks and oscillations that are not easily appreciated or quantified by routine clinical or diagnostic approaches. Whereas epilepsy may involve a hyper-connected state causing abnormal oscillations, the dementias may involve the opposite situation – disconnected networks causing impaired oscillations.

Many studies have demonstrated abnormal EEG and MEG oscillations in normal aging as well as fronto-temporal dementia [37] and Alzheimer's dementia [38-46]. Small-world network metrics are altered in fMRI [47] and MEG [48] data from patients with Alzheimer's disease, and these features correlated with mini-mental status test scores [38]. Measurements of oscillation coherence are also abnormal in patients with mild cognitive impairment [49-50]. Furthermore, there is growing interest in abnormalities of the default network in aging and dementia [21, 45]. This functional work is paralleled by structural network approaches that also show abnormalities in Alzheimer's disease [51]. Network approaches may thus represent a new set of diagnostic procedures that could be used to predict the development of Alzheimer's disease [52], and perhaps aid in the design of therapeutic interventions, and in monitoring disease progression.

The high sensitivity of T2-weighted MRI sequences for detecting white matter abnormalities has sparked interest in potential clinical correlations of these abnormal signals to cognition and dementia. Although clinical MRI reports commonly describe such T2-signal abnormalities as nonspecific, the tools of network analysis may dovetail well with the recent emergence of white matter tractography to improve diagnostic specificity. Anatomical and functional connectivity measurements may provide valuable information relevant to disease states extending beyond the gross structural information of routine MRI. For example, one recent study demonstrated abnormal MEG oscillations in adolescents with periventricular white matter disease [53].

Parkinson's Disease

The rhythmic tremor of Parkinson's disease (PD) represents an easily visualized clinical manifestation of abnormal oscillatory behavior in the brain. The frequency of the tremor correlates with the frequency of sub-thalamic nucleus (STN) oscillations during invasive human recording. Increased thalamo-cortical theta frequency coherence has been implicated specifically in bradykinesia [54]. Beta and gamma frequency oscillations have been implicated in the manifestation of bradykinesia as well, with gamma replacing beta oscillations during the normal transition from movement planning to execution. The persistence of beta oscillation may thus underlie the bradykinesia of PD patients. Treatments that improve bradykinesia (dopaminergic agents, STN stimulation and STN lesions) improve the abnormal delay transitioning from beta to gamma oscillations [30]. The correlations between oscillations and clinical symptoms may extend to other movement disorders as well [14].

Pain

Network approaches and oscillations have been applied toward understanding pain syndromes such as compressive radiculopathy, primary neurogenic pain (such as trigeminal neuralgia), and migraine. Abnormal oscillations in theta and beta frequencies, as well as increased thalamo-cortical coherence, have been reported in these settings [55-57]. Painful cutaneous stimulation has been shown to suppress spontaneous thalamo-cortical oscillations [58]. Surgical treatment (stimulation or ablation) that provides clinical benefit for chronic pain is accompanied by resolution of abnormal burst firing patterns during invasive thalamic recordings [59]. Such recordings from patients suffering from pain syndromes have revealed thalamic firing patterns consistent with a "dysrhythmia" of thalamo-cortical oscillations, which may be a general theme for several neurological and psychiatric disorders [60]. Altered neuronal network architecture has been demonstrated in migraine patients using EEG [61]. The practical clinical utility of network correlates of central pain mechanisms remains largely unexplored.

Malignancy

Although brain tumors tend to cause symptoms referable to their location or to compression of adjacent structures, they have also been shown to disrupt both local and distant connectivity [62-65], and the effects of treatment are also being investigated [66]. Understanding tumor-mediated network disruption may provide insight into susceptibility of neuro-oncology patients to network-level clinical complications, such as seizures, psychotropic drug side effects, or encephalopathy from systemic abnormalities (infection, dehydration, metabolic derangements).

Psychiatric Disorders

Investigation of network and oscillatory pathology has proven fruitful in evaluating psychiatric disorders that lack focal lesions in the traditional neurological sense [30]. Patients with schizophrenia, for example, exhibit altered beta frequency synchrony and decreased fMRI coherence measures during certain cognitive tasks. Structural imaging demonstrated decreased long-range connectivity and enhanced local connectivity, and suggested the latter as a mechanism contributing to sensory hallucinations. Similarly, abnormal coupling patterns were found in MEG-defined functional networks of schizophrenics compared to healthy controls during a facial emotion task [67]. Sleep-related networks measured by routine EEG appear to be disrupted in depressed patients [68].

In autism, there is a known increased forebrain white-to-gray matter volumetric ratio. This finding is now complemented by studies revealing altered gamma frequency oscillations and decreased functional connectivity (fMRI) during cognitive tasks [30]. Thalamo-cortical firing patterns, which can influence the cortical (and therefore EEG) expression of electrical oscillations, is altered in patients with affective disorders who underwent invasive monitoring [59]. Whether and how psychotropic medications, electro-convulsive therapy, or other interventions influence neural processing assessed by these techniques remains to be investigated, as well as the potential to predict therapeutic response or relapse.

Toward a Pathophysiology Framework

The studies outlined here are converging on a common theme for neurological disease of altered network connectivity as well as altered oscillations - two intricately linked features of neuronal circuits. Certainly, linear cause-and-effect concepts of neurological disorders have paved many pathophysiological roads, for example, from

Table 1.2. Examples of Reported Network and Oscillation Analysis Among CNS Disorders

	EEG/MEG	MRI/fMRI
Seizures	-Altered synchrony -Pre-ictal decrease in β synchrony -Pre-ictal increase in γ synchrony	-Abnormal default network
PD	-Enhanced β oscillation in normal movement planning -β gives way to γ oscillation during movement execution -Increased β is seen with akinesia in PD patients -STN stimulation and lesions reduce β and facilitate γ -DA treatments reduce β and facilitate γ -STN oscillation frequency matches tremor frequency	-Limited network studies
AD	-Increased θ and δ during wakefulness -Decreased β and α (α correlates with dementia severity) -Decreased γ power in resting state -ACh projections important for β and γ oscillations	-Reduced connectivity between PFC and hippocampus -Altered connectivity in MCI patients -Decreased white matter tracts by DTI -Abnormal default network
Pain	-Altered thalamic firing patterns and thalamocortical coherence during invasive recordings -Altered theta and beta oscillations on EEG	-Limited network studies
Migraine	-Altered network dynamics *via* EEG studies	-Limited network studies
Tumor	-altered network structure in resting state MEG	--Limited network studies
Autism	-Lack of γ synchrony during visual (face) stimuli	-Decreased connectivity -Abnormal default network
Schizo-phrenia	-Reduced β and γ (but not lower freq) in visual and auditory stimulation. -Reduced β and normal γ for mooney faces (suggests local synchrony breakdown)	-Reduced fMRI coherence -Decreased long-range connectivity -Increased local connectivity (proposed relation to hallucinations)

thrombo-embolism to stroke syndrome and from antibody to myasthenic weakness. However, connecting complex neuronal processes with molecular substrates is less straightforward, despite routine invocation of seemingly direct links, such as altered serotonin levels and mood, dysfunctional ion channels and epilepsy, or decreased acetylcholine signaling and dementia. Network approaches offer a potential mechanism to capture this complexity that complements traditional localization and pathophysiology (Table **1.2**).

The utility of network approaches for clinical goals such as prognosis and guidance of therapy remains to be rigorously tested. One major challenge involves optimizing the technology for reliable use in the individual patient, taking into account their particular clinical features and co-morbidities. Ultimately, the potential for these tools to improve our capacity to diagnose, treat and monitor patients over time is enhanced by the widespread availability of these technologies and the rapidly growing knowledge base generated by their application to a variety of neurological conditions. Emerging applications include developmental changes [69-70] (also see Chapter 3), multiple sclerosis [71], chronic systemic disease (diabetes [72]), and even spinal cord injury [73-74].

The most immediate practical application for these new approaches may be to improve our diagnostic armamentarium, including sub-classification or phenotyping patients across the clinical spectrum of disease presentations, and to evaluate potential links between co-morbid diseases often encountered clinically (for example, epilepsy and mood disorders, Parkinsonism and sleep disorders, pain and depression, sleep and pain). Increased awareness of these developments will accelerate further bench-to-bedside translation ultimately to routine patient care.

GLOSSARY

Cluster Coefficient: A network metric describing the extent to which immediate neighbors of a node (based on single connection, rather than physical distance necessarily) are also connected to one another (social network analogy: "how many of my friends are also friends with each other?"). See references 4 and 5 for mathematical details.

Coupling: Coordinated activity between discreet regions; can be measured by various algorithms applied to pairs of EEG or MEG electrodes (or fMRI voxels) reflecting brain activity patterns. Synchrony, coherence, correlation, and covariance have variable mathematical meanings in the literature, but have been used to describe particular patterns of coupling, and hence, presumed functional connectivity.

Oscillation: Rhythmic fluctuations of a biological signal, characterized by frequency and amplitude. EEG, MEG, and fMRI techniques detect oscillations of different types of signals, with distinct spatio-temporal resolution [15].

Path Length: A network metric reflecting the smallest number of nodes that must be traversed to connect any two nodes in a network (social network analogy: "what is the minimum number of hand-shakes between any two people in a population?"). See references 4 and 5 for mathematical details.

Small–World Network: a graph theory term referring to the structure of a network with 1) highly connected local clusters of nodes, and 2) relatively few "long range" connections between clusters. This pattern yields a relatively high clustering coefficient, and low mean path length [4]. Small world architecture lies between the two extremes designated by, on one hand, regular or ordered graphs (with only local connectivity, high cluster coefficients, and high path lengths), and on the other hand, random networks (similar frequency of local and distant connections, low cluster coefficients, and low path lengths). See references 4 and 5 for mathematical details.

REFERENCES

[1]   Matthews PM, Honey GD, Bullmore ET. Applications of fMRI in translational medicine and clinical practice. Nat Rev Neurosci 2006; 7(9): 732-44.
[2]   Ramnani N, Behrens TE, Penny W, Matthews PM. New approaches for exploring anatomical and functional connectivity in the human brain. Biol Psychiatry 2004; 56(9): 613-9.
[3]   Reijneveld JC, Ponten SC, Berendse HW, Stam CJ. The application of graph theoretical analysis to complex networks in the brain. Clin Neurophysiol 2007; 118(11): 2317-31.
[4]   Watts DJ, Strogatz SH. Collective dynamics of 'small-world' networks. Nature 1998; 393(6684): 440-2.
[5]   Bassett DS, Bullmore E. Small-world brain networks. Neuroscientist 2006; 12(6): 512-23.
[6]   Sporns O, Kotter R. Motifs in brain networks. PLoS Biol 2004; 2(11): e369.
[7]   Hagmann P, Thiran JP, Jonasson L, *et al.* DTI mapping of human brain connectivity: statistical fibre tracking and virtual dissection. Neuroimage 2003; 19(3): 545-54.
[8]   Faugeras O, Adde G, Charpiat G, *et al.* Variational, geometric, and statistical methods for modeling brain anatomy and function. Neuroimage 2004; 23 Suppl 1: S46-55.
[9]   Hagmann P, Kurant M, Gigandet X, *et al.* Mapping human whole-brain structural networks with diffusion MRI. PLoS ONE 2007; 2(7): e597.

[10]   Ioannides AA. Dynamic functional connectivity. Curr Opin Neurobiol 2007; 17(2): 161-70.

[11]   He BJ, Snyder AZ, Zempel JM, Smyth MD, Raichle ME. Electrophysiological correlates of the brain's intrinsic large-scale functional architecture. Proc Natl Acad Sci USA 2008; 105(41): 16039-44.

[12]   Hagmann P, Cammoun L, Gigandet X, *et al*. Mapping the structural core of human cerebral cortex. PLoS Biol 2008; 6(7): e159.

[13]   Greicius MD, Supekar K, Menon V, Dougherty RF. Resting-State Functional Connectivity Reflects Structural Connectivity in the Default Mode Network. Cereb Cortex 2008 Apr 9.

[14]   Schnitzler A, Gross J. Normal and pathological oscillatory communication in the brain. Nat Rev Neurosci 2005; 6(4): 285-96.

[15]   Buzsáki G. Rhythms of the brain. Oxford ; New York: Oxford University Press; 2006.

[16]   Hochberg LR. Turning thought into action. N Engl J Med 2008; 359(11): 1175-7.

[17]   Sederberg PB, Schulze-Bonhage A, Madsen JR, *et al*. Hippocampal and neocortical gamma oscillations predict memory formation in humans. Cereb Cortex 2007; 17(5): 1190-6.

[18]   Palop JJ, Chin J, Mucke L. A network dysfunction perspective on neurodegenerative diseases. Nature 2006; 443(7113): 768-73.

[19]   Fries P. A mechanism for cognitive dynamics: neuronal communication through neuronal coherence. Trends Cogn Sci 2005; 9(10): 474-80.

[20]   Damoiseaux JS, Rombouts SA, Barkhof F, *et al*. Consistent resting-state networks across healthy subjects. Proc Natl Acad Sci USA 2006; 103(37): 13848-53.

[21]   Buckner RL, Andrews-Hanna JR, Schacter DL. The brain's default network: anatomy, function, and relevance to disease. Ann N Y Acad Sci 2008; 1124: 1-38.

[22]   Guggisberg AG, Honma SM, Findlay AM, *et al*. Mapping functional connectivity in patients with brain lesions. Ann Neurol 2008; 63(2): 193-203.

[23]   Damoiseaux JS, Beckmann CF, Arigita EJ, *et al*. Reduced resting-state brain activity in the "default network" in normal aging. Cereb Cortex 2008; 18(8): 1856-64.

[24]   Ferri R, Rundo F, Bruni O, Terzano MG, Stam CJ. The functional connectivity of different EEG bands moves towards small-world network organization during sleep. Clin Neurophysiol 2008; 119(9): 2026-36.

[25]   Thomas RJ, Mietus JE, Peng CK, Goldberger AL. An electrocardiogram-based technique to assess cardiopulmonary coupling during sleep. Sleep 2005; 28(9): 1151-61.

[26]   Goldberger AL. Non-linear dynamics for clinicians: chaos theory, fractals, and complexity at the bedside. Lancet 1996; 347(9011): 1312-4.

[27]   Morgan RJ, Soltesz I. Nonrandom connectivity of the epileptic dentate gyrus predicts a major role for neuronal hubs in seizures. Proc Natl Acad Sci USA 2008; 105(16): 6179-84.

[28]   Netoff TI, Clewley R, Arno S, Keck T, White JA. Epilepsy in small-world networks. J Neurosci 2004; 24(37): 8075-83.

[29]   Ponten SC, Bartolomei F, Stam CJ. Small-world networks and epilepsy: graph theoretical analysis of intracerebrally recorded mesial temporal lobe seizures. Clin Neurophysiol 2007; 118(4): 918-27.

[30]   Uhlhaas PJ, Singer W. Neural synchrony in brain disorders: relevance for cognitive dysfunctions and pathophysiology. Neuron 2006; 52(1): 155-68.

[31]   Staba RJ, Frighetto L, Behnke EJ, *et al*. Increased fast ripple to ripple ratios correlate with reduced hippocampal volumes and neuron loss in temporal lobe epilepsy patients. Epilepsia 2007; 48(11): 2130-8.

[32]   Worrell GA, Gardner AB, Stead SM, *et al*. High-frequency oscillations in human temporal lobe: simultaneous microwire and clinical macroelectrode recordings. Brain 2008; 131(Pt 4): 928-37.

[33]   Bartolomei F, Wendling F, Bellanger JJ, Regis J, Chauvel P. Neural networks involving the medial temporal structures in temporal lobe epilepsy. Clin Neurophysiol 2001; 112(9): 1746-60.

[34]   Guye M, Regis J, Tamura M, *et al*. The role of corticothalamic coupling in human temporal lobe epilepsy. Brain 2006; 129(Pt 7): 1917-28.

[35]   Kramer MA, Kolaczyk ED, Kirsch HE. Emergent network topology at seizure onset in humans. Epilepsy Res 2008; 79(2-3): 173-86.

[36]   Douw L, de Groot M, van Dellen E, *et al*. 'Functional connectivity' is a sensitive predictor of epilepsy diagnosis after the first seizure. PLoS ONE 2010; 5(5): e10839.

[37]   de Haan W, Pijnenburg YA, Strijers RL, *et al*. Functional neural network analysis in frontotemporal dementia and Alzheimer's disease using EEG and graph theory. BMC Neurosci 2009; 10: 101.

[38.   Stam CJ, Jones BF, Manshanden I, *et al*. Magnetoencephalographic evaluation of resting-state functional connectivity in Alzheimer's disease. Neuroimage 2006; 32(3): 1335-44.

[39]   Stam CJ, Jones BF, Nolte G, Breakspear M, Scheltens P. Small-world networks and functional connectivity in Alzheimer's disease. Cereb Cortex 2007; 17(1): 92-9.

[40]   Stam CJ, Montez T, Jones BF, *et al*. Disturbed fluctuations of resting state EEG synchronization in Alzheimer's disease. Clin Neurophysiol 2005; 116(3): 708-15.

[41]   Stam CJ, van der Made Y, Pijnenburg YA, Scheltens P. EEG synchronization in mild cognitive impairment and Alzheimer's disease. Acta Neurol Scand 2003; 108(2): 90-6.

[42]   Supekar K, Menon V, Rubin D, Musen M, Greicius MD. Network analysis of intrinsic functional brain connectivity in Alzheimer's disease. PLoS Comput Biol 2008; 4(6): e1000100.

[43]   Rossini PM, Rossi S, Babiloni C, Polich J. Clinical neurophysiology of aging brain: from normal aging to neurodegeneration. Prog Neurobiol 2007; 83(6): 375-400.

[44]   Jeong J. EEG dynamics in patients with Alzheimer's disease. Clin Neurophysiol 2004 ; 115(7): 1490-505.

[45]   Andrews-Hanna JR, Snyder AZ, Vincent JL, *et al.* Disruption of large-scale brain systems in advanced aging. Neuron 2007; 56(5): 924-35.

[46]   Montez T, Poil SS, Jones BF, *et al.* Altered temporal correlations in parietal alpha and prefrontal theta oscillations in early-stage Alzheimer disease. Proc Natl Acad Sci USA 2009; 106(5): 1614-9.

[47]   Supekar K, Uddin LQ, Prater K, Amin H, Greicius MD, Menon V. Development of functional and structural connectivity within the default mode network in young children. Neuroimage 2010; 52(1): 290-301.

[48]   Stam CJ, de Haan W, Daffertshofer A, *et al.* Graph theoretical analysis of magnetoencephalographic functional connectivity in Alzheimer's disease. Brain 2009; 132(Pt 1): 213-24.

[49]   Kramer MA, Chang FL, Cohen ME, Hudson D, Szeri AJ. Synchronization measures of the scalp electroencephalogram can discriminate healthy from Alzheimer's subjects. Int J Neural Syst 2007; 17(2): 61-9.

[50]   Koenig T, Prichep L, Dierks T, *et al.* Decreased EEG synchronization in Alzheimer's disease and mild cognitive impairment. Neurobiol Aging 2005; 26(2): 165-71.

[51]   He Y, Chen Z, Evans A. Structural insights into aberrant topological patterns of large-scale cortical networks in Alzheimer's disease. J Neurosci 2008; 28(18): 4756-66.

[52]   Lehmann C, Koenig T, Jelic V, *et al.* Application and comparison of classification algorithms for recognition of Alzheimer's disease in electrical brain activity (EEG). J Neurosci Methods 2007; 161(2): 342-50.

[53]   Pavlova M, Lutzenberger W, Sokolov AN, Birbaumer N, Krageloh-Mann I. Oscillatory MEG response to human locomotion is modulated by periventricular lesions. Neuroimage 2007; 35(3): 1256-63.

[54]   Sarnthein J, Jeanmonod D. High thalamocortical theta coherence in patients with Parkinson's disease. J Neurosci 2007; 27(1): 124-31.

[55]   Sarnthein J, Jeanmonod D. High thalamocortical theta coherence in patients with neurogenic pain. Neuroimage 2008; 39(4): 1910-7.

[56]   Stern J, Jeanmonod D, Sarnthein J. Persistent EEG overactivation in the cortical pain matrix of neurogenic pain patients. Neuroimage 2006; 31(2): 721-31.

[57]   Walton KD, Dubois M, Llinas RR. Abnormal thalamocortical activity in patients with Complex Regional Pain Syndrome (CRPS) Type I. Pain 2010 Mar 23.

[58]   Ploner M, Gross J, Timmermann L, Pollok B, Schnitzler A. Pain suppresses spontaneous brain rhythms. Cereb Cortex 2006; 16(4): 537-40.

[59]   Jeanmonod D, Schulman J, Ramirez R, *et al.* Neuropsychiatric thalamocortical dysrhythmia: surgical implications. Neurosurg Clin N Am 2003; 14(2): 251-65.

[60]   Llinas RR, Ribary U, Jeanmonod D, Kronberg E, Mitra PP. Thalamocortical dysrhythmia: A neurological and neuropsychiatric syndrome characterized by magnetoencephalography. Proc Natl Acad Sci USA 1999; 96(26): 15222-7.

[61]   Strenge H, Fritzer G, Goder R, Niederberger U, Gerber WD, Aldenhoff J. Non-linear electroencephalogram dynamics in patients with spontaneous nocturnal migraine attacks. Neurosci Lett 2001; 309(2): 105-8.

[62]   Bartolomei F, Bosma I, Klein M, *et al.* Disturbed functional connectivity in brain tumour patients: evaluation by graph analysis of synchronization matrices. Clin Neurophysiol 2006; 117(9): 2039-49.

[63]   Bosma I, Douw L, Bartolomei F, *et al.* Synchronized brain activity and neurocognitive function in patients with low-grade glioma: a magnetoencephalography study. Neuro Oncol 2008; 10(5): 734-44.

[64]   Bosma I, Reijneveld JC, Klein M, *et al.* Disturbed functional brain networks and neurocognitive function in low-grade glioma patients: a graph theoretical analysis of resting-state MEG. Nonlinear Biomed Phys 2009; 3(1): 9.

[65]   Bosma I, Stam CJ, Douw L, *et al.* The influence of low-grade glioma on resting state oscillatory brain activity: a magnetoencephalography study. J Neurooncol 2008; 88(1): 77-85.

[66]   Douw L, Baayen H, Bosma I, *et al.* Treatment-related changes in functional connectivity in brain tumor patients: a magnetoencephalography study. Exp Neurol 2008; 212(2): 285-90.

[67]   Ioannides AA, Poghosyan V, Dammers J, Streit M. Real-time neural activity and connectivity in healthy individuals and schizophrenia patients. Neuroimage 2004; 23(2): 473-82.

[68]   Leistedt SJ, Coumans N, Dumont M, Lanquart JP, Stam CJ, Linkowski P. Altered sleep brain functional connectivity in acutely depressed patients. Hum Brain Mapp 2009 ; 30(7): 2207-19.

[69]   Micheloyannis S, Vourkas M, Tsirka V, Karakonstantaki E, Kanatsouli K, Stam CJ. The influence of ageing on complex brain networks: a graph theoretical analysis. Hum Brain Mapp 2009 ; 30(1): 200-8.

[70]   Smit DJ, Boersma M, van Beijsterveldt CE, *et al.* Endophenotypes in a dynamically connected brain. Behav Genet 2010; 40(2): 167-77.

[71]   He Y, Dagher A, Chen Z, *et al.* Impaired small-world efficiency in structural cortical networks in multiple sclerosis associated with white matter lesion load. Brain 2009; 132(Pt 12): 3366-79.

[72]   van Duinkerken E, Klein M, Schoonenboom NS, *et al.* Functional brain connectivity and neurocognitive functioning in patients with long-standing type 1 diabetes with and without microvascular complications: a magnetoencephalography study. Diabetes 2009; 58(10): 2335-43.

[73]   De Vico Fallani F, Astolfi L, Cincotti F, *et al.* Cortical functional connectivity networks in normal and spinal cord injured patients: Evaluation by graph analysis. Hum Brain Mapp 2007; 28(12): 1334-46.

[74]   De Vico Fallani F, Astolfi L, Cincotti F, *et al.* Brain connectivity structure in spinal cord injured: evaluation by graph analysis. Conf Proc IEEE Eng Med Biol Soc 2006; 1: 988-91.

	CHAPTER 2

A Primer on Networks in Neuroscience

Mark A. Kramer[*]

Department of Mathematics and Statistics, Boston University, 111 Cummington St, Boston MA 02215, USA

Abstract: Networks now play a prominent role in neuroscience research, supported by new data acquisition and analysis techniques. In this chapter we provide a brief introduction to this emerging field, with particular emphasis on methods to create (structural or functional) networks from neuronal data to characterize structural network properties. We also outline three simple models of networks, including the small-world network. The concepts introduced in this chapter provide a basic foundation to begin further exploration of networks in neuroscience, neurology and psychiatry. These clinical topics are covered in substantially more detail in the remaining chapters of the book.

Keywords: Node, edge, graph, path length, clustering coefficient, small world, functional connectivity.

INTRODUCTION

The appearance of networks in neuroscience has grown tremendously in the past decade, supported by new data acquisition and analysis techniques. To summarize this expanding field is a daunting task and not the goal of this chapter. Instead, we will consider a brief introduction to network analysis, with emphasis on the application of networks to problems in neuroscience. We will focus on techniques to create networks (either functional or structural) from data, tools to analyze networks, and methods to construct simple network models. The goal of this chapter is to introduce these concepts and provide the reader with a basic background applicable in later chapters and for further exploration of this emerging field. More detailed discussions of networks and their applications may be found in the references [1-5] and in the remaining chapters.

STRUCTURAL AND FUNCTIONAL NETWORKS

Many examples of networks exist in the world. These include structural networks (e.g., the network of roads that connect cities and towns), social networks (e.g., the networks of film actors that collaborate in movies), and biological networks (e.g., a network of neurons connected with synapses or gap junctions). In each case, we can divide the network into two fundamental components: *nodes* (the cities, actors, or neurons) and *edges* (the roads, films, or synapses) that connect node pairs. In what follows, we will focus on *binary, undirected* networks. In these simplified networks, an edge either exists between two nodes or does not, and the presence of an edge provides no directional (i.e., no causal) information.

In neuroscience, networks are typically divided into two categories: structural networks and functional networks [4]. In *structural* networks, the edges represent physical connections between nodes. At the microscopic spatial scale, these include synaptic or gap junction connections between individual neurons. In neuroscience, the only complete structural network mapped at this scale is for the nematode worm *C. elegans* [6-7]. At the macroscopic spatial scale, white matter tracts are used to infer synaptic connections between brain regions and construct structural networks in humans [8-10].

Functional (or "effective") networks rely on the coupling between dynamic activity recorded from separate brain areas. For example, we illustrate in Fig. (**2.1A**) simulated electroencephalogram (EEG) data recorded from two electrodes placed on the scalp surface of a human subject. EEG data is an example of what is commonly referred to as time series data, reflecting the temporal information contained in the sampled data points. To construct a simple functional network from EEG time series data (consisting of only two nodes), we determine how closely the EEG signals recorded at the two electrodes are related. Many measures exist to characterize this "match" (or coupling) between EEG signals [11]. Here we will employ a very simple measure: the cross correlation. The idea of this meas-

*Address correspondence to Mark A. Kramer: Department of Mathematics and Statistics, Boston University, 111 Cummington St, Boston MA 02215, USA; Email: mak@bu.edu

ure is to compare the two time series and see how well the voltage traces align. In doing so, we compare the signals both directly and shifted in time with respect to one another. Examining how the signals align over different time shifts allows us to detect if one signal is simply a delayed version of another. When the alignment between the two signals is good the cross correlation approaches 1; when the alignment is poor the cross correlation approaches 0. If two signals are completely out of phase (e.g., when one reaches its maximum, the other reaches its minimum, and vice versa) the cross correlation approaches -1. Depending on the time shift between the two signals, we may observe any of the three types of correlation, as we now describe.

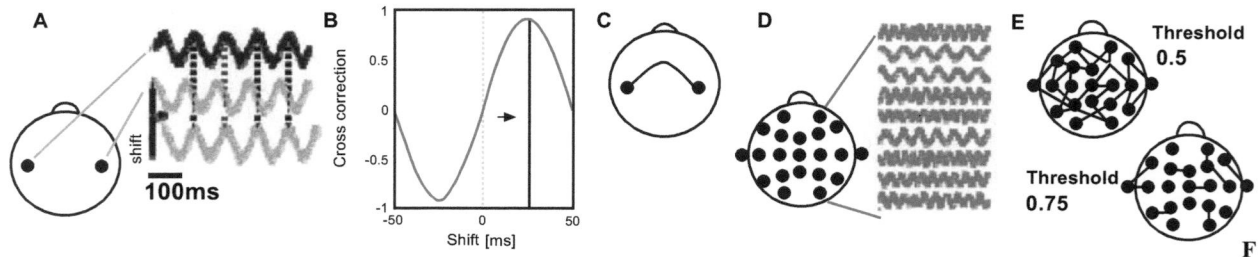

Fig. (2.1). Example method to construct functional networks from voltage data. In this simulated example (panel **A**), EEG data are recorded from two electrodes on the scalp surface. The EEG data (black and upper gray curve) are simple sinusoids with added noise, and the lower gray trace is the middle trace shifted to the right by ~25ms - this time advance of the EEG signal causes it to align phase with the top (black) trace, indicated by the vertical dashed lines. The cross correlation between the two electrodes is large when we shift the EEG data from one electrode by 25 ms (panel **B**). Because the cross correlation is strong enough, we link the two electrodes with an edge (black line) and thus form a simple two-node network (panel **C**). Simulated multivariate data recorded from many EEG electrodes (panel **D**), results in a much more complicated network in which the number of edges depends upon the choice of coupling threshold (panel **E**).

The cross correlation between the two simulated EEG recordings varies between -1 and 1 (Fig. **2.1B**). With no shift in the signals, the cross correlation is small (near 0). If we delay one signal backwards in time by 25 ms, the two EEG recordings "anti-correlate" (i.e., when one signal peaks, the other troughs) and the cross correlation approaches -1. When we advance one signal (gray in Fig. **2.1A**) forward in time by 25 ms, the two EEG recordings align and the cross correlation reaches 0.9. This last result indicates that the voltage activity observed at the two electrodes is coupled: the EEG data exhibit a strong correlation at a specific time shift. We represent this graphically by connecting the two electrodes with an edge (Fig. **2.1C**). In doing so, we have created a simple, 2-node network with one edge. The two nodes represent the two EEG electrodes, and the edge indicates sufficiently strong coupling between the voltage activity recorded from the two electrodes.

This procedure extends to any number of electrodes obtained for clinical or research purposes (for example the ~20 electrodes typically used in the 10-20 electrode configuration). In this case, we compute the coupling between the voltage data recorded for all electrode pairs (Fig. **2.1D**). We then connect electrode pairs whose coupling exceeds a threshold value (e.g., 0.5) with an edge. As we show in Fig. (**2.1E**), the connectivity becomes much more difficult to visualize as the number of nodes increases. In fact, as the number of nodes increases, the maximum number of possible edges increases dramatically: a 21-node network could support over 200 edges compared to 1 possible edge in the 2-node network. Simple visual inspection of the network structure, which sufficed for the 2-node network (Fig. **2.1C**), becomes inadequate for this larger, more complicated network. Methods for compressing this mass of relationships are discussed below.

Two subtleties exist in constructing functional networks from time series data. First, what coupling measure is most appropriate? Different measures exist that focus on linear interactions [12-14], nonlinear interactions [15], wavelet coherence [16], causality [17], and many other methods [11]. Each measure provides a different view of the coupling and requires different processing methods and assumptions (e.g., filtering the data in a specific frequency band to extract phase information, or choice of embedding dimension). Recent studies suggest that linear and nonlinear coupling measures perform equally well when applied to macroscopic voltage data, although subtle changes in the physiological state of the brain may require more sophisticated coupling measures [18-23]. Second, how do we determine the appropriate coupling threshold? In Fig. (**2.1**) we connected electrode pairs with edges whose coupling measure (in this case the cross correlation) exceeded a threshold value (e.g, 0.5). No technique yet exists to choose the most appropriate coupling threshold. One approach is to examine the networks produced for a variety of threshold values and seek consistent results [15, 24-30]. However, we may find that different threshold values produce extremely different networks (compare the two networks in Fig. **2.1E**).Another approach to defining a coupling threshold is first to apply an appropriate statistical hypothesis test to the coupling result computed for each electrode pair. Doing so, we may then assign a p-value to each edge and threshold these p-values rather than the original coupling measure [31]. An advantage of this approach is that multiple comparisons (a p-value exists for each electrode pair) may be addressed using sophisticated statistical techniques [32], and a measure of network uncertainty can be deduced, namely the number of spurious edges in the network [31]. One difficulty of this approach is the development of an appropriate method to determine the statistical significance of the coupling measure. For classical linear measures (such as the coherence or cross correlation), analytic techniques exist to determine the statistical significance of the measure, although these typically require specific assumptions about the data (e.g., the asymptotic case of extremely large sample sizes). For modern nonlinear measures, no such analytic methods to assess statistical significance exist. Instead one might employ a bootstrapping procedure. However, bootstrapping techniques are computationally expensive and typically not tractable for large networks.

SIMPLE MEASURES TO CHARACTERIZE NETWORK STRUCTURE

Typically, after constructing a functional network, we analyze its structure. A useful, first analysis is visual inspection of the network (e.g., visual inspection of the networks in Fig. **2.1E**). But, as mentioned above, as the number of nodes in a network increases, so does the number of possible edges, and visual inspection becomes less useful. For a network of N nodes, the maximum possible number of edges is $N(N-1)/2$. When N is large (e.g., in a high density EEG recording with 128 electrodes or a multi-electrode array with 100 contacts) the networks typically become much too complicated for visual inspection (Fig. **2A,B**). To go beyond visual inspection and characterize the structure of these large networks, many measures exist [1,3,5]. In this section, we consider three of these measures: the degree, path length, and clustering coefficient.

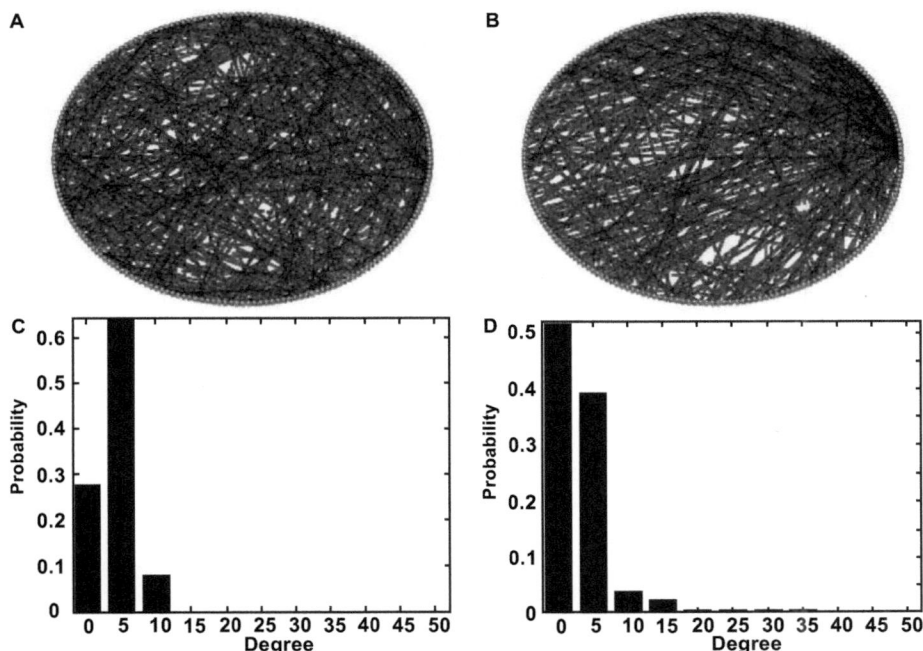

Fig. (2.2). Two large networks consisting of 200 nodes (**A**, **B**). We arrange the nodes (gray) in the network as a ring, although this does not imply a literal spatial location in the "real" experiment. Each node represents an individual electrode or sensor, and each edge (black line) indicates sufficiently strong coupling between activity recorded simultaneously at two nodes. For such large networks, the network structure becomes much more difficult to characterize through visual inspection. The degree distributions for each network are shown in panels **C** and **D**. For the network in (**A**) most of the nodes have a degree near 5. For the network in (**B**), most of the nodes have a degree less than five, but some nodes have a high degree (up to 35 edges). This is a substantial difference in the architecture of the network, which is not readily apparent upon visual inspection.

The *degree* (*d*) of a node is simply the number of edges that touches it. In Fig. (**2.3**), we show a five node network, and list the degree of each node (in this case a value of either 2 or 4). To summarize the degree values of the entire network, we compute the average degree (*D*) of all nodes, and find in this case a value of 2.4. For much larger networks, the distribution of degree values is a useful measure that illustrates the probability of observing a node of degree *d* (such as shown in Fig. **2.2C**). In many real-world networks (including the film actor network and neural networks [33]), the degree distribution exhibits a power law: the probability of observing a node of degree *d* decreases as $1/d^{\alpha}$ where α is a positive number (Fig. **2.2D**) [2]. In these networks high degree nodes (which appear less frequently than the low degree nodes) may serve important functional roles in the network (i.e., may act as hubs) although this is not always the case [34]. Degree distributions with power law behavior are also known as scale-free because the degree distribution looks the same (just scaled by a constant value) if we multiply the value of *d* by a constant.

The *path length* (*l*) is the minimum number of edges traversed to go from one node to another in the network. We assume here that each node is reachable from any other node; when this is not the case, care must be taken to account for unreachable nodes. In the example 5-node network (Fig. **2.3A**), the path length from node *i* to any other node is 1; node *i* can reach any other node by traversing 1 edge. Nodes *ii-v* can reach any other node in 1 or 2 steps. We note that many different paths exist between nodes. For example, we can travel directly from node *ii* to node *iii*, or we can pass through node *i* on the way to node *iii*. When computing the path length between any two nodes, by convention we always choose the shortest path between them. The *average path length* (*L*) is calculated from the path length between each node and all other nodes in the network; for the 5-node network, the average path length is 1.4.

The final measure we consider is the *clustering coefficient* (*c*). The clustering coefficient of a node is the number of connections that exist between the nearest neighbors of a node, expressed as a proportion of the maximum number of possible connections between the nearest neighbors of the node. This definition is perhaps best illustrated through an example. In the 5-node network, choose node *ii* and notice that this node has two neighbors (i.e., two nodes directly connected to node *ii* by a single edge, nodes *i* and *iii* in Fig. **2.3B**). We now examine whether an edge exists between the two neighbor nodes. In this example, it does (see Fig. **2.3A**) so we complete a triangle or cluster in the network. In social networks, clustering is typically high; the friends (nearest neighbors) of an individual (the chosen node) also tend to be friends (i.e., edges connect the nearest neighbors of the chosen node). The formula to compute the clustering coefficient for a node *n* is,

$$c_n = \frac{E(\Gamma_n)}{k_n(k_n - 1)/2}$$

Here, Γn is a list of the nearest neighbors of node *n*, $E(\Gamma n)$ is the number of edges between the nearest neighbors of *n* (but does not include edges that connect to node *n* directly), and k_n is the number of nodes in Γn. For *n=i* in the example 5-node network, $\Gamma i = \{ii,iii,iv,v\}$ and $k_n=4$. Two edges exist within this neighborhood (between nodes *ii* and *iii*, and between nodes *iv* and *v*), so $E(\Gamma i) = 2$. Plugging into the equation above, we find $c_i=2/6=1/3$. This result indicates that of all the possible completed triangles between the nearest neighbors of node *i*, only one-third exist. To complete all of the triangles between the nearest neighbors of node *i* would require additional connections between nodes *ii* and *iv*, nodes *ii* and *v*, nodes *iii* and *iv*, and nodes *iii* and *v*. For the other nodes, the clustering coefficient equals 1. All possible triangles between the nearest neighbors of these other nodes do exist. The *average clustering coefficient* (*C*) is the average of *c* between all nodes in the network; for the 5-node network *C* is 13/15.

In this section we described three measures of network structure. These measures provide simple numeric summaries to characterize complex networks, consisting of many nodes and edges. As an example of the application of these measures, we consider the nervous system of *C. elegans*, which has been completely mapped at the cellular level. The network consists of *N*=282 nodes (or neurons). The average degree *D*=14, average path length *L*=2.65, and average clustering coefficient *C*=0.28 [33]. Already these results reveal some interesting aspects about the network structure (for example, we can travel from one neuron to any other in 3 steps, on average). To further interpret these results, we consider three reference networks described in the next section.

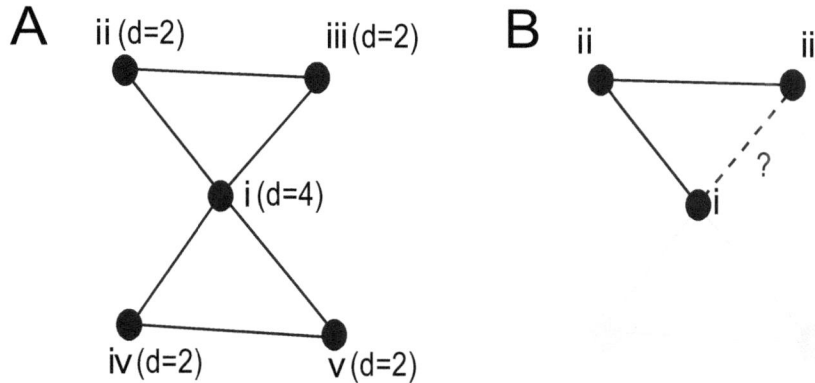

Fig. (2.3). An example 5-node network to illustrate the simple measures of network structure. We label the 5-nodes (circles) with roman numerals and connect the nodes with edges (lines; (**A**). The number in parentheses next to each node indicates its degree (*d*). To determine the clustering coefficient of node *ii*, we first determine its nearest neighbors (the other two nodes in the network are grayed out; (**B**). We then determine if an edge exists between these neighbors (the dotted line). Because this edge exists in panel A, the three nodes form a triangle or cluster.

SIMPLE NETWORK MODELS

In the previous section, we considered three measures to summarize observed (or constructed) networks. In this section, we consider three simple models to generate networks. For each network, we outline the construction method and provide approximate formulas for the average degree, average path length, and average clustering coefficient.

We start with a *regular network*, in which we arrange the nodes as a ring and connect each node to the k closest nodes on the ring (Fig. **2.4A**). The result is a network with mesh-like connections between neighboring nodes. For a regular network of N nodes, approximate formulas exist for the average degree, average path length, and average clustering coefficient. The expression for the average degree is simply $\underline{D}=k$. In a regular network, the same number of edges is connected to each node. The expression for the average path length is $\underline{L} \sim N/(2k)$. As the number of nodes (N) increases, so does the average path length; in a large network we must travel many edges (from neighbor to neighbor around the circumference of the circle in Fig. **2.4A**) to reach our destination. Finally, the average clustering coefficient is a constant: $\underline{C} \sim 3/4$ for large k. In the regular network, the mesh-like connections between nodes establish many clusters (or triangles).

The second model network we consider is a traditional *random network*. In this network, we connect each pair of nodes with probability p. To construct this network, we imagine flipping a (perhaps biased) coin for each node pair. If the coin flip results in heads, we connect the two nodes with an edge, otherwise we do not (Fig. **2.4C**). Approximate formulas for the network measures exist for a random network of N nodes as well. The average degree is $\underline{D} \sim p(N-1)$, the probability of success (p) multiplied by the number of times we flip the biased coin for each node (note that, in a network of N nodes with no self connections, each node can connect to $N-1$ other nodes). The average path length, $\underline{L} \sim \ln(N)/\ln(\underline{D})$, increases as the number of nodes increases, although not as quickly as in the regular network. Finally, the average clustering coefficient, $\underline{C} \sim \underline{D}/N$, decreases as the number of nodes N increases; clusters (or triangles) appear infrequently in random networks.

To illustrate the differences between a regular and random network, consider $N=20$ nodes and $\underline{D}=4$. Using the formulas above, we find a larger average path length for the regular network ($\underline{L} \sim 2.5$) compared to the random network ($\underline{L} \sim 2.16$). To travel from one node to another in the regular network, we might imagine proceeding from neighboring node to neighboring node around the circumference of a circle (Fig. **2.4A**). Travel in the random network typically requires fewer steps because connections span the middle of the circle; no longer is travel restricted to the circle circumference (Fig. **2.4C**). For this same example ($N=20$ nodes and $\underline{D}=4$), we find a much larger clustering coefficient for the regular network ($\underline{C} \sim 0.75$) compared to the random network ($\underline{C} \sim 0.2$). In the random network, the nearest neighbors of a node are no more likely to be connected than any other nodes; the probability that a node's "friends" are also friends in a random network is simply p (that is, the baseline probability of any two nodes being connected). In the regular network, the mesh-like structure of the connections supports completed triangles (i.e., clusters).

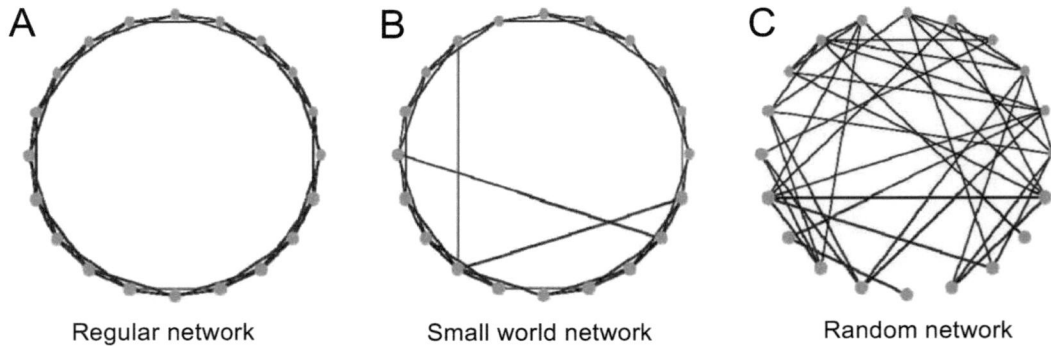

Regular network   Small world network   Random network

Fig. (2.4). Examples of a regular network, small world network, and random network (N=20 and $\underline{D}$=4). In the regular network (**A**), mesh-like connections occur between neighboring nodes. In the small world network (**B**), most connections are local, but a few long distance connections exist. These few shortcuts dramatically decrease the average path length of the network, without impacting the clustering coefficient substantially. In the random network (**C**), edges occur between node pairs with equal probability.

Is either the regular or random network a good approximation to the *C. elegans* neural network? To address this, we fix N=282 and $\underline{D}$=14 (the values for *C. elegans* [33]), compute the average path length and average clustering coefficients for the corresponding regular and random networks, and compare these values to those determined for the observed neural network in Table **2.1**.

Table 2.1. The Average Path Length ($\underline{L}$) and Average Clustering Coefficient ($\underline{D}$) for the *C. elegans* Neural Network, as Well as a Regular and a Random Network with the Same Number of Nodes and Average Degree [33]

	C. elegans	Regular	Random
L	2.65	10	2.13
D	0.28	0.75	0.05

These calculations suggest that the average path length of the *C. elegans* network is better approximated by a random network; the average path length of both networks is considerably shorter than that for a regular network. Yet, we find that the clustering coefficient of the *C. elegans* network is poorly approximated by the random network. The *C. elegans* network possesses a higher clustering coefficient, which is better approximated by the regular network. We conclude that neither the regular nor random network accurately represents both the clustering coefficient and average path length calculated for the *C. elegans* network. Each model captures only one important aspect of the network topology.

The final model we consider — the small world network — provides a better approximation to the *C. elegans* network. Like this neural network, the small world network possesses both a small average path length and a large average clustering coefficient. We construct the small world network in the following way [33]. First, we begin with a regular network of N nodes each with k edges. We then rewire each edge with probability p. More specifically, we choose an edge, flip a biased coin (with a probability of success p), and if the flip is successful, we disconnect one end of the edge and reconnect it to another node chosen at random (with uniform probability) from all other nodes. When p is small, the result is a rewiring of a few network edges (Fig. **2.4B**). These edges typically serve as network shortcuts; we can follow these edges to quickly move from one side of the network to the other. The result of these few shortcuts is a dramatic decrease in the average path length. However, because we rewire only a few edges, the average clustering coefficient of the network remains large. These are the characteristics of a small world network: a few shortcuts create a network with small average path length and large average clustering coefficient. Brain networks (both structural and functional) appear frequently to possess small world structure [35-38]. We might interpret these observations as the brain seeking to balance segregation of information processing to local structures and integration of this processing between distant structures [4]. In attempting to achieve this balance, perhaps the brain seeks to minimize wiring (therefore making most connections local) and maximize efficiency (so that signals may travel quickly from one brain region to another through a minority of large distance connections). These reasonable arguments make the small world network a compelling model of brain networks.

We conclude with suggested questions to consider when examining networks in neuroscience literature (Table **2.2**). Each question focuses on topics considered in this primer, which provides only a brief introduction to the field of networks. Many other network measures exist beyond the three discussed here (e.g., betweenness or assortativity). Similarly, other network models exist (e.g., preferential attachment) beyond the regular, random, and small world networks. Nevertheless, we hope this brief introduction has prepared (and motivated) readers to pursue further study in this growing field.

Table 2.2. Questions to Consider when Reading Literature on Networks

1. Is the network *structural* or *functional*?
2. If the network is functional:
a. What coupling method determined node connectivity?
b. What coupling *threshold* defined the edges?
3. What is the average degree, average path length, and average clustering coefficient?
4. Is the network approximately *regular*, *random*, or *small world*?

CONCLUSIONS

The application of networks to problems in neuroscience is rapidly expanding. The emergence of new technology (e.g., high-density multi-electrode array recordings from thin slices of brain tissue *in vitro*, or diffusion tensor imaging of white matter tracks *in vivo*) permits unprecedented collection of neuronal network data. Characterizing these networks — and understanding their implications for brain function — will require the continued development of mathematical tools and theory.

In this chapter, we considered two types of networks studied in neuroscience: structural networks and functional networks. Both types of networks undoubtedly serve important roles in the brain. Structural networks form the backbone of neural connectivity, while functional networks make dynamic use of this backbone and transiently unite disparate brain regions. Although we distinguished between these two types of networks, dynamic brain activity (resulting in functional connections) alters brain structural connectivity (through plasticity mechanisms, for example); in other words, brain structural connectivity and functional connectivity are interrelated.

REFERENCES

[1]   Wasserman S, Faust K. Social Network Analysis: Methods and Applications. Cambridge University Press; 1994.
[2]   Albert R, Barabási A. Statistical mechanics of complex networks. Rev Mod Phys 2002; 74: 47–97.
[3]   Newman M. The structure and function of complex networks. SIAM Rev 2003; 45(2): 167.
[4]   Bullmore E, Sporns O. Complex brain networks: graph theoretical analysis of structural and functional systems. Nat Rev Neurosci 2009; 10(3): 186–98.
[5]   Kolaczyk ED. Statistical Analysis of Network Data: Methods and Models. Springer; 2009.
[6]   White J, Southgate E, Thomson J, Brenner S. The structure of the nervous system of the nematode caenorhabditis elegans. Philos T Roy Soc B 1986; 314(1165): 1–340.
[7]   Achacoso TB, Yamamoto WS. AYs Neuroanatomy of C Elegans for Computation. CRC-Press; 1992.
[8]   Iturria-Medina Y, Canales-Rodríguez EJ, Melie-García L, *et al.* Characterizing brain anatomical connections using diffusion weighted MRI and graph theory. Neuroimage 2007; 36(3): 645–60.
[9]   Iturria-Medina Y, Sotero RC, Canales-Rodríguez EJ, Alemán-Gómez Y, Melie-García L. Studying the human brain anatomical network via diffusion-weighted MRI and Graph Theory. Neuroimage 2008; 40(3): 1064–76.
[10]   Hagmann P, Cammoun L, Gigandet X, *et al.* Mapping the structural core of human cerebral cortex. PLoS Biology 2008; 6(7): e159 EP.
[11]   Pereda E, Quiroga R, Bhattacharya J. Nonlinear multivariate analysis of neurophysiological signals. Prog Neurobiol 2005; 77: 1–37.

[12] Brazier MA. Electrical seizure discharge within the humn brain: the problem of spread. In: Braizer MA, editor. Epilepsy, its phenomenon in man. Academic Press; 1973.

[13] Tharp BR, Gersch W. Spectral analysis of seizures in humans. Comput Biomed Res 1975; 8(6): 503–21.

[14] Mitra P, Bokil H. Observed Brain Dynamics. Oxford University Press; 2008.

[15] Ponten SC, Bartolomei F, Stam CJ. Small-world networks and epilepsy: graph theoretical analysis of intracerebrally recorded mesial temporal lobe seizures. Clin Neurophysiol 2007; 118(4): 918–27.

[16] Lachaux JP, Lutz A, Rudrauf D, *et al.* Estimating the time-course of coherence between single-trial brain signals: an introduction to wavelet coherence. Clin Neurophysiol 2002; 32(3): 157–174.

[17] Kamiski M, Ding M, Truccolo WA, Bressler SL. Evaluating causal relations in neural systems: granger causality, directed transfer function and statistical assessment of significance. Biol Cybern 2001; 85(2): 145–57.

[18] Aarabi A, Wallois F, Grebe R. Does spatiotemporal synchronization of EEG change prior to absence seizures? Brain Res 2008; 1188: 207–221.

[19] Ansari-Asl K, Senhadji L, Bellanger JJ, Wendling F. Quantitative evaluation of linear and nonlinear methods characterizing interdependencies between brain signals. Phys Rev E 2006; 74(3 Pt 1): 031916.

[20] Kreuz T, Mormann F, Andrzejak R, Kraskov A, Lehnertz K, Grassberger P. Measuring synchronization in coupled model systems: A comparison of different approaches. Physica D 2007; 225(1): 29–42.

[21] Mormann F, Kreuz T, Rieke C, Andrzejak R, Kraskov A, David P, *et al.* On the predictability of epileptic seizures. Clin Neurophysiol 2005; 116(3): 569–587.

[22] Osterhage H, Mormann F, Staniek M, Lehnertz K. Measuring synchronization in the epileptic brain: A comparison of different approaches. Int J Bifurcat Chaos 2007; 17(10): 3539–3544.

[23] Quiroga RQ, Kraskov A, Kreuz T, Grassberger P. Performance of different synchronization measures in real data: a case study on electroencephalographic signals. Phys Rev E 2002; 65(4 Pt 1): 041903.

[24] Stam CJ. Functional connectivity patterns of human magnetoencephalographic recordings: a 'small-world' network? Neurosci Lett 2004; 355(1-2): 25–8.

[25] Micheloyannis S, Pachou E, Stam CJ, Vourkas M, Erimaki S, Tsirka V. Using graph theoretical analysis of multi channel EEG to evaluate the neural efficiency hypothesis. Neurosci Lett 2006; 402(3): 273–7.

[26] Srinivas K, Jain R, Saurav S, Sikdar S. Small-world network topology of hippocampal neuronal network is lost, in an in vitro glutamate injury model of epilepsy. Eur J Neurosci 2007; 25(11): 3276–86.

[27] Stam CJ, Jones BF, Nolte G, Breakspear M, Scheltens P. Small-world networks and functional connectivity in Alzheimer's disease. Cereb Cortex 2007; 17(1): 92–9.

[28] Kramer MA, Kolaczyk ED, Kirsch HE. Emergent network topology at seizure onset in humans. Epilepsy Res 2008; 79(2-3): 173–86.

[29] Supekar K, Menon V, Rubin D, Musen M, Greicius M. Network Analysis of Intrinsic Functional Brain Connectivity in Alzheimer's Disease. PLoS Comp Bio 2008; 4(6): e1000100 EP.

[30] Yamasaki K, Gozolchiani A, Havlin S. Climate networks around the globe are significantly affected by El Niño. Phys Rev Lett 2008; 100(22): 228501.

[31] Kramer MA, Eden UT, Cash SS, Kolaczyk ED. Network inference with confidence from multivariate time series. Phys Rev E 2009; 79(6 Pt 1): 061916.

[32] Storey JD, Tibshirani R. Statistical significance for genomewide studies. Proc Natl Acad Sci 2003; 100(16): 9440–9445.

[33] Watts DJ, Strogatz SH. Collective dynamics of small-world networks. Nature 1998; 393(6684): 440–2.

[34] Doyle J, Alderson D, Li L, Low S, Roughan M, Shalunov S, *et al.* The "robust yet fragile" nature of the Internet. Proc Natl Acad Sci USA 2005; 102(41): 14497–14502.

[35] Song S, Sjöström PJ, Reigl M, Nelson S, Chklovskii DB. Highly nonrandom features of synaptic connectivity in local cortical circuits. PLoS Biol 2005; 3(3): e68.

[36] Kaiser M, Hilgetag CC. Nonoptimal component placement, but short processing paths, due to long-distance projections in neural systems. PLoS Comput Biol 2006; 2(7): e95.

[37] Achard S, Salvador R, Whitcher B, Suckling J, Bullmore E. A resilient, low-frequency, small-world human brain functional network with highly connected association cortical hubs. J Neurosci 2006; 26(1): 63–72.

[38] Bassett DS, Bullmore E. Small-world brain networks. The Neuroscientist : a review journal bringing neurobiology, neurology and psychiatry 2006; 12(6): 512–23.

CHAPTER 3

Neural Networks in the Developing Human Brain

Catherine J. Chu-Shore[1,*], Verne S. Caviness[2] and Sydney S. Cash[2]

[1]Divisions of Pediatric Neurology and Neurophysiology, Department of Neurology, Massachusetts General Hospital, 175 Cambridge Street, Suite 340, Boston, MA 02114, USA and [2]Neurology Department, 55 Fruit Street, Wang 7, Massachusetts General Hospital, Boston, MA, 02114, USA

Abstract: The brain undergoes massive and exquisitely controlled age-specific anatomical and physiological changes throughout development. The network paradigms discussed in this chapter provide a rich new method to track these dynamic interregional relationships and describe global properties of the developing system as a whole. Here, as background, we review the primary events of anatomical and physiological neurodevelopment from gestation through adolescence. We then describe early work elucidating the presence and evolution of age-specific functional brain networks in normal neurodevelopment. Finally, we discuss work aimed at understanding how these relationships may be altered in disease, and perhaps even rectified with treatment. Although much remains to be done, the application of the network model to the developing human brain holds tremendous promise for future discovery.

Keywords: Pruning, maturation, neuroanatomy, default network, epilepsy, autism.

INTRODUCTION

The paradigm of network approaches provides a rich means of analyzing the dynamic interdependencies in what is surely one of the most complex, integrated and plastic systems - the developing human brain. Historically, study of the development of the nervous system has largely been explicitly reductionist. While certainly valuable, these piecemeal approaches may overlook the unique and emergent properties that are evident when evaluating a system as an integrated whole. The study of networks, however, provides a framework for capturing the global properties and interrelationships inherent in the human brain. Network methods are expected to become invaluable for child neurologists, as we attempt to track the development and self-organization of the human brain as it matures.

From the embryonic process of primary neurulation to the elaboration of a mature central nervous system, anatomical and functional neural networks grow from a few countable connections to the complex networks present in the mature human brain. This neurodevelopmental process involves the enactment of determined genetic templates as well as responses to expected as well as unpredictable environmental experiences. Understanding the earliest foundation and development of the brain's neural networks provides insights into the anatomical and functional relationships seen in the mature human brain. Furthermore, understanding the ontogeny of neural networks through normal fetal, neonatal, and infant connectivity patterns yields insights into the manner and timing of potential pathology, spanning the range of subtle to devastating neurodevelopmental consequences. Here, we outline the principal histogenetic events and sequences of developmental neurobiology that help shape developmental networks, as well as highlight some of the recent findings explicitly describing anatomical and functional connectivity in this new and rapidly expanding area of scientific inquiry. Much of the basic work in this field comes from experiments in animals, notably rodents and non-human primates. The overview we present here draws upon this experimental work but, where available, is based upon observations in the developing human nervous system.

ANATOMICAL DEVELOPMENT

The human brain undergoes dramatic changes throughout childhood. At birth, the human brain weighs 300-350g and approximately doubles in size over the first year. Although total brain size reaches approximately 1350-1500g by age 6 years and does not increase significantly after that, ongoing structural and functional changes are thought to occur in a near-equilibrium of progressive and regressive events throughout life [1,2].

---

*Address correspondence to Catherine J. Chu-Shore: Divisions of Pediatric Neurology and Neurophysiology, Department of Neurology, Massachusetts General Hospital, 175 Cambridge Street, Suite 340, Boston, MA 02114, USA; Email: cchushore@partners.org

The familiar laminated architecture of the human cortex [3,4] develops primarily over the course of fetal development. At the cellular level, precursors of projection neurons [5,6] in the ventricular zone (adjacent to the ventricles) [7-10], amplified by secondary divisions in the subventricular zone [11,12], undergo massive proliferation in the first 2-6 months of gestation [13]. Overlapping with this period, neuronal precursors migrate radially along a glial scaffolding to form the early cortical plate where they distribute primarily in an inside to outside pattern with respect to time of origin [9,10]. Interneurons, by contrast, arise in the ganglionic eminences to converge upon the developing cortex by tangential migrations [5,6]. Continuing migration and post migration rearrangements position the neuronal somata in the five laminar arrays so distinctive of the neocortex. Subsequently, the elaboration of dendritic and axonal neuropil, in architectonic and laminar distinctive patterns ultimately is associated with the emergence of the 6-layered mature human cortex by 8 months gestation [10], with each step coinciding with the expression of critical regulatory genes [14]. At a macroscopic level, the brain is simultaneously undergoing significant gyral folding during this time. The fetal brain initially has a smooth cortical surface with only a single intra-hemispheric fissure at 10 weeks. Primary sulci are evident by 6-7 months gestation and secondary and tertiary sulcation are completed shortly after birth [15-17].

Cerebral cortical development continues to evolve dramatically throughout infancy through early adolescence in a non-linear and heterochronic fashion. Serial MRI studies reveal that cortical gray matter volume increases initially prior to puberty followed by a net loss post-puberty [18]. This predictable sequence is observed in cortical regions associated with primary motor and sensory functions prior to association cortices and regions such as prefrontal cortex, felt to be involved in executive functions [19,20].

Many underlying cellular and ultrastructural processes are thought to account for the inverted U-shaped pattern of cortical volume [21] (see Fig. **3.1**). Early fetal brain development is a time of initial massive neuronal proliferation followed by subsequent selective cell death where differential architectonic field and laminar cell death appears to confer the essential architectonic pattern to each field [13, 22-25]. Heightened synaptogenesis initiates in the third trimester and continues through the first 2 years of life, followed by a prolonged period of dendritic pruning during childhood and adolescence, during which synaptic density decreases by approximately 40% of maximum. Similar to patterns of cortical volume change, synaptic density reaches a maximum in primary sensory cortical regions prior to association cortices. For example, from the work of Huttenlocher and associates, maximal synaptic density in the primary auditory cortex and visual cortices are observed around 3 months of age, compared to approximately 15 months in the prefrontal cortex [23]. Variation between cortical layers is also observed, such that deeper cortical layers receiving primary afferent input (layer 4) and giving rise to efferent fibers (layers 5 and 6) develop more rapidly than more superficial layers (2 and 3) [23]. Selective dendritic pruning and consolidation of remaining synaptic connections continues through childhood and extends in some regions into puberty. The timing of the gross cortical volume loss evident on MRI appears to correlate with increased synaptic pruning demonstrated at the ultrastructural level in normal pathology specimens.

Whereas axon number as with neuron number undergoes a massive elaboration and pruning sequence in the early phase of cerebral maturation [27,28], white matter volume increases continuously with age, in large part due myelination of cortico-cortical fibers. White matter myelination creates a near-constant conduction latency between brain regions, irrespective of distance [29]. Oligodendrocytic myelination of neuronal axons begins during the second trimester of fetal development with continued dramatic increases seen in the first 2 years of life [30], and continues at slower rates throughout the first 3 decades of life [31]. Perhaps by no coincidence, white matter myelination follows a similar sequence observed in cortical maturation, with fibers mediating primary sensory then motor systems myelinated first in infants, followed by white matter underlying temporal and parietal association cortices, and subsequently prefrontal and lateral temporal cortices in the brain in young children [32,33]. Distinction between gray and white matter can be difficult using standard MRI techniques, owing in part to ambiguity of signal defined gray-white boundaries in the fetal and early postnatal brain in early stages of myelination [10]. Diffusion tensor imaging (DTI), which employs fractional anisotropy (FA) as a measure of the preferred direction of diffusion of water molecules, and by inference, of the pattern of white matter connectivity, offers one possible alternative [34]. This technique can be used to infer the anatomy of white matter tracts in all ages, including largely unmyelinated immature brains. Longitudinal work evaluating DTI and white matter tractography across infant and

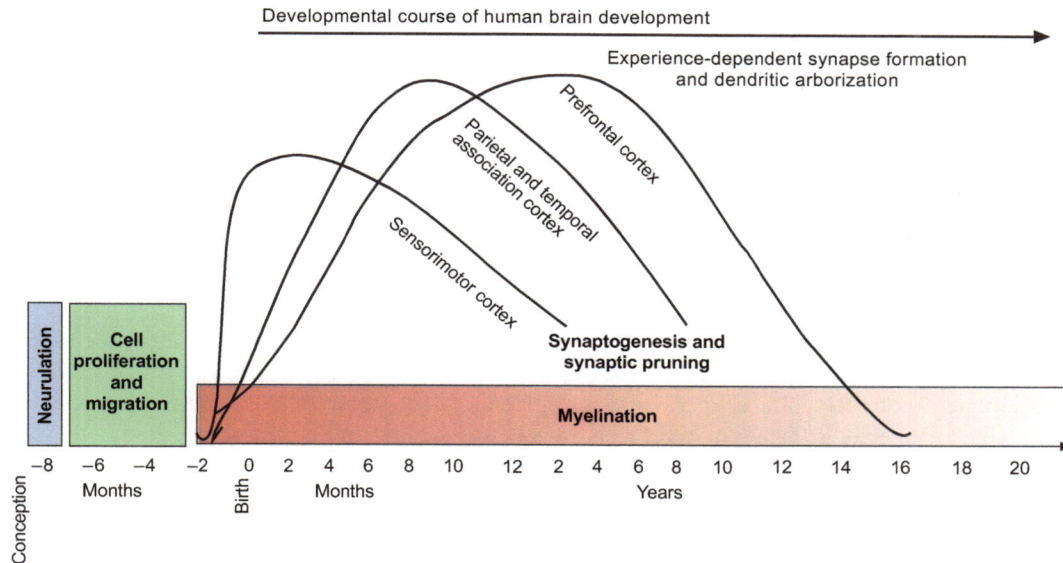

Fig. (3.1). The observed timeline of some of the progressive and regressive structural changes present over the course of prenatal through adolescent brain development (reprinted with permission from reference [21]). This figure may be taken to represent the general hierarchical elaboration of forebrain neural systems where the events in primary representations anticipate those in successively more integrative regions [26].

child development reveals that nearly all prominent white matter tracts can be identified at birth, although the tracts appear thinner and with lower FA values at younger ages [35,36]. FA values increase dramatically in the first 24 months and resemble typical adult values by 48 months, reflecting increased myelination and corresponding restriction of directional water molecule mobility. Interestingly, the major interhemispheric pathways of the corpus callosum and anterior commissure are present in newborns, but association fibers such as the superior longitudinal fasciculus, inferior longitudinal fasciculus, and inferior fronto-occipital fasciculus are not apparent until 3-12 months of age (see Fig. **3.2**). These very early anatomical connections appear to mirror patterns of functional connectivity seen in young infants (see below).

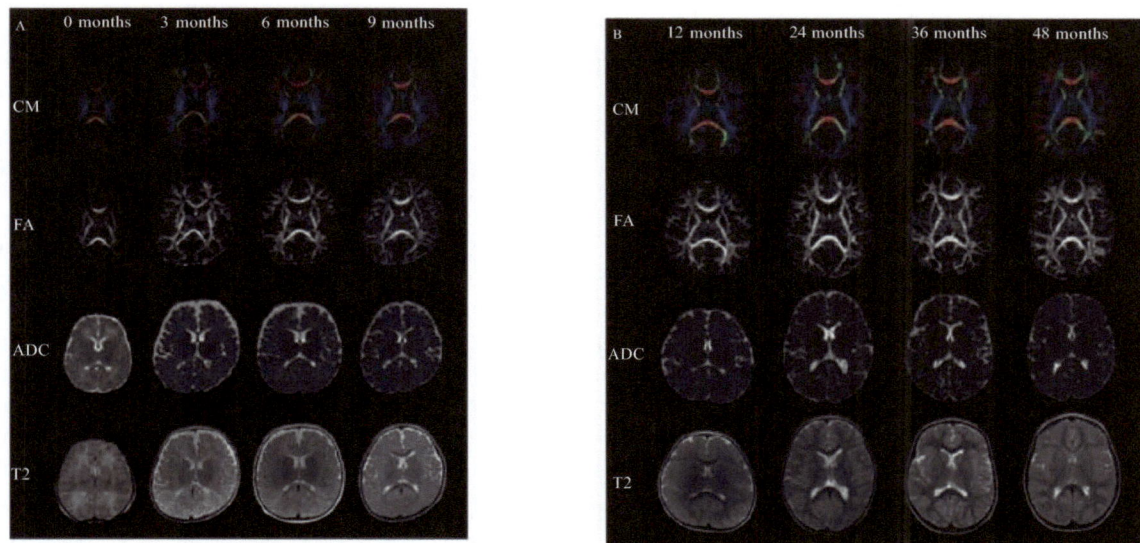

Fig. (3.2). Representative axial color maps (CM), diffusion tensor maps (FA), ADC and T2 sequences at 0, 3, 6, 9, 12, 24, 36, and 48 months (reprinted with permission from reference 35).

PHYSIOLOGICAL DEVELOPMENT

Anatomical and physiological relationships in the brain are clearly related, but not synonymous. Physiological connections are undoubtedly influenced and constrained to some extent by structural frameworks [37]. Likewise, neural activity, directed initially by spontaneous activity and subsequently environmental experiences, serves to guide all aspects of architectural development, from neurogenesis, neuronal differentiation and migration, to synaptogenesis and dendritic pruning [38-45]. Thus, anatomy and physiology interdependently direct the development and stabilization of cortical networks. Coinciding with the development of the anatomical framework described above, here we describe some stable, age-specific, physiological patterns that have been observed over the course of brain development.

An early positron emission tomography (PET) study evaluated 29 children with transient neurological episodes who turned out to have unrevealing clinical evaluations and subsequently normal neurodevelopment. The imaging showed regional patterns of metabolic changes that were similar to patterns of anatomical development [46]. Specifically, the cerebral metabolic rates for glucose (CMRG) was highest initially in the sensorimotor cortex in newborns (<5 weeks), increased in parietal, temporal and occipital cortices by 3 months, followed by increases in the frontal and dorso-lateral occipital cortical regions by 6-8 months. Absolute values of CMRG followed an inverted U-shape curve: initially low at birth and reaching adult values by 2 years, but continuing to increase beyond adult values until approximately 9 years of age, at which point they declined again, returning to adult values in the second decade. This metabolic peak lags well behind the timing of peak synaptic densities, but grossly correlates with changes in cortical volume [13, 23]. The evolving regions of heightened metabolism in infancy were similar to known myelination patterns, and the brain metabolic changes in childhood are postulated to reflect the overlapping processes of cell death, dendritic arborization, synaptogenesis and subsequent dendritic pruning.

Scalp electroencephalography (EEG) primarily measures voltage changes from summated post synaptic potentials of large cortical neuronal populations. EEG rhythms dramatically change from the prenatal period through development to adulthood [47]. Common features in fetal and newborn sleep EEGs include periods of low amplitude background (tracé discontinue or tracé alternant) alternating with prolonged periods of rapid eye movement (REM) sleep [48,49]. Continuous periods are characterized by greater asynchrony of waveforms between regions and hemispheres and dominated by delta range (0.3-1.5 Hz) asynchronous activities with overriding faster (8-22 Hz) frequencies, termed delta brushes. The duration of discontinuous periods ("interburst intervals") decreases with age and the EEG patterns mature to a continuous background over the first few weeks of life [49].

In infants age 0-24 months during quiet sleep, lower frequencies are consistently more prominent than higher frequencies [50]. Longitudinally, delta (0-4 Hz) and theta (4-7 Hz) power increases through late gestation and early infancy, followed by a plateau that initiates around 2 months and 4 months of age, respectively. From 0-4 months of age, spectral power of alpha (8-12 Hz) and beta (13-19 Hz) frequencies declines followed by subsequent increase with a peak at 12-16 weeks [50].

Well-characterized sleep rhythms also evolve over the first year. Asynchronous and prolonged 11-15 Hz sleep spindles are first evident in the bilateral fronto-central regions at 6-9 weeks of age and gradually shorten and become more synchronous between hemispheres within the first year of life [51,52]. In children, independent sleep spindles of slightly different frequencies are present in the frontal regions (11-12.75 Hz) and the centro-parietal regions (13-14.75 Hz) [52]. Greater interhemispheric synchrony between waveforms is evident by 6 months of age, however asynchronous spindles persist through the first 2 years of life [49]. Symmetric, high amplitude frontal predominant K-complexes are evident in by 5-6 months of life and clearly recognizable midline and central vertex sharp waves are present by 16 months [49]. The emergence of these paroxysmal sleep rhythms is thought to reflect the underlying maturation of thalamocortical circuits [53]. REM sleep is evident at birth and decreases over the first 2 years of life, while the percentage of sleep time spent in quiet sleep simultaneously increases [48]. Slow wave sleep epochs are evident by 4-5 months of age and continue to mature toward adult patterns through childhood [49].

The spatial organization and dominant frequencies of EEG rhythms during wakefulness likewise matures with age. A dominant amplitude posterior alpha rhythm is reliably present in the majority of adults during quiet wakefulness and is suppressed by eye opening or certain mental activities [47]. During wakefulness, a slower, sinusoidal theta rhythm over posterior regions is present in early infancy and matures to a reactive, posterior dominant alpha rhythm by 3 years of age [52]. The frequency of the posterior dominant rhythm increases linearly with age, reaching 10 Hz by age 15 years, and the amplitude peaks at near 60 uV by age 6-9 years [54]. Rhythmic posterior delta activity (termed posterior slowing of youth) is also evident in pediatric EEGs. This episodic rhythm is present at 1 year, peaking in amplitude between 5-7 years and persists until early teenage years [55].

FUNCTIONAL CONNECTIVITY

Functional connectivity analytical techniques infer connections between components of a system by identifying patterns between the physiological activities of the components. These connections are then used to generate networks for further analysis such as graph theory metrics (described in Chapter 2). Work evaluating functional connectivity network patterns in infants and children and longitudinal evolution over time has been sparse, but is gaining recent attention. As graph theory and network science provide tractable means to analyze dynamic, integrated systems, work in this area offers immense promise from diagnostics and phenotyping to natural history and treatment planning.

Early studies evaluating physiological inter-relationships calculated coherence between EEG signals obtained from individual channels in different frequency bands. Phase-locked coherence between spatially separated EEG channels may reflect underlying physiological connectivity between large populations of cortical neurons. In one study, the spatial patterns of coherence between EEG channels in alpha range frequencies were compared between school-age children and adults using a 128 channel electrode array [56]. Although short-range coherence was not different between adults and school-age children, there was increased coherence between more distant anterior and posterior electrodes in adults. These changes were thought to reflect the increased anatomical connectivity of longer range cortical connections with age through maturation of myelination of long-distance axons and fasciculi.

Stimulus evoked oscillatory signals and phase synchronization of signals between different EEG electrode channels has also been investigated across development. Interestingly, somatotopically organized delta brushes in the sensorimotor cortex appear to be triggered by contralateral sensory stimulation, either through spontaneous movements or tactile stimulation in premature infants, possibly reflecting early organization of sensory neural circuits [57]. By 8 months of age and thereafter, characteristic 40 Hz gamma band oscillations are evident in the left frontal region in response to visual stimuli [58]. These oscillations are felt to represent a neuronal binding mechanism involved in the development of complex visual processing. Age-specific maturation of evoked gamma band oscillations in response to complex visual phenomena has been demonstrated in occipital and parietal regions, from childhood through young adulthood [39, 59]. Using a 62 electrode scalp array in 68 participants aged 6-21 years, one group demonstrated age-specific patterns of phase synchrony between EEG signals in response to visual stimuli in multiple frequency bands [60]. Interestingly, phase synchronization in the beta band was noted to follow an age-specific topography, with initially widespread synchronization followed by a period of desynchronization, preceding more focal synchronization patterns. These processes correlated with reaction times and detection rates to stimulus onset, with worsened performance and decreased synchrony noted during adolescence. These findings may reflect the non-linear, complex processes underlying the normal maturation of functional cortical networks.

Recent work evaluating developmental functional connectivity patterns has been performed using resting state functional connectivity MRI (rs-fcMRI). This method uses fMRI to measure the correlation of low frequency (<0.1Hz) blood oxygenation level-dependent (BOLD) signal fluctuations between selected brain regions of interest (ROI) occurring at rest (that is, awake and with no task, usually with eyes closed). BOLD fluctuations in the resting state are thought to indirectly reflect "spontaneous" neural activity. Cortical areas are divided into ROIs by any number of methods, and regions with correlated activity are inferred to be functionally connected. These regions and their connections are interpreted as the nodes and links in networks for further analysis (described further in Chapter 2).

A proposed "resting state" or "default mode" network, which is active during quiet wakefulness but shows decreased activity during some goal-oriented tasks, has been described in adults using rs-fcMRI [61,64], although there is ongoing discussion of the definition and meaning of such networks [65]. The evolution of this proposed adult network has been evaluated across infancy and through adolescence. Rs-fcMRI study in 12 preterm infants at term during 10 minutes of sleep identified five networks with consistent coherence patterns across all infants [66]. The areas with coherent BOLD fMRI signal changes were seen symmetrically in homotopic cortical regions, including: the bilateral medial sections of the occipital lobes, somatomotor cortices, posterior temporal cortices, anterior prefrontal cortices, and the medial and lateral parts of the posterior parietal cortices. The authors hypothesize that the interhemispheric functional connections seen between homologous brain regions may reflect the relatively early presence and maturation of underlying transcallosal white matter tracts. Considered collectively, these networks largely resembled the described default-mode network in adults and the authors suggested that the infant network may represent a predecessor "proto-default-mode network." A separate group recently evaluated longitudinal rs-fcMRI from preterm infants through term. This group also identified a precursor to the adult resting state default network in full-term control infants. However, this putative precursor network was not evident in preterm infants at term equivalent [67]. Emphasizing the likely age-specific pattern of development of the default network, another group demonstrated that the described adult default network shows an intermediate profile in school age children between the early pattern seen in infancy and the mature form of adulthood [68].

More recently, patterns of cerebral activity have been probed with another indirect technique, near-infrared spectroscopy (NIRS), which measures cerebral blood oxygenation *via* hemoglobin saturation content. The temporal correlation between regional fluctuations using NIRS was employed to infer functional connectivity networks in infants 0-6 months of age during presumed sleep. Inter-hemispheric connectivity between temporal regions was evident by 3 months of age and persisted through 6 months. In addition, some intra-hemispheric (left parieto-temporal) connectivity patterns were discernable by 6 months of age, which the authors hypothesized was related to the maturation of the left arcuate fasciculus and early language needs. Frontal regions demonstrated a decrease in connectivity over the three time points, and anterior-posterior connections revealed a U-shaped curve, perhaps

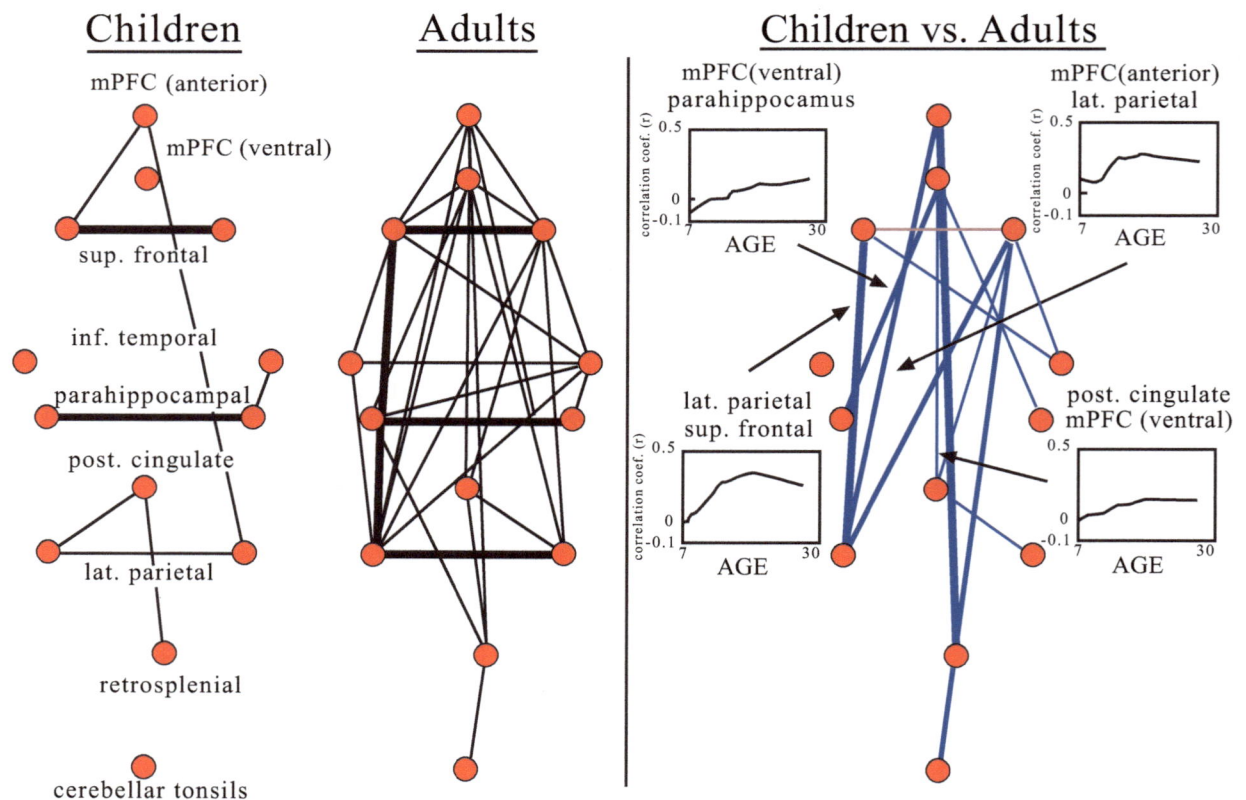

Fig. (3.3). A graph visualization of the correlation between default network regions in children (aged 7-9 years) and in adults (aged 21-31 years) represented in pseudo-anatomical organization. Statistically significant differences in functional connectivity between children and adults are highlighted in the right panel. (Adapted with permission from reference [58]).

reflecting more complex processes including selective organization with synaptic pruning and stabilization [69].

School age children have been studied with rs-fcMRI as well. Prior work in adults demonstrated two distinct fronto-parietal and cingulo-opercular networks thought to be involved in initiating and controlling attention in tasks. In the resting state, strong intra-network connectivity and minimal inter-network connectivity was observed in healthy adults [70]. Using a similar paradigm, school-age children were found to have decreased segregation of these two distinct adult networks as well as decreased connectivity within each network [71]. Adolescents (age 10-15 years) showed an intermediate network structure. Within these networks, overall, there was also an increase in long-range connections and a decrease in short-range connections with age (see Fig. **3.3**). As performance on control tasks thought to be mediated by these networks improves with age, these authors hypothesized that the age-dependent remodeling of these two networks represents the underlying developing learning mechanism for task controlling behaviors.

Large-scale network properties based on the increasingly popular graph theory approach have been evaluated in school-age children and young adults using rs-fcMRI [72]. This work found that small world properties were present in both children (ages 7-9 years) and young adults (ages 19-22 years). There was no statistical difference between the children and young adult groups for several metrics: mean path length, mean clustering coefficient, mean small-world property (characterized by high clustering coefficient and low characteristic path length), or measures of global efficiency (the harmonic mean of the minimum path length between each pair of nodes). Children demonstrated relative increased subcortical-cortical connectivity, whereas young adults were found to have higher levels of hierarchical network organization (characterized by high degree nodes that exhibit lower clustering and vice versa) and stronger cortico-cortical connections, suggesting the development of increased, specialized, functional cortical connectivity patterns with age. In this work, children were more likely to demonstrate functional connectivity between nearby anatomical regions compared with young adults. These authors hypothesized that increased long-range functional integration occurs with age and is related to processes of myelination as well as relative weakening of local, nonspecific connections.

Although small world network characteristics may not clearly vary with age, there may be some component of genetic variation. Interestingly, one study found that mean path length and clustering coefficient metrics derived from EEG functional networks may have a heritable component based on evaluation of a large adult twin and sibling cohort [73].

A more recent study evaluated both the phase difference and coherence of beta rhythms between limited EEG channels in 485 healthy subjects ranging from infants to adolescents. EEG recordings were obtained from four locations in each hemisphere (frontal, central, parietal, and occipital), each 6 cm apart [74]. The coherence between channel pairs as well as the phase lag was calculated in the anterior-posterior and posterior-anterior directions. This study found an initial increase in coherence at all inter-electrode distances in both directions in the first 2-3 years, followed by a sharp decline to near-baseline before age years and then steady increases in only shorter-range (6-12 cm) connections. Phase delays were found to have a similar inflection before 4 years and then steady increase between longer-range (18-24 cm) connections. The authors postulated that, since conduction velocity should remain stable or decrease with age, given known myelination maturation, these findings may reflect increased synaptic connections in local domains that increased short-range coherence and increased processing time or phase delay between longer-distance connections.

The relative decrease in long-distance functional connectivity over age found by Thatcher and colleagues [74] appears to contrast with known myelination patterns and rs-fcMRI work above [71,72,75]. This discrepancy highlights the difficulty in comparing EEG- and fMRI-derived network structures. These two methodologies generate functional networks through related, but distinct physiological measures in non-overlapping frequency ranges (high temporal resolution measures of neural activity in EEG versus high spatial resolution measures of oxygen consumption patterns in fMRI). In the above EEG study, Thatcher and colleagues averaged all connections of similar distance for comparison, possibly obscuring the development of selected, consolidated connections, whereas rs-fcMRI studies evaluate only specific regions of interest among all possible connections. Further studies to validate these early fMRI and EEG results are needed and future work evaluating simultaneous EEG and fMRI connectivity patterns will be useful to help clarify the relationship between these two methodologies.

CLINICAL IMPLICATIONS

Work delineating the normal development of anatomical and functional networks in the brain reveals many finely-tuned, complex patterns of normal maturation. At any point along this temporal axis, problems can emerge with potentially significant neurodevelopmental consequences. Measurements of functional and anatomical network relationships in pediatric disease states may provide new insights into how large and small alterations in anatomy and physiology can impact the connectivity patterns and distributed processing in brain networks and the clinical consequences of these changes.

Prior studies evaluating the altered functional connectivity patterns in children have employed both resting state and task-oriented functional connectivity MRI and DTI methods, primarily evaluating alterations in connectivity in patients with neurocognitive disorders. In one study, 8 year-old children who were born prematurely and had lower intelligence scores on standard neuropsychological testing underwent fMRI scanning during a passive auditory listening task [76]. Affected children were found to have increased functional connectivity between regions associated with language processing (Wernicke's area, right inferior frontal gyrus, left and right supramarginal gyri and components of the inferior parietal lobules) compared with normal controls, suggesting that children born prematurely and who have lower intelligence may have altered systems for language processing compared with controls. Whether the connectivity findings are causative of the cognitive impairment, result from it, or are an epiphenomenon remains uncertain.

Adolescents with Tourette syndrome have been shown to have more immature fronto-parietal and cingulo-opercular networks, which are hypothesized to be involved in impulse control, compared to age-matched controls [77]. Similarly, work evaluating rs-fcMRI and task-related fcMRI patterns in children with untreated attention deficit disorder compared to normal controls found decreased functional connectivity between multiple regions in the cortical-striatal-thalamic circuit as well as increased connectivity in the orbitofrontal and superior temporal cortices compared to controls [78]. Interestingly, these findings were mitigated or normalized with stimulant treatment [79], emphasizing not only the pathological relevance of network analysis in this population, but also the potential for using functional imaging to predict and/or monitor treatment responsiveness.

Much energy has been devoted to understanding altered connectivity patterns that may underlie the pervasive cognitive dysfunctions seen in autism spectrum disorders (ASD) [80]. DTI techniques have shown that white matter integrity may be altered in the corpus callosum, superior temporal gyrus, and temporal stem in patients with ASD [81,82]. Evaluation of rs-fcMRI networks in adolescents and adults with ASD revealed overall weaker functional connectivity across the expected default network, and during a social task that required attributing mental states to animated cartoons, compared to controls [83]. Furthermore, evaluation of symptom severity revealed that measurements of worse social impairment, more restricted behaviors, and poorer verbal and non-verbal communication skills each correlated with altered connectivity patterns between the posterior cingulate cortex and multiple regions of the described default network [84,85].

CONCLUSIONS

The human brain undergoes massive inter-related anatomical and physiological changes throughout development and yet maintains functionality as an integrated complex system at each stage of development. Investigation of developmental brain networks is exploding, due in part to the availability of new technologies that allow for precise characterization of functional and anatomical networks in the immature brain. Network science allows for an evaluation and comparison of the unique age-dependent global and interdependent properties of this complex and dynamic system. Much work remains to be done yet this approach is certain to continue to grow rapidly and lead to new insights into the complex interplay between anatomical and functional networks. Further work will help us to better understand the age-dependent clinical consequences of focal and global network disruptions in the developing brain and how these processes may be modified by genetics, experience, disease, and perhaps guided clinical interventions. Ultimately these insights may offer new opportunities for early detection and prognostication in a variety of neurodevelopmental disorders, and may potentially reveal new opportunities for therapies that improve ultimate neurocognitive outcomes in children, and the adults that they become.

REFERENCES

[1]   Caviness VS, Jr., Kennedy DN, Richelme C, Rademacher J, Filipek PA. The human brain age 7-11 years: a volumetric analysis based on magnetic resonance images. Cereb Cortex 1996; 6(5): 726-36.

[2]   Koop M, Rilling G, Herrmann A, Kretschmann HJ. Volumetric development of the fetal telencephalon, cerebral cortex, diencephalon, and rhombencephalon including the cerebellum in man. Bibl Anat 1986; (28): 53-78.

[3]   Brodmann K. Vergleichende Lokalisationslehre der Grosshirnrinde. Leipzig: Barth; 1909.

[4]   von Economo C, Koskinas GN. Die Cytoarchitektonik der Hirnrinde des erwaschsenen Menschen. Berlin: Springer-Verlag; 1925.

[5]   Anderson SA, Kaznowski CE, Horn C, Rubenstein JL, McConnell SK. Distinct origins of neocortical projection neurons and interneurons in vivo. Cereb Cortex 2002; 12(7): 702-9.

[6]   Kriegstein AR. Constructing circuits: neurogenesis and migration in the developing neocortex. Epilepsia 2005; 46(Suppl 7): 15-21.

[7]   His W. Die Entwicklung des Menschlichen Gehirns wahrend der ersten Monate. Leipzig: von S. Hirzel; 1904.

[8]   Sauer FC. Mitosis in the neural tube. J Comp Neurol 1935; 62(2): 377-405.

[9]   Sidman RL, Miale IL, Feder N. Cell proliferation and migration in the primitive ependymal zone; An autoradiographic study of histogenesis in the nervous system. Exp Neurol [doi: DOI: 10.1016/0014-4886(59)90024-X] 1959; 1(4): 322-33.

[10]   Sidman RL, Rakic P. Development of the human central nervous system. In: Haymaker W, Adams RD, editors. Histology and Histopathology of the Nervous System. Springfield: Charles C Thomas; 1982; p. 3-145.

[11]   Kowalczyk T, Pontious A, Englund C, *et al.* Intermediate Neuronal Progenitors (Basal Progenitors) Produce Pyramidal-Projection Neurons for All Layers of Cerebral Cortex. Cereb Cortex 2009 19(10): 2439-50.

[12]   Noctor SC, Martinez-Cerdeno V, Ivic L, Kriegstein AR. Cortical neurons arise in symmetric and asymmetric division zones and migrate through specific phases. Nat Neurosci 2004; 7(2): 136-44.

[13]   Herschkowitz N. Brain development in the fetus, neonate and infant. Biol Neonate 1988; 54(1): 1-19.

[14]   Osheroff H, Hatten ME. Gene expression profiling of preplate neurons destined for the subplate: genes involved in transcription, axon extension, neurotransmitter regulation, steroid hormone signaling, and neuronal survival. Cereb Cortex 2009; 19(Suppl 1): i126-34.

[15]   Gilles FH, Leviton A, Dooling EC. The Developing Human Brain. Boston, MA: John Wright, PSG Inc; 1983.

[16]   van der Knaap MS, van Wezel-Meijler G, Barth PG, Barkhof F, Ader HJ, Valk J. Normal gyration and sulcation in preterm and term neonates: appearance on MR images. Radiology 1996; 200(2): 389-96.

[17]   Lan LM, Yamashita Y, Tang Y, *et al.* Normal fetal brain development: MR imaging with a half-Fourier rapid acquisition with relaxation enhancement sequence. Radiology 2000; 215(1): 205-10.

[18]   Giedd JN, Blumenthal J, Jeffries NO, *et al.* Brain development during childhood and adolescence: a longitudinal MRI study. Nat Neurosci 1999; 2(10): 861-3.

[19]   Durston S, Hulshoff Pol HE, Casey BJ, Giedd JN, Buitelaar JK, van Engeland H. Anatomical MRI of the developing human brain: what have we learned? J Am Acad Child Adolesc Psychiatry 2001; 40(9): 1012-20.

[20]   Gogtay N, Giedd JN, Lusk L, *et al.* Dynamic mapping of human cortical development during childhood through early adulthood. Proc Natl Acad Sci USA 2004; 101(21): 8174-9.

[21]   Casey BJ, Tottenham N, Liston C, Durston S. Imaging the developing brain: what have we learned about cognitive development? Trends Cogn Sci 2005; 9(3): 104-10.

[22]   Finlay BL, Wikler KC, Sengelaub DR. Regressive events in brain development and scenarios for vertebrate brain evolution. Brain Behav Evol 1987; 30(1-2): 102-17.

[23]   Huttenlocher PR, Dabholkar AS. Regional differences in synaptogenesis in human cerebral cortex. J Comp Neurol 1997; 387(2): 167-78.

[24]   Finlay BL, Slattery M. Local differences in the amount of early cell death in neocortex predict adult local specializations. Science 1983; 219(4590): 1349-51.

[25]   Verney C, Takahashi T, Bhide PG, Nowakowski RS, Caviness VS, Jr. Independent controls for neocortical neuron production and histogenetic cell death. Dev Neurosci 2000; 22(1-2): 125-38.

[26]   Mesulam M. Neurocognitive networks and selectively distributed processing. Rev Neurol (Paris) 1994; 150(8-9): 564-9.

[27]   LaMantia AS, Rakic P. Axon overproduction and elimination in the anterior commissure of the developing rhesus monkey. J Comp Neurol 1994; 340(3): 328-36.

[28]   LaMantia AS, Rakic P. Axon overproduction and elimination in the corpus callosum of the developing rhesus monkey. J Neurosci 1990; 10(7): 2156-75.

[29]   Salami M, Itami C, Tsumoto T, Kimura F. Change of conduction velocity by regional myelination yields constant latency irrespective of distance between thalamus and cortex. Proc Natl Acad Sci USA 2003; 100(10): 6174-9.

[30]   Barkovich AJ, Kjos BO, Jackson DE, Jr., Norman D. Normal maturation of the neonatal and infant brain: MR imaging at 1.5 T. Radiology 1988; 166(1 Pt 1): 173-80.

[31]   Ashtari M, Cervellione KL, Hasan KM, *et al*. White matter development during late adolescence in healthy males: a cross-sectional diffusion tensor imaging study. Neuroimage 2007; 35(2): 501-10.

[32]   Grodd W. Normal and abnormal patterns of myelin development of the fetal and infantile human brain using magnetic resonance imaging. Curr Opin Neurol Neurosurg 1993; 6(3): 393-7.

[33]   Thompson PM, Giedd JN, Woods RP, MacDonald D, Evans AC, Toga AW. Growth patterns in the developing brain detected by using continuum mechanical tensor maps. Nature 2000; 404(6774): 190-3.

[34]   Sundgren PC, Dong Q, Gomez-Hassan D, Mukherji SK, Maly P, Welsh R. Diffusion tensor imaging of the brain: review of clinical applications. Neuroradiology 2004; 46(5): 339-50.

[35]   Hermoye L, Saint-Martin C, Cosnard G, *et al*. Pediatric diffusion tensor imaging: normal database and observation of the white matter maturation in early childhood. Neuroimage 2006; 29(2): 493-504.

[36]   Dubois J, Dehaene-Lambertz G, Perrin M, *et al*. Asynchrony of the early maturation of white matter bundles in healthy infants: quantitative landmarks revealed noninvasively by diffusion tensor imaging. Hum Brain Mapp 2008; 29(1): 14-27.

[37]   Ponten SC, Daffertshofer A, Hillebrand A, Stam CJ. The relationship between structural and functional connectivity: Graph theoretical analysis of an EEG neural mass model. Neuroimage 2010; 52(3): 985-94.

[38]   Hubel DH, Wiesel TN, LeVay S. Plasticity of ocular dominance columns in monkey striate cortex. Philos Trans R Soc Lond B Biol Sci 1977; 278(961): 377-409.

[39]   Uhlhaas PJ, Roux F, Rodriguez E, Rotarska-Jagiela A, Singer W. Neural synchrony and the development of cortical networks. Trends Cogn Sci 2010; 14(2): 72-80.

[40]   Hebb D. The organization of behavior: a neuropsychological theory: Wiley; 1949.

[41]   Chu CJ, Jones TA. Experience-dependent structural plasticity in cortex heterotopic to focal sensorimotor cortical damage. Exp Neurol 2000; 166(2): 403-14.

[42]   Komuro H, Rakic P. Modulation of neuronal migration by NMDA receptors. Science 1993; 260(5104): 95-7.

[43]   Rakic P, Komuro H. The role of receptor/channel activity in neuronal cell migration. J Neurobiol 1995; 26(3): 299-315.

[44]   Katz LC, Shatz CJ. Synaptic activity and the construction of cortical circuits. Science 1996; 274(5290): 1133-8.

[45]   Holmes GL, McCabe B. Brain development and generation of brain pathologies. Int Rev Neurobiol 2001; 45: 17-41.

[46]   Chugani HT, Phelps ME, Mazziotta JC. Positron emission tomography study of human brain functional development. Ann Neurol 1987; 22(4): 487-97.

[47]   Silva ENEaFLd, editor. Electroencephalography: basic principles, clinical applications, and related fields: Lippincott Williams & Wilkins; 2004.

[48]   Louis J, Cannard C, Bastuji H, Challamel MJ. Sleep ontogenesis revisited: a longitudinal 24-hour home polygraphic study on 15 normal infants during the first two years of life. Sleep 1997; 20(5): 323-33.

[49]   Nunes ML, Da Costa JC, Moura-Ribeiro MV. Polysomnographic quantification of bioelectrical maturation in preterm and fullterm newborns at matched conceptional ages. Electroencephalogr Clin Neurophysiol 1997; 102(3): 186-91.

[50]   Sterman MB, Harper RM, Havens B, Hoppenbrouwers T, McGinty DJ, Hodgman JE. Quantitative analysis of infant EEG development during quiet sleep. Electroencephalogr Clin Neurophysiol 1977; 43(3): 371-85.

[51]   Louis J, Zhang JX, Revol M, Debilly G, Challamel MJ. Ontogenesis of nocturnal organization of sleep spindles: a longitudinal study during the first 6 months of life. Electroencephalogr Clin Neurophysiol 1992; 83(5): 289-96.

[52]   Grigg-Damberger M, Gozal D, Marcus CL, *et al*. The visual scoring of sleep and arousal in infants and children. J Clin Sleep Med 2007; 3(2): 201-40.

[53]   Scher MS, Loparo KA. Neonatal EEG/sleep state analyses: a complex phenotype of developmental neural plasticity. Dev Neurosci 2009; 31(4): 259-75.

[54]   Eeg-Oloffson IPaO. The development of the electroencephalogram in normal children from the age of 1 through 15 years: non-paroxysmal activity. Neuropaediatrie 1971; 2(3): 247-304.

[55]   O PIaE-O. The development of the electroencephalogram in normal children from the age of 1 through 15 years: non-paroxysmal activity. Neuropaediatrie 1971; 2(3): 247-304.

[56]   Srinivasan R. Spatial structure of the human alpha rhythm: global correlation in adults and local correlation in children. Clin Neurophysiol 1999; 110(8): 1351-62.

[57]   Milh M, Kaminska A, Huon C, Lapillonne A, Ben-Ari Y, Khazipov R. Rapid cortical oscillations and early motor activity in premature human neonate. Cereb Cortex 2007; 17(7): 1582-94.

[58]   Csibra G, Davis G, Spratling MW, Johnson MH. Gamma oscillations and object processing in the infant brain. Science 2000; 290(5496): 1582-5.

[59]   Werkle-Bergner M, Shing YL, Muller V, Li SC, Lindenberger U. EEG gamma-band synchronization in visual coding from childhood to old age: evidence from evoked power and inter-trial phase locking. Clin Neurophysiol 2009; 120(7): 1291-302.

[60]   Uhlhaas PJ, Roux F, Singer W, Haenschel C, Sireteanu R, Rodriguez E. The development of neural synchrony reflects late maturation and restructuring of functional networks in humans. Proc Natl Acad Sci USA 2009; 106(24): 9866-71.

[61]   Buckner RL, Andrews-Hanna JR, Schacter DL. The brain's default network: anatomy, function, and relevance to disease. Ann N Y Acad Sci 2008; 1124: 1-38.

[62]   Kennedy DP, Courchesne E. Functional abnormalities of the default network during self- and other-reflection in autism. Soc Cogn Affect Neurosci 2008; 3(2): 177-90.

[63]   Damoiseaux JS, Rombouts SA, Barkhof F, *et al.* Consistent resting-state networks across healthy subjects. Proc Natl Acad Sci USA 2006; 103(37): 13848-53.

[64]   Greicius MD, Krasnow B, Reiss AL, Menon V. Functional connectivity in the resting brain: a network analysis of the default mode hypothesis. Proc Natl Acad Sci USA 2003; 100(1): 253-8.

[65]   Cole DM, Smith SM, Beckmann CF. Advances and pitfalls in the analysis and interpretation of resting-state FMRI data. Front Syst Neurosci 2010; 4: 8.

[66]   Fransson P, Skiold B, Horsch S, *et al.* Resting-state networks in the infant brain. Proc Natl Acad Sci USA 2007; 104(39): 15531-6.

[67]   Smyser CD, Inder TE, Shimony JS, *et al.* Longitudinal analysis of neural network development in preterm infants. Cereb Cortex 2010 20(12): 2852-62.

[68]   Fair DA, Cohen AL, Dosenbach NU, *et al.* The maturing architecture of the brain's default network. Proc Natl Acad Sci USA 2008; 105(10): 4028-32.

[69]   Homae F, Watanabe H, Otobe T, *et al.* Development of global cortical networks in early infancy. J Neurosci 2010; 30(14): 4877-82.

[70]   Dosenbach NU, Fair DA, Miezin FM, *et al.* Distinct brain networks for adaptive and stable task control in humans. Proc Natl Acad Sci USA 2007; 104(26): 11073-8.

[71]   Fair DA, Dosenbach NU, Church JA, *et al.* Development of distinct control networks through segregation and integration. Proc Natl Acad Sci USA 2007; 104(33): 13507-12.

[72]   Supekar K, Musen M, Menon V. Development of large-scale functional brain networks in children. PLoS Biol 2009; 7(7): e1000157.

[73]   Smit DJ, Stam CJ, Posthuma D, Boomsma DI, de Geus EJ. Heritability of "small-world" networks in the brain: a graph theoretical analysis of resting-state EEG functional connectivity. Hum Brain Mapp 2008; 29(12): 1368-78.

[74]   Thatcher RW, North DM, Biver CJ. Development of cortical connections as measured by EEG coherence and phase delays. Hum Brain Mapp 2008; 29(12): 1400-15.

[75]   Fair DA, Cohen AL, Power JD, *et al.* Functional brain networks develop from a "local to distributed" organization. PLoS Comput Biol 2009; 5(5): e1000381.

[76]   Gozzo Y, Vohr B, Lacadie C, *et al.* Alterations in neural connectivity in preterm children at school age. Neuroimage 2009; 48(2): 458-63.

[77]   Church JA, Fair DA, Dosenbach NU, *et al.* Control networks in paediatric Tourette syndrome show immature and anomalous patterns of functional connectivity. Brain 2009; 132(Pt 1): 225-38.

[78]   Cao X, Cao Q, Long X, *et al.* Abnormal resting-state functional connectivity patterns of the putamen in medication-naive children with attention deficit hyperactivity disorder. Brain Res 2009; 1303: 195-206.

[79]   Rubia K, Halari R, Cubillo A, Mohammad AM, Brammer M, Taylor E. Methylphenidate normalises activation and functional connectivity deficits in attention and motivation networks in medication-naive children with ADHD during a rewarded continuous performance task. Neuropharmacology 2009; 57(7-8): 640-52.

[80]   Minshew NJ, Keller TA. The nature of brain dysfunction in autism: functional brain imaging studies. Curr Opin Neurol 2010; 23(2): 124-30.

[81]   Alexander AL, Lee JE, Lazar M, *et al.* Diffusion tensor imaging of the corpus callosum in Autism. Neuroimage 2007; 34(1): 61-73.

[82]   Lee JE, Bigler ED, Alexander AL, *et al.* Diffusion tensor imaging of white matter in the superior temporal gyrus and temporal stem in autism. Neurosci Lett 2007; 424(2): 127-32.

[83]   Kana RK, Keller TA, Cherkassky VL, Minshew NJ, Just MA. Atypical frontal-posterior synchronization of Theory of Mind regions in autism during mental state attribution. Soc Neurosci 2009; 4(2): 135-52.

[84]   Monk CS, Peltier SJ, Wiggins JL, *et al.* Abnormalities of intrinsic functional connectivity in autism spectrum disorders. Neuroimage 2009; 47(2): 764-72.

[85]   Weng SJ, Wiggins JL, Peltier SJ, *et al.* Alterations of resting state functional connectivity in the default network in adolescents with autism spectrum disorders. Brain Res 2010; 1313: 202-14.

CHAPTER 4

Brain Anatomy and Small-World Networks

Danielle S. Bassett[1,2*] and Edward T. Bullmore[2]

[1]*Biological and Soft Systems, Department of Physics, University of Cambridge, UK and* [2]*Brain Mapping Unit, Department of Psychiatry, University of Cambridge, UK*

Abstract: Network analysis of neural and other information-processing systems has recently provided unique insights into the large-scale cohesive organization of subcomponents at many scales of space and time. In this chapter, we describe the network analysis of neural systems in general and that of the healthy and diseased human brain in particular. We present evidence from a variety of species and data modalities that neural systems show the so-called "small-world" network phenomenon which also ubiquitously characterizes social groups, scientific collaborations, the world wide web, transportation networks, power grids, etc. We attempt to provide reasons why this property might have been selected in brain evolution, and to explain its functional significance, while delineating the methodological intricacies of network analysis of neuroimaging data.

Keywords: Network construction, scale-free, exponential, power law, human, monkey, cortical thickness, degree distribution, small world, modularity, tractography.

SMALL-WORLD NETWORKS

In 1929, a Hungarian novelist by the name of Frigyes Karinthy published a short story entitled "Chains" in which he explored his belief in a shrinking modern world in which human friendship networks spanned larger and larger physical distances [1]. In the 1960s, both empirical and theoretical work by Gurevish, de Sola, and Kochen [2], describing the structure of social networks, suggested that indeed two randomly chosen individuals in the USA could contact each other with the help of at least two friends. The experimental studies of Stanley Milgram in 1967 showed that the average social distance between any two people in the United States was equal to three. In sociology, the small-world network as a social construct began to be investigated while the physics and mathematics communities produced random network theory (dating back to Erdös and Rényi) [3, 4]. In an article in Nature in 1998, Watts and Strogatz proposed a simple model to bridge the gap between random network theory and small-world networks, thus connecting two disparate academic worlds; see Fig. (4.1) [5]. In the following years, the statistical physics of non-random or complex networks has turned out to be relevant to many sciences besides sociology, including economics, computer science, epidemiology and neuroscience.

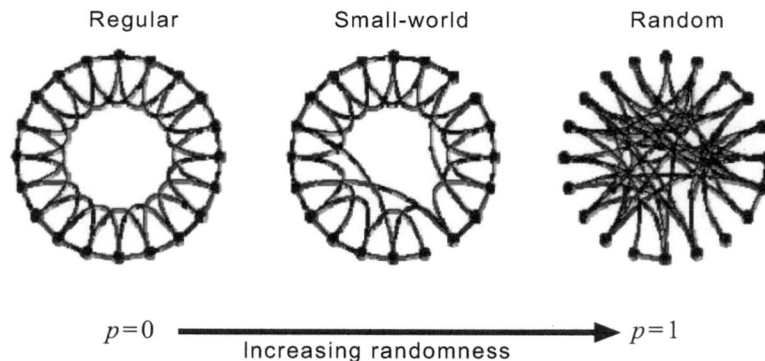

Regular   Small-world   Random

$p=0$ ──────── Increasing randomness ────────▶ $p=1$

Fig. (4.1). The concept of "small-worldness". In 1998, Watts and Strogatz published the first generative small-world model. They began with a regular lattice network in the shape of a ring. Then, they rewired the edges with probability p where p was allowed to range between 0 and 1. When the rewiring probability was $p = 0$, the network remained a regular lattice: high clustering, C, and high path-length, L. When the probability was $p = 1$, the network had a perfect random topology: low clustering, C, and short path-length, L. For intermediate values of p, a small-world topology emerged where the clustering was high, similar to a regular lattice, but the path-length was short, similar to a random network. (This figure was reproduced with permission from [5]).

*****Address correspondence to Danielle S. Bassett:** Brain Mapping Unit, Department of Psychiatry and Biological and Soft Systems, Department of Physics, University of Cambridge, UK; Email: dbassett@physics.ucsb.edu

Matt T. Bianchi, Verne S. Caviness and Sydney S. Cash (Eds.)

This chapter is focused on the study of complex brain networks over a wide range of species and spatial scales: from the neuronal connectome of the nematode *C. elegans* to the pattern of white matter tracts in the human brain. We will begin with a description of network analysis and a brief exposition of the reasons why we might expect nervous system networks to be small-world. The following section will provide the current evidence for small-world architecture of anatomical connectivity in the brain, further reporting additional organizational principles that have recently become evident. In closing we will briefly summarize a few methodological points and suggest further lines of inquiry. Additional information about graph theoretic network analysis can also be found in Chapter 2.

INTRODUCTORY CONCEPTS

Networks are made up of *nodes* (*e.g.* people in social networks or cortical regions in brain networks) and *edges* (*e.g.* friendships in social networks or white matter tracts in anatomical brain networks); see Fig. (**4.2**). Edges can be defined as either directed or undirected; undirected edges indicate that 'A' connects to 'B' just as 'B' connects to 'A' while directed edges are necessary to indicate that 'A' may be connected to 'B' in a different way (*e.g.*, more or less strongly) than 'B' is connected to 'A'. A *neighbor* in network terms is defined as any node that is connected to a given node by one edge (*e.g.* a direct acquaintance rather than a friend of a friend). Small-world networks are characterized by two properties: 1) a large amount of *clustering*, C, where neighbors of a given node are likely connected to each other (*e.g.*, your friends are more likely to know each other than not) and 2) a short *path length*, L, where transmission of information or goods between any two nodes of the network requires only a few connections. This second property of a short path length has been popularized in the media by the idea of the "Six Degrees of Kevin Bacon", whereby any actor can be connected through their film roles to Kevin Bacon within six co-star associations.

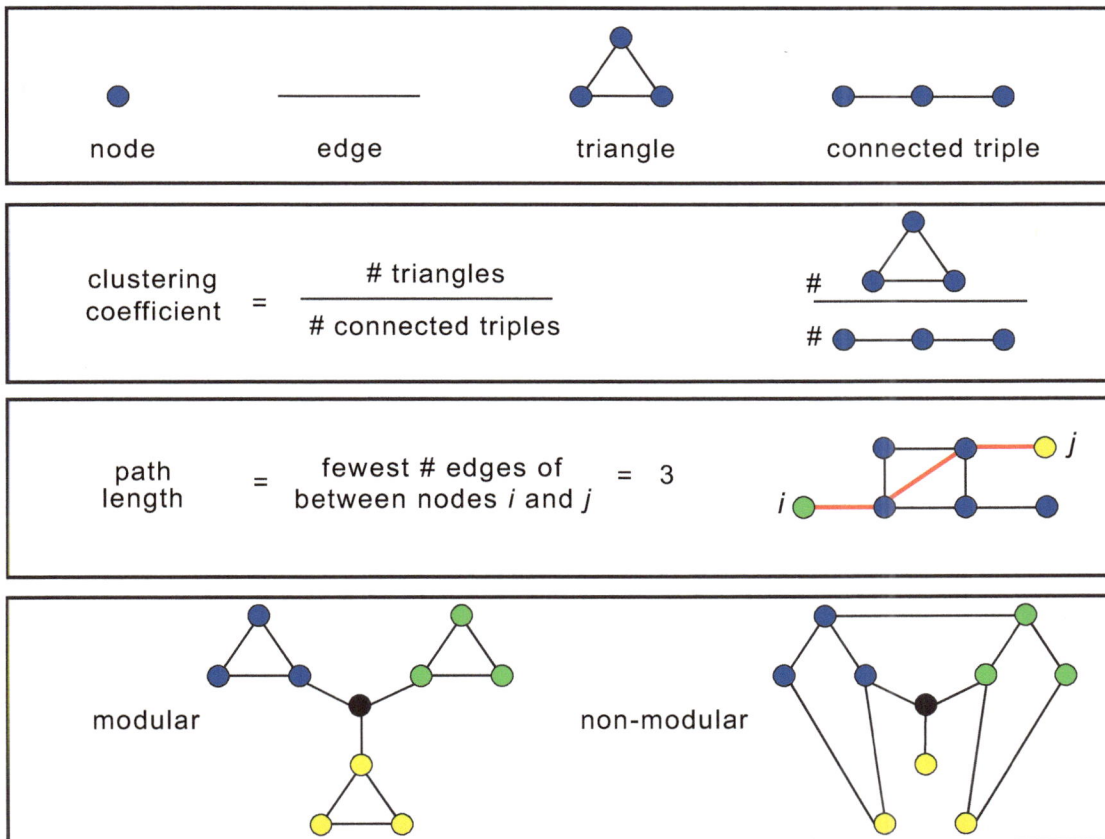

Fig. (4.2). A basic tutorial of network concepts. Definitions for a node, an edge, a triangle, and a connected triple are given in the top panel. The clustering coefficient, C, is given by the ratio of the number of connected triangles to the number of connected triples (second panel). The path length, L, is given by the fewest number of edges linking one node, *i*, to another node, *j* (third panel). A modular network structure occurs when there are more connections within a module than between modules. In this schematic, modules are given by distinct colors, *e.g.*, blue, green, and yellow (bottom panel). (This figure is reproduced with permission from [95]).

In an anatomical brain network, the short path length property would indicate that information can be transferred from one region to any other region by traversing only a few major white matter tracts; see Fig. (**4.3**) for a schematic of brain network construction. Similarly at the neuronal level, in the network of *C. elegans* a short path length indicates that any two neurons can communicate by the transmission of signals over just a few synapses. This illustrates the general principle that some key brain network properties, like short path length, may be conserved across different species and across micro and macro scales of space (and time). This scale-invariance is sometimes described as a fractal or self-similar aspect of brain network organization, because similar patterns are seen at different levels of observation.

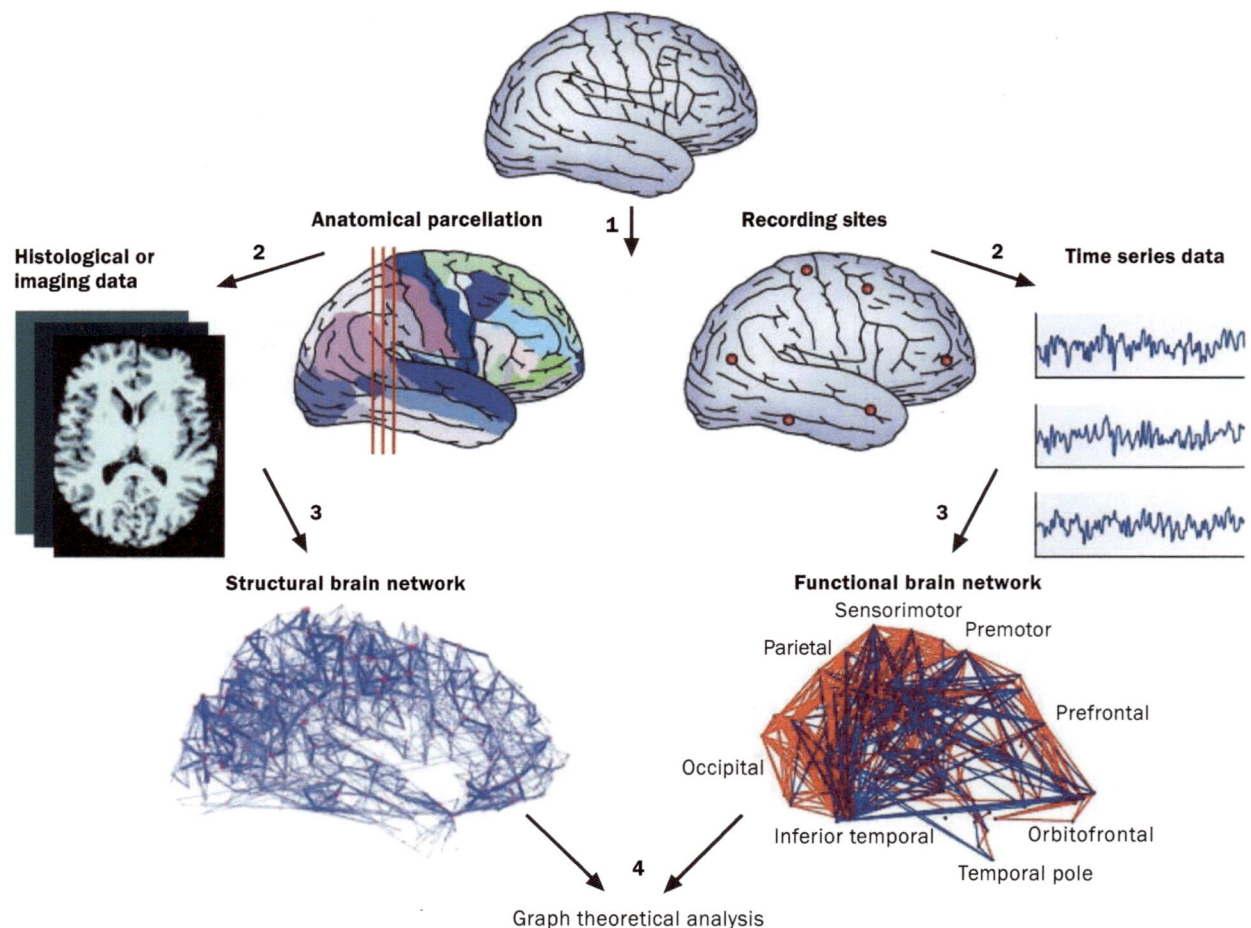

Fig. (4.3). A schematic description of brain network construction. Types of brain networks include both anatomical and functional. During the construction of an anatomical brain network (left-most portion of the figure), the cortex is usually subdivided into a number of regions (usually on the order of 100-1000) using one of many possible parcellation schemes. This parcellation is applied to histological or imaging data from which pair-wise regional connections are estimated. The resultant anatomical brain network is then analyzed using metrics originating from graph theory. (This figure is reproduced with permission from [53]).

Small-world properties are usually compared to benchmark networks: a small-world network has a clustering coefficient, C, larger than a regular network and a path length, L, similar to a random network. A regular network is one in which nodes are connected to all of their nearest neighbors within certain distance away from them (all connectivity is local); these networks show very high clustering coefficients but very long path lengths (no long range connections). A random network is one in which nodes are randomly wired together such that the clustering coefficient is small and the path length is short (short- and long-range connections are equally likely). An important sub-categorization of small-world networks is according to their *degree distribution* [6]. The *degree*, k, of a node is equal to the number of edges connected to it. The distribution of degrees across all nodes in a network may be a complex function containing many "regimes". A regime of a degree distribution is a range of degrees over which the degree distribution can be fit by a simple function such as a line (in which case it is called a power-law regime), a quadratic, or an exponential. A power-law regime indicates that there are not only relative highly connected nodes but also relatively poorly connected nodes and the full spectrum of connected nodes in between, with no "typical" level of connectivity; this lack of a preferred or typical level (or scale) of connectivity leads to the descriptive term "scale-free". A near perfect power-law over the *entire* degree range indicates that the whole network is "scale-free," indicating that the network has a large number of nodes with relatively high degree, also known as *hubs*. A regime of scaling behavior in the degree distribution combined with regimes of exponential or other non-scaling (*e.g.*, non-linear portions of the degree distribution) behavior is known as "broad-scale". Brain networks have largely been found to follow an exponentially truncated power-law, indicating that these networks are "broad scale" and not "scale-free" [6]. It is plausible that evolutionary and metabolic constraints on wiring in the brain have precluded the multiple localized connections necessary to construct the very highly connected hubs of a scale-free distribution. The relationship between the degree of a node and its local connectivity or *clustering* is defined as the *hierarchy*: the hierarchy parameter, β, is defined as the slope on a log-log plot of the nodal clustering coefficients and the degrees across all nodes in the network [7].

In the pages that follow, these and other terms given in italics will be defined in further detail in the Appendix, "Glossary of Terms," at the end of this chapter.

WHY WOULD WE EXPECT BRAIN ANATOMY TO SHOW SMALL-WORLD PROPERTIES?

We can draw lines of argument from both function and anatomy to suggest that we might expect small-world properties in the connectivity networks of human brains. Firstly, convergent evidence over the last several decades suggests that human brain activity is characterized by both segregation and integration of function [8-10]. For example, Fodor's primarily functional analysis distinguished modular or informationally encapsulated mental functions, which have a specialized and localized neural representation, from so-called isotropic Quineian processes, which are represented by more globally distributed and less specialized neural systems[1].

Anatomically it is well known that the brain is a heterogeneous, non-random structure at both macro and micro scales. Brodmann was the first to exploit these structural heterogeneities to subdivide the brain into large cortical sub-regions with distinct cyto-architectures [11]. The seminal work of Mountcastle, who discovered and characterized the columnar organization of the cortex, followed by Hubel and Wiesel, who extended our understanding of columnar organization specifically in the visual cortex, underscored the concept of a modular brain [12-13]. The laminar organization of cortical regions, the segregation of white and gray matter, the separation of visual cortical areas, the organization of the basal ganglia, the existence of topographic maps [14], and ocular dominance patterns, the organization of cortical columns, and the symmetric modular structure of genetic expression all provide evidence for the importance of physical or spatial segregation in brain architecture [9]. Mounting evidence suggests that this inherent modular structure maximizes the efficiency, adaptability, and evolvability of the system [15, 16] as had been philosophically postulated decades ago by Herbert Simon, a political scientist, economist and psychologist who was among the founding fathers of artificial intelligence and the science of complex systems [17].

In both localized or segregated systems, and distributed or integrated systems, it is thought that individual processing units are coordinated by rhythmic electrical oscillations. Coherence of more spatially distributed systems is mediated by lower frequency, e.g. β-band (12-30 Hz) and lower oscillations [18]. Conversely, cognitive binding, or the multimodal integration of information into a coherent perception, over shorter physical distances is thought to be mediated by high frequency γ-band oscillations ($\geq$ 40 Hz) [19-21]. This combination of functional segregation and integration over short and long distances as mediated by different frequency bands suggests an abstract functional architecture that contains a high topological clustering (functional modules which are to some degree segregated from each other and from the whole system) as well as a short topological path length (functional modules are interconnected or integrated enough to allow the system to function as a whole). In the sense that form (or anatomy) follows or mirrors function, this combination of segregation and integration of function suggests a

---

[1]Fodor, Jerry A. (1983). Modularity of Mind: An Essay on Faculty Psychology. Cambridge, Mass.: MIT Press. ISBN 0-262-56025-9

small-world anatomical topology where clustering (segregation) and short path length (integration) are further intricately combined.

Secondly, we can hypothesize that the brain has evolved to optimize information transfer. Quick, efficient, and adaptive processing of external events is necessary for the continuation of life and therefore it is probable that natural selection exerted a positive selection pressure on this trait. Work in the physics community has shown that the topology of small-world networks maximizes the possibility of efficient information transfer characterized by both fast responses and coherent oscillations that provide better computational power than other benchmark network topologies [22-25]. A strong relationship between small world topology and dynamic complexity is confirmed by many other studies: robust yet controlled synchronizability of these systems is associated with a small-world topology, marking a critical point in the dynamics of generic systems of coupled oscillators, from disordered to globally coherent oscillations [23, 26-27]. Preliminary studies indicate that its functional connectivity architecture places the healthy human brain in a meta-stable state (or at a critical point) where a wide dynamic range of distributed functions is possible without the potential for uncontrolled global synchronizability, as would perhaps be characteristic of epileptic seizures [20]. There is evidence for the criticality of nervous system dynamics at both micro (cellular) and macro (neuroimaging) scales of spatial resolution [28-29].

In addition to the suggestive properties described above, there may be further reasons to expect small-world brain architecture that we will learn as we apply network theory to brain anatomical data in the coming years.

WHAT OTHER PATTERNS MIGHT WE EXPECT?

Small-worldness isn't everything. Given the ubiquity of small-world properties in many systems throughout disparate disciplines, it is useful to ask the question: "What other network patterns would we expect to find in anatomical brain networks that might be more specific to neural systems?"

The small-world property as originally described by Watts and Strogatz [5] and quantified by Humphries [30], is a purely topological property, meaning that it is an organizational property of the brain's pattern of connections independent of where the connections are located in physical space. However, we know that the brain is characterized by a physically structured organization, *e.g.*, as evidenced by its spatial modularization into cortical micro-columns and lamina. Thus, we may expect brain networks to have specific spatial structures that distinguish them from the networks of other systems.

Perhaps one of the most well-studied physical properties of the connectivity in the brain is the minimization of wiring length on multiple spatial scales [31-32].

It is thought that positive selection for minimization of wiring in the evolutionary process is driven by an energy efficiency constraint [33]. Several aspects of brain structure are compatible with this selection pressure: the segregation of white and gray matter, separation of visual cortical areas, scaling of number of areas/ neuronal density with brain size [34-35], organization of cortical areas and basal ganglia, existence of topographic maps, ocular dominance patterns, dimensions of axonal and dendritic arbors, and the fraction of gray matter occupied by axons and dendrites [36-38] have all been found to minimize wiring. However, if minimization of wiring were the only constraint, local connections would dominate the network [39] and long-distance connections would disappear, leading to delayed information transfer and resultant metabolic energy depletion [40-41]. Thus the brain must have a counteracting constraint such as the minimization of energy costs induced by adding a few long distance connections, creating a small-world network [42]. The simultaneous minimization of wiring and energy costs may explain the modular structure found throughout neural systems [9, 39, 41, 43-44].

EVIDENCE FOR SMALL-WORLD BRAIN ORGANIZATION

We can now move from the question of "why would we expect brain anatomical networks theoretically to have small-world properties" to the question of "what have we actually found empirically?" Here, we will present evidence from both anatomy and function to suggest that the brain is wired in a small-world manner.

FROM ANATOMY - ANIMAL STUDIES

Throughout the past decades, structural organization of neural systems has proved to be largely scale-invariant over a range of spatial resolutions from the connectivity between the neurons in the nematode worm to the large white matter tracts bridging the entire human cortex. The quantification of anatomical network properties began in non-human mammals in the 1990s and was particularly dependent on the distillation by Van Essen, Felleman, Young, Scannell and others, of whole-brain connectivity maps from original tract tracing studies in both the macaque and cat cortex [45-49].

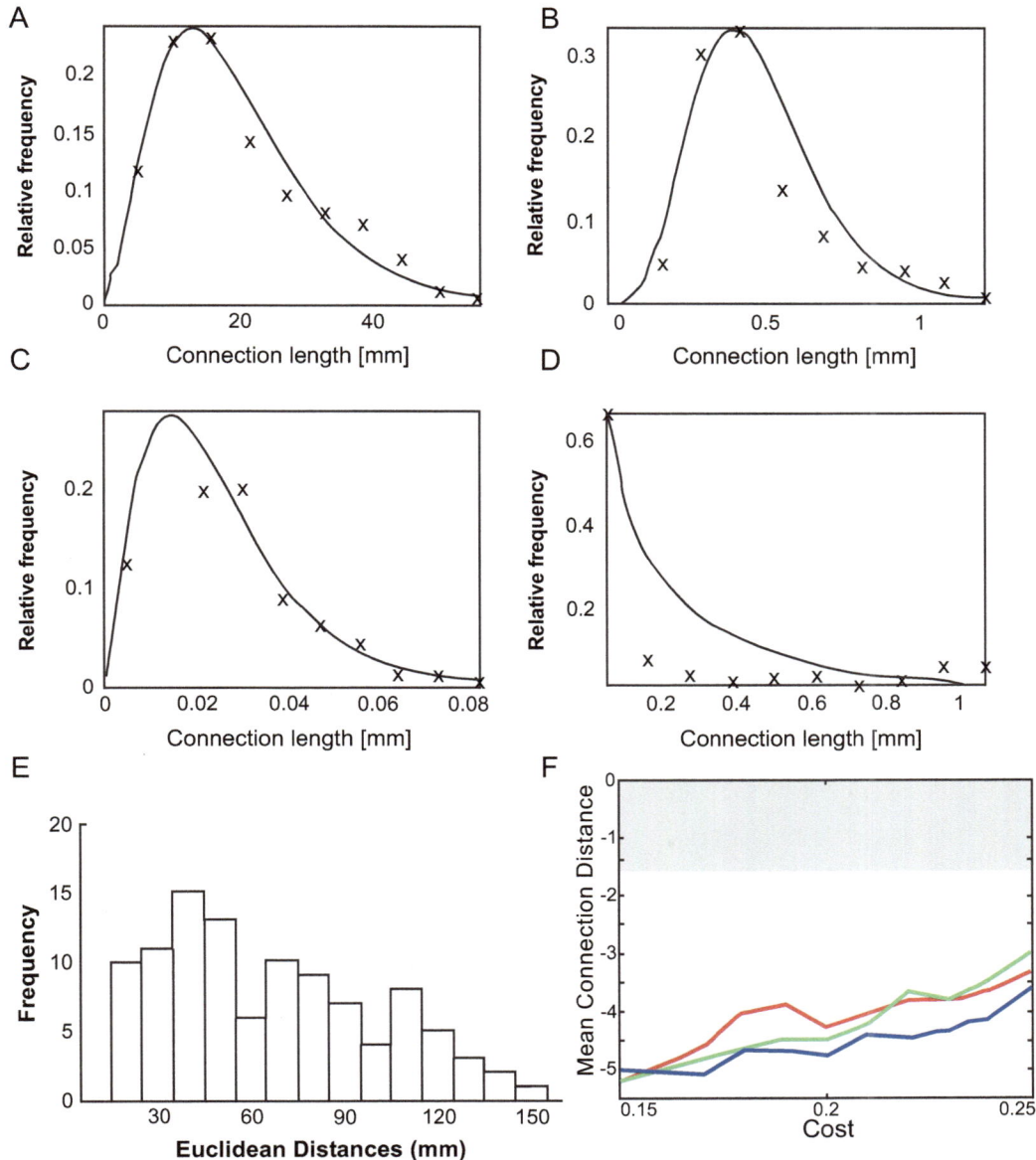

Fig. (4.4). Connection lengths in different nervous system networks. Panel **A** shows the connection length distributions for the Macaque cortical network derived from tract tracing studies, while that of the rat supragranular neuronal network is in panel **B** [108]. The *C. elegans* frontal (**C**) and complete network (**D**) are also shown. Each distribution shows a preference for shorter distance connections, significantly different from the Gaussian distribution expected from a random connectivity pattern between network components. Panel **E** is the connection length distribution for a human anatomical network derived from covariation in cortical thickness [56]. Z-score for the mean connections distance of the unimodal (green), multimodal (blue), and transmodal (red) cortices of a human anatomical network derived from covariation in gray matter volume is shown in panel **F** [71]; gray section indicates the mean connection length expected for a random distribution of connections. Note the human network connections lengths are significantly below that expected from a random distribution. (This figure is reproduced with permission from [56, 71, 82]).

Subsequent work by Watts and Strogatz in 1998 showed that the neuronal system of *C. elegans* had small-world properties including a clustering coefficient similar to a regular network and a path length similar to a random network [5]. Later, the nematode's neuronal wiring diagram was also found to display a hierarchical modularity with direct relationships to functional subsystems [50]. This work was quickly followed by Hilgetag and Sporns, who showed that the connectivity matrices derived from the tract tracing data of the macaque and cat also had small-world properties [43, 51] (see Table 4.1 for exact values and [52-53] for reviews). More recently, these connectivity matrices based on tract tracing have been used to identify anatomical network hubs, which are consistently found to be polysensory or multimodal in function across a range of mammalian species [54].

Table 4.1. Small World Parameters in Anatomical Connectivity Matrices

Data	N	L	C	λ	γ
Neuronal Networks					
C. elegans	282	2.65	0.28	1.17	5.60
Tract Tracing Studies					
Macaque Visual Cortex	30	1.73	0.53	1.04	1.47
Macaque Whole Cortex	71	2.38	0.46	1.17	3.06
Cat Cortex	52	1.81	0.55	1.06	1.77
Human Neuroimaging					
Hagmann et al. (2006, DSI)	748	2.34	0.031	1.19	3.92
Hagmann et al. (2006, DSI)	4522	3.33	0.011	1.15	16.17
He et al. (2007, sMRI)	54	3.05	0.30	1.15	2.36
Iturria-Medina et al. (2008, DW-MRI)	90	~	~	1.12	1.85
Gong et al. (2009, DTI)	78	2.32	0.49	1.15	4.08

Macaque visual cortex and whole cortex data are similar to those introduced by Felleman and Van Essen and Young; cat cortex data are similar to those introduced by Scannell *et al.* [45-49]. Classical small world parameters, path length *L* and clustering *C* (λ and γ after scaling by random network parameters) are as summarized by Sporns and Zwi [51]; *N* indicates the number of nodes in the network. Human neuroimaging data are as presented in references [55-58].

HUMAN ANATOMICAL NETWORKS: CORTICAL THICKNESS AND GRAY MATTER VOLUME IN HEALTH AND DISEASE

Large-scale human anatomical networks were first studied in 2006 (DTI) [56] and 2007 (cortical thickness) [56]; see Fig. (**4.3**) for a schematic of brain network construction and Fig. (**4.5**) for some initial results. In 2007, He and colleagues constructed a human anatomical network based on cortical thickness measurements in a large group of 124 healthy adults of both genders (71 male) [56]. The cortical thickness measurements were averaged within 54 regions of interest inclusively covering the whole brain. For all possible pairs of regions, a correlation, $r_{i,j}$, was determined between the average cortical thickness in region *i* and the average cortical thickness in region *j* across subjects. The pairwise correlations, *r*, were subsequently thresholded for statistical significance such that any correlation that was above the threshold for significance was taken to indicate a true connection - and was drawn as an edge on the graph of the anatomical network – while those below the threshold for significance were not included as edges in the graph. The resulting network contained 104 connections out of a maximum possible number of 2862, indicating a sparsity level or *cost* of 7.3%, and connected 45 regions out of the total 54. This large connected component showed robust small world properties, a predominance of short range connections consistent with a minimization of wiring constraint, an exponentially truncated power-law degree distribution (i.e., a degree distribution which contains a power-law scaling regime which then falls off exponentially at very high degree) indicating that the network was broad-scale [59] (see Fig. **4.6**), and the presence of hubs predominantly located in association cortex as had been previously found in resting state functional magnetic resonance imaging (fMRI) networks [60]. The term "resting state" refers to the state of the brain when a person is at rest, most often studied by placing people in a scanner with their eyes either open or closed and asking them to think of nothing in particular. Resting state studies are assumed to measure endogenous brain activity, characterized in fMRI by what is called the "default network" [61], composed of areas of the brain that consistently function coherently in the resting state.

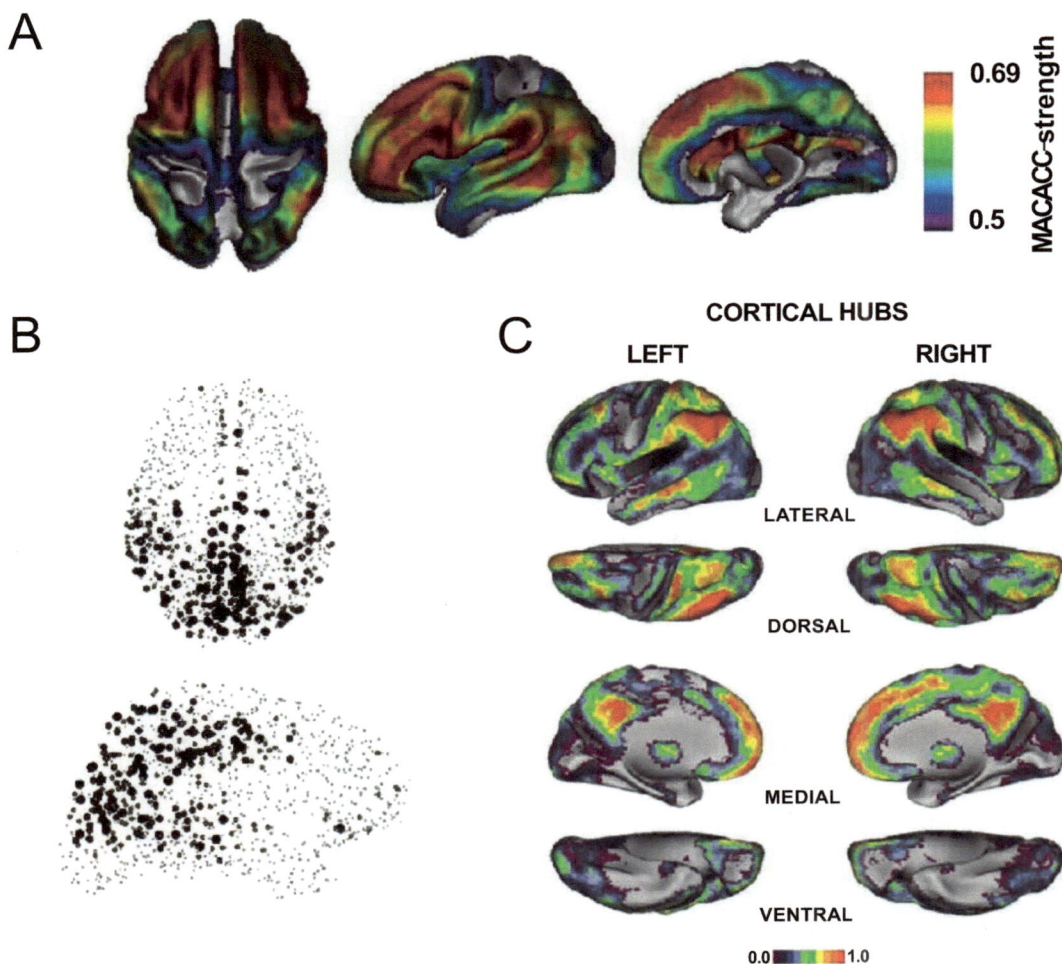

Fig. (4.5) The distribution of estimated average connection strengths in human cortical networks. The strength of connections to other regions in an anatomical network derived from covariation in cortical thickness over subjects are estimated over the whole brain with strongest connected regions (association regions in frontal and inferior temporal cortex) shown in red [92] (panel **A**). Panel **B** shows that regions with the highest strength in an anatomical network derived from diffusion spectrum imaging (DSI) are located in the precuneus and visual areas [79]. Panel **C** shows that regions with highest strength in functional resting state (fMRI) data are located in both frontal and precuneus/visual cortex, seemingly a combination of the findings in panels **A** and **B** [102]. This figure is reproduced with permission from [92, 79, 102].

The same data was further analyzed to show the modular structure of the anatomical brain network [62]; see Fig. (**4.7**). Chen *et al.* found that the anatomical brain network derived in healthy controls from cortical thickness measurements was organized into six topological modules: nodes inside a given module were highly connected to other nodes inside that module but less connected to nodes in other modules (for details of estimation algorithms for *modularity*, see [63-64]). Importantly, these six modules were closely aligned with known functional domains such as auditory/language, strategic/executive, sensorimotor, visual, and mnemonic processing suggesting a direct relationship between distinct functions and highly structured anatomical connectivity. Interestingly, large-scale functional networks derived from human fMRI studies are similarly structured in a modular fashion with largely overlapping modules [65-66].

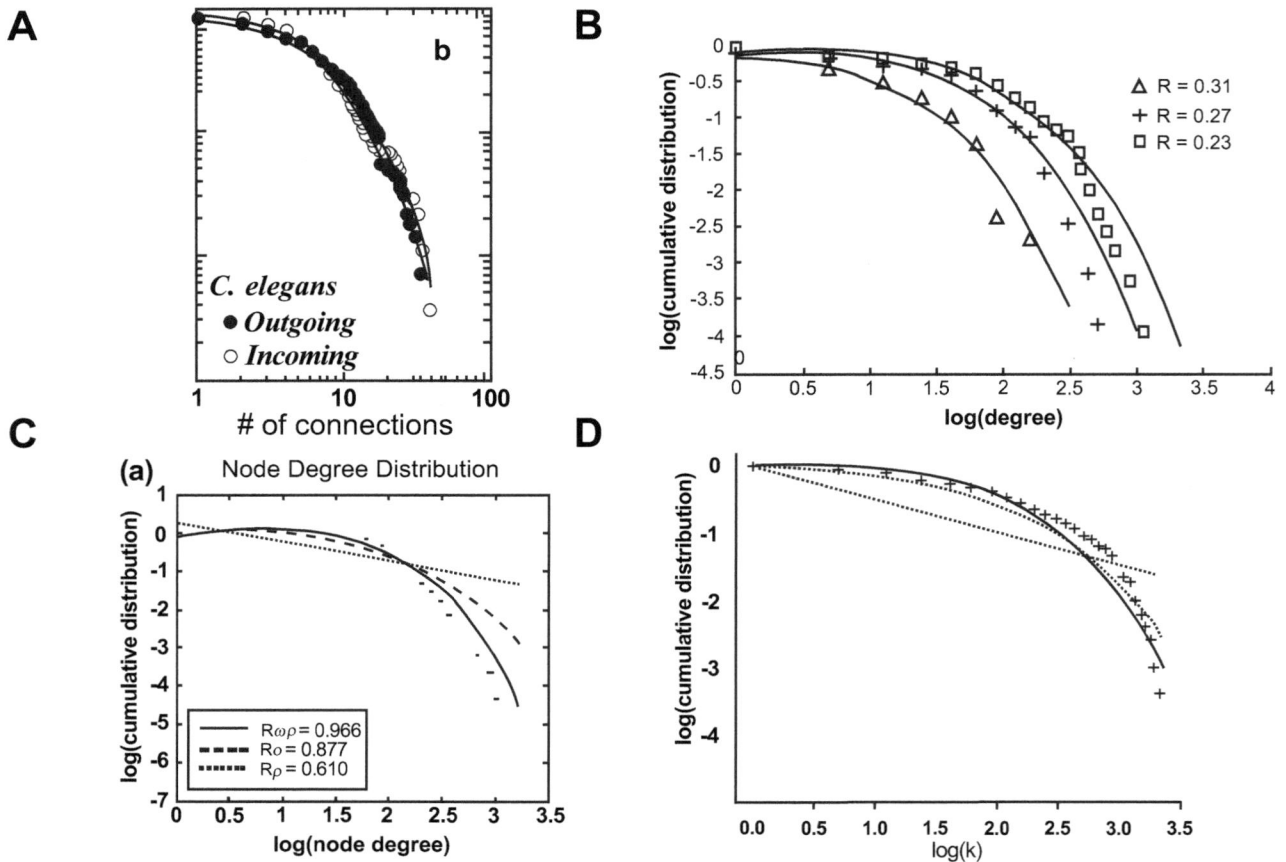

Fig. (4.6). The degree distributions in anatomical neural networks. The cumulative degree distributions are given for *C. elegans* (panel **A**) [6], the human anatomical network derived from covariation in cortical thickness (panel **B**) [56], the human anatomical network derived from diffusion spectrum imaging (panel **C**) [58], and a human functional resting state network (panel **D**) [60]. Note that all degree distributions are exponentially truncated and therefore do not follow a power-law; these networks are therefore not scale-free [59]. This figure is reproduced with permission from [6, 56, 58, 60].

In addition to the description of the healthy brain, two recent studies have extended these methods to both Alzheimer's disease and multiple sclerosis [67-68]. In the Alzheimer's study, the network derived from 92 patients was compared to that derived from 97 matched controls [67]. While remaining largely small-world, the diseased network showed altered small-world properties including a larger clustering coefficient (indicating abnormally high local efficiency) and longer path-length (indicating decreased global efficiency) than the healthy network, in addition to a decreased hypothetical robustness to targeted lesioning of the network hubs. Robustness to attack is a general measure of network stability and resilience. Two types of robustness have been defined: robustness to random attack or lesioning and robustness to targeted attack or lesioning. To measure robustness, the connectivity of the network is measured as nodes are removed from the network either randomly (random attack) or in order of degree (highest to lowest, i.e., a targeted attack on the network hubs). Robust networks are those that retain global connectivity, as measured by the size of the largest connected component of the network, even after removal of several nodes. See Achard *et al.* [60] for an application of the robustness measure to human brain functional resting state networks.

In addition to these global changes, He *et al.* found strong regional variation between the groups using a property known as *centrality* which measures an index region's relative importance to communication in the network by looking at how many of the shortest paths between other regions must pass through that index region [69]. The occipital cortices in the Alzheimer's network showed abnormally high centrality while regions of the temporal and parietal heteromodal association cortices were significantly less central than they were in the healthy brain.

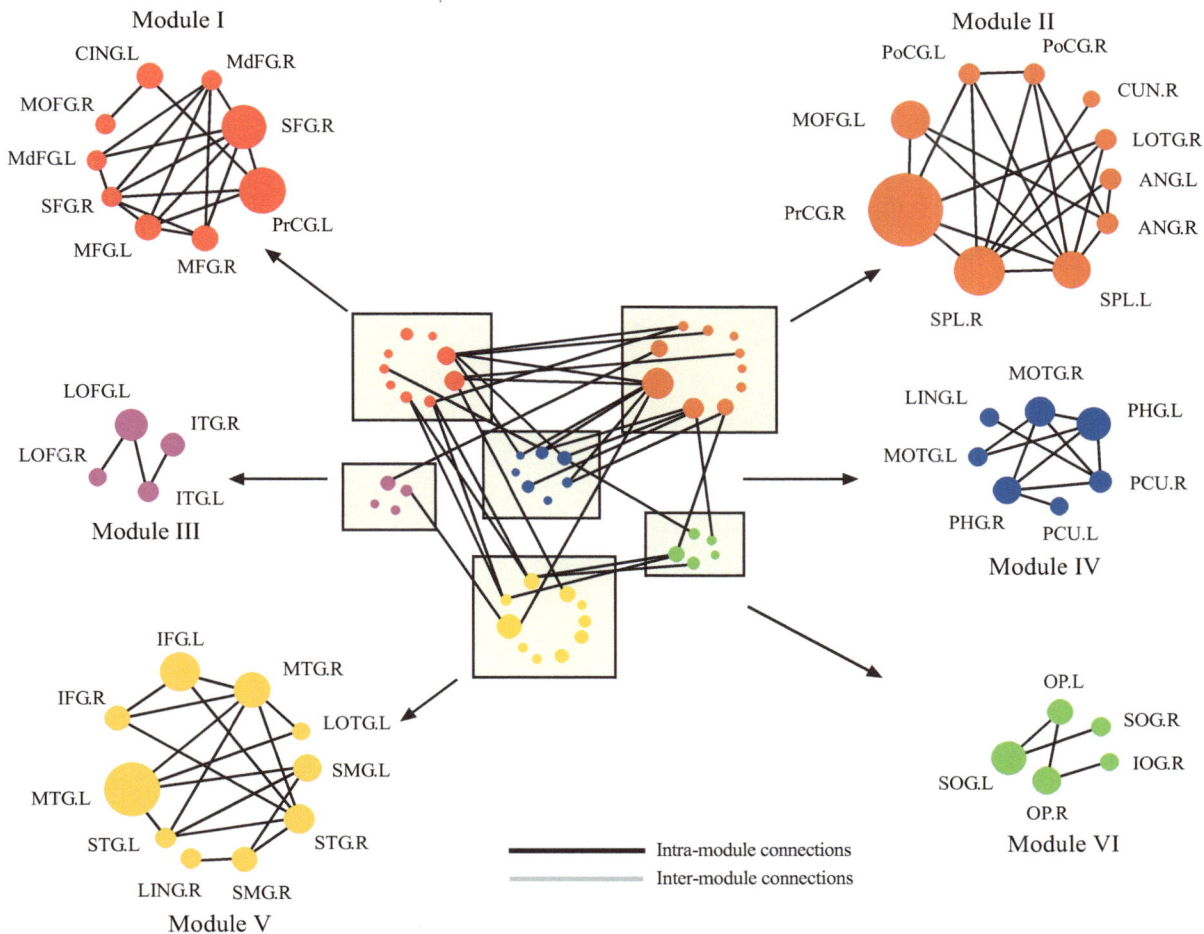

Fig. (4.7). A schematic illustrating modularity in human anatomical networks. The human anatomical network derived from covariation in cortical thickness [56] shows a distinct modular structure. In all, six anatomical modules can be described which closely align with known functional domains such as auditory/language (yellow), strategic/executive (red), sensorimotor (orange), visual (green), and mnemonic processing (blue). This figure is reproduced with permission from [62].

Subsequent work categorized 303 multiple sclerosis patients into 6 groups according to the severity of their white matter lesions [68]. The small-world properties of each group's cortical-thickness based network were measured using the *global efficiency*, which had been previously defined by Latora and Marchiori as the inverse of the network's average path-length [70]. Remarkably, global network efficiency was directly correlated with the white matter lesion severity across the 6 patient groups with significant regional inefficiencies apparent in the insula, precentral gyrus, prefrontal and temporal association cortices, providing evidence for a dysconnection hypothesis of multiple sclerosis in which aberrant neuronal connectivity encompasses widely distributed brain regions.

While the above studies all derived networks from cortical thickness measurements, such group anatomical networks may also be derived from other structural measurements including gray matter volume measurements. Bassett *et al.* performed such a study in 259 healthy controls and 203 people with schizophrenia [71]. Instead of characterizing whole brain networks of the two groups, this study separated the cortical regions (approximately representing Brodmann areas) into Mesulam's three classical categories of cortex: unimodal (primary and secondary association cortices), multimodal (heteromodal association cortices), and transmodal (including the extended limbic system) [72]. Robust group differences were found specifically in the multimodal sub-network where the schizophrenic population showed a larger average connection distance, suggesting spatially inefficient wiring patterns, and an inverse hierarchical topology [7]; see Fig. (**4.8**). Regional differences as measured by degree, clustering and betweenness centrality also pointed to well-accepted areas of abnormal regional anatomy in schizophrenia, including the prefrontal and inferior temporal cortices.

a Healthy volunteers   **b People with schizophrenia**

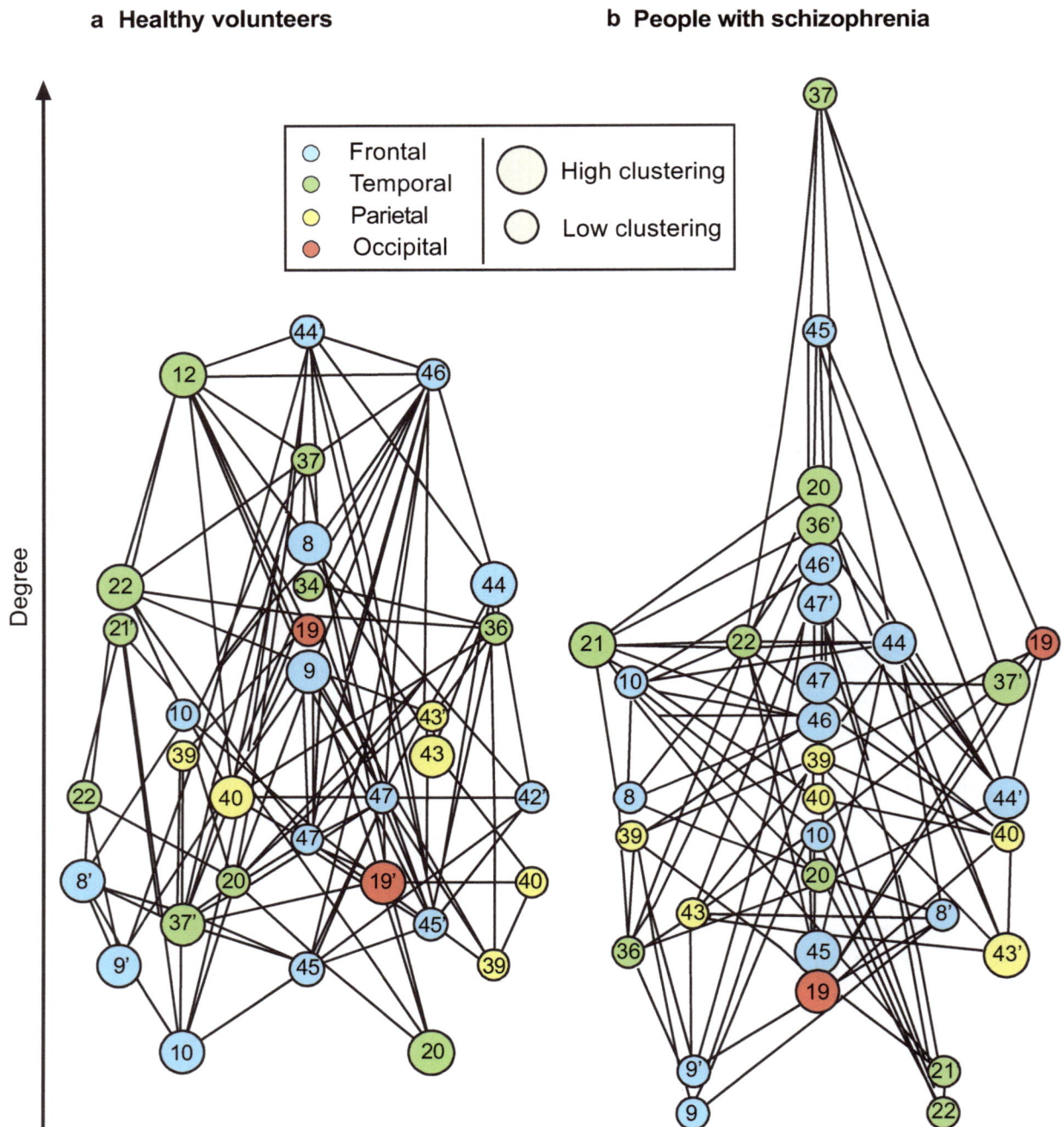

Fig. (4.8). The concept of hierarchical organization in health compared to schizophrenia. Nodes are indicated by circles and represent Brodmann areas of the heteromodal association cortex, given by the number in their centers; apostrophes denote areas in the left-hemisphere. The larger the circle, the higher the clustering of that node; color indicates the approximate anatomical location of the area by lobe. An edge indicates a strong covariation in gray matter volumes of two regions over subjects in a given group: healthy controls on the left and schizophrenic patients on the right. The nodes are organized by ascending degree; hubs are located at the top of the figure while non-hubs are located towards the bottom. This relationship between degree and clustering indicates the hierarchical organization of the cortical sub-network: the healthy hierarchical organization is characterized by hubs with low clustering while the schizophrenic brain shows an inverted relationship between degree and clustering where hubs have lower clustering than other nodes in the network [71]. This figure was reproduced with permission from [53, 71].

The networks discussed thus far in this article have defined connections simply based on the estimated strength of their actual presence in a real brain. However, one can imagine many other ways to define a "connection" that could open new avenues of inquiry. Wright *et al.* suggested studying the genetic contributions to anatomical connectivity between gray matter regions in a set of 10 monozygotic and 10 dizygotic twins [73]. Schmitt *et al.* built upon this idea by studying network edges or connections based on how strongly they were mediated by genetics [74] and found that networks derived from these connections also displayed a small-world architecture. These genetically mediated networks contained somatomotor, visual, and temporal-insular-orbital modules and showed a stronger clustering within frontal cortices than had been seen in other networks; see Fig. (**4.9**). It is important to note in this context that the small-world architecture of functional resting state networks derived from encephalography (EEG) data has also recently been shown to be strongly heritable in a large cohort of 574 twin pairs [75].

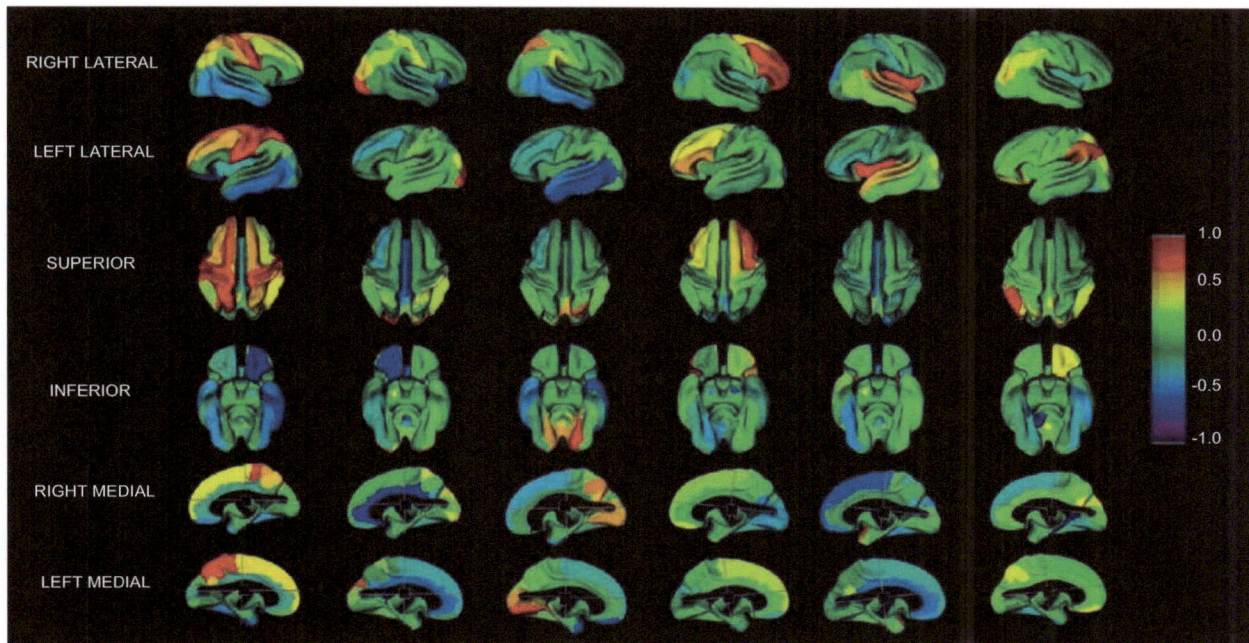

Fig. (4.9). Genetically mediated human cortical networks. Schmitt *et al.* determined the strength of genetic mediation of the correlation between the cortical thickness in any two regions over subjects. The first six principal components of this genetically mediated covariation matrix indicate networks containing somatomotor, visual, and temporal-insular-orbital modules. This figure is reproduced with permission from [74].

HUMAN ANATOMICAL NETWORKS: DIFFUSION IMAGING

The discovery that magnetic resonance imaging could be used to study water diffusion in the cortex occurred in the 1970s but it was not until twenty years later that diffusion tensor imaging (DTI) was proposed to characterize the distribution of water diffusion in space as a voxel-wise tensor [76]. Around the turn of the century, the tensor model was used to reconstruct white matter pathways [77]. With recent advances in diffusion imaging methods, several groups have begun to study individualized networks where connections are defined by pathways along which water diffuses with a definite trajectory within the cortex [55, 57-58, 78-79]. Tractography is the name given to the tracking of these trajectories of water diffusion in the cortex, and as a method, it allows us to estimate a probability of two areas being connected by a white matter tract for any given person. This is in contrast to the volumetric methods introduced in the previous section where we gain a probability of two areas being correlated or "connected" for a given group of people rather than a single person. Tools capable of providing network metrics for individuals is critical for clinical applications, where decisions are made based on data from individual patients. In DTI, we therefore have a simpler interpretation of anatomical network edges or "connectivity": the actual presence, size, and integrity of white matter tracts.

In the first such study, Hagmann *et al.* used diffusion spectrum tractography to construct fine-grained (N=748 and N=4522) anatomical networks of a single healthy human subject [55] (followed by a second subject in a methodological paper published a year later [80]). Hagmann shows that specific architectural properties, such as small-worldness, are consistent across varying spatial resolutions, indicating a connectivity pattern which is fractal in space. Hagmann also reports a hierarchical or modular architecture of the anatomical connections consistent with gross-scale cortical lobes and smaller-scale known functional units. These preliminary findings were confirmed by Iturria *et al.* who studied 20 healthy young adults using diffusion weighted magnetic resonance imaging (DW-MRI) and a more coarse-grained parcellation scheme containing only 90 regions (a similar order of magnitude to the cortical thickness and gray matter networks described in the previous section) [57, 78]. An important consistent finding in diffusion imaging studies is the presence of hubs in the medial posterior cortices; specifically in the precuneus, superior parietal, superior frontal, putamen, and insula as first reported by Iturria [57]. These hub positions are in contrast to the locations of hubs in both volumetric anatomical and resting state functional networks, which tend to be more evenly distributed across association cortex [56, 60].

Hagmann followed up his original analysis in a single person with a larger study in 6 healthy volunteers again using DSI and a fine-grained parcellation scheme of 998 regions [79]; see Fig. (**4.5B**). The purpose of this article was to describe the structural core of the human brain's anatomy. As such, the authors began with a deterministic tractography algorithm and subsequently defined the "connectivity backbone" of the network by determining a *minimum spanning tree* with a maximized sum of edge weights. Additional connections were added (edges with the greatest tractography probability added first) until the average degree of each node was 4. This procedure is more complicated than simply thresholding the connection matrix as had been done in previous studies, but may produce a more accurate picture of the whole brain's structural core. The hubs of this network, consistent with the work by Iturria, were concentrated in the medial posterior cortex, *e.g.*, posterior cingulate, precuneus, cuneus, and paracentral lobule, suggesting their role in functional integration. This article provides a helpful scientific addition to the field in its visualizations of single subject networks, showing a large amount of inter-subject variability not depicted as clearly elsewhere in the literature. Understanding this variability will be critical for translation of these methods into clinical use.

In the largest diffusion network study to date, Gong and colleagues [58] performed diffusion tensor imaging (DTI) tractography on 80 healthy right-handed subjects (38 male) between the ages of 18 and 31 and constructed a group network (using a prior anatomical template, N=78) by including those tracks which were identified consistently across all 80 individuals. After confirming the presence of small-world characteristics and an exponentially truncated power-law degree distribution in agreement with all previous anatomical studies in the human, macaque, cat, and *C. elegans*, Gong and colleagues [58] list the hubs of their networks as precuneus, medial occipital gyrus, superior frontal, and superior occipital and calcarine cortex. In addition to finding pivotal nodes, the authors also discovered the central edges or connections which often linked one of the hubs to other areas of the network suggesting a role for these "bridging connections" in multimodal integration of association cortex. As shown in Fig. (**4.5**), it is interesting to note that the various flavors of network construction lead to somewhat different end results. In particular, the presence of frontal hubs in the DTI study by Gong *et al.* [58], which are lacking in the DSI studies by Hagmann *et al.* [55, 79-80], may stem from the inclusion by Gong *et al.* of edges which were replicable between all subjects. This constraint of replicability may give preference to important frontal connections that have lower tractography probabilities than other portions of the brain closer to the center of the head.

The advent of network analysis of brain imaging data has allowed the community to address the question of wiring minimization from a complementary perspective. In the first study based on DSI data, Hagmann *et al.* [55] showed that the distribution of anatomical connections followed an exponentially truncated power-law, *e.g.* the anatomical brain network at this gross scale was dominated by short distance connections while maintaining a few longer distance connections, mirroring the fact that, at lower scales, neurons are most likely to connect to their nearest neighbors [9]. The predominance of short distance connections was confirmed by following studies in healthy subjects from other imaging modalities [56, 71] and further agrees with estimation of anatomical length distributions of fiber tracts in the macaque, cat, rat, and *C. elegans* [81-82]. A study of the interplay between the small-world topology and the ubiquitous predominance of short range connections has yet to be more fully characterized [83].

METHODOLOGICAL CONSIDERATIONS

Network analysis depends on two apparently simple but theoretically loaded definitions: the definition of the nodes and the definition of the edges [84]. For the *C. elegans* neural network these definitions are relatively straightforward: a node is a neuron and an edge is a (chemical or electrical) synapse between two neurons. Other systems such as the global air transport network also have simple definitions: a node is a city and an edge is a (scheduled) flight between any two cities. However, for brain networks constructed at a coarser scale, by statistical analysis of neuroimaging data, these definitions become hazier.

We have previously said that nodes are brain regions but we have not discussed the question of how to choose these brain regions. How many regions should there be? Should the regions respect cytoarchitectonic boundaries? Similarly, we have described several methodologies to define an edge based on regional covariations in thickness or volume, white matter tract integrity, or genetic variability. With each distinct definition we create a distinct network. To what degree should we expect these networks to be the same? To what degree and how should we expect them to be different? One of the current challenges to the field, therefore, is to characterize the repercussions of alterations in these basic definitions. An understanding of the finer-grained spatial organization of individual neurons or groups of neurons in the brain of a given species, such as those proposed by the Human Connectome [85] and Blue Brain [86] projects, may help us in this endeavor. However, it is possible that while low inter-subject variability in some simpler systems such as *C. elegans* suggests that studying a single system's network is reasonable, the inter-subject variability in the human or other mammalian brains will likely be considerably greater than in the nematode and will need to be carefully handled in the construction of canonical maps of the human brain connectome.

In the course of these excursions into the study of whole brain human anatomical networks, several methodological limitations in each imaging modality have come to light. These weaknesses are differential, i.e., the three types of networks based on tract tracing, diffusion spectrum imaging, and volumetric data each have methodological issues distinct from the others. It is therefore important to realize that while we do not have any "perfect" anatomical connectivity descriptions, the evidence from all lines of inquiry robustly support small-world network architecture of anatomical brain networks throughout the animal kingdom.

As described earlier in this chapter, the first anatomical brain networks were derived from tract tracing studies in non-human primates. Each connection in these networks was gleaned from a near-exhaustive search of the tract-tracing literature where each reported tract could come from a different monkey under different injection methods and localized using different anatomical templates [87]. The experimental variation in these tract-tracing studies can be large. In addition, it is possible that the subsequent whole-brain connectivity matrix may be significantly biased by which tracts scientists have studied most and in which areas of the cortex they were located. Further, these mammalian networks based on tract-tracing studies provide only single hemisphere information; network parameters of a single hemisphere are likely very different than those from a whole brain of two interconnected hemispheres. In light of these difficulties, the even earlier *C. elegans* network is perhaps our strongest representative, in which neurons, locations, and synapses have been largely reproduced in several individual animals [88-89].

The use of correlations in volumetric data to infer connectivity between brain regions over human subjects is necessarily indirect, being based on the probability that axonal connectivity confers a mutually trophic effect on the growth of connected regions, thus inducing a correlation in cortical thickness or other volumetric quantities over subjects [90-91]. Lerch and Worsley confirmed that these correlation values were indirect measurements of anatomical connectivity between two regions as evidenced by their agreement with diffusion tensor imaging (DTI) measurements of axonal pathways [92]; see Fig. (**4.5A**). However, it is not yet clear whether a particular morphological measure, whether it be cortical thickness, gray matter volume, or some other measure, is most sensitive to this effect. It is also as yet unclear how variability in a given subject population will alter the connectivity matrix differentially. Further work is necessary to clarify the effects of these and other methodological perturbations on the resultant anatomical network. More fundamentally, it is unfortunate that as yet these networks do not retain individual variation: a large subject pool is necessary to create a single group network subsequently devoid of subject-specific information. Therefore, relationships between anatomical network measures and cognitive or neuropsychological variables cannot be probed directly using this method.

Finally, the imaging modality that does provide individualized anatomical networks, *e.g.* diffusion tensor/spectrum imaging, is plagued by what is known as a "distance bias": long-distance connections are more difficult to track than short-distance connections. Therefore, anatomical networks derived from these types of data will likely be biased towards shorter-distance connections and a higher average clustering of those connections in a small physical neighborhood. Several *post hoc* corrections for this bias have been suggested [79-80] though none are definitive. While the existence of a distance bias is clear from the technical analysis of tracking algorithms, experimental evidence for its extent is conflicting. Daugeut and colleagues compared fiber tracts derived from DTI tractography with histologically derived tract tracing in a macaque brain [93]. While the agreement between the two methods was generally good, the ability of DTI tractography to describe connections to regions remote from the seed location was hampered. On the other hand, it has been suggested that distance bias apparent in interhemispheric connections was in fact biological, another reflection of wiring constraint, as shown by a comparison of DTI in healthy young subjects and postmortem brain tissue studies [94]. Greater understanding of the technical and biological biases operating against appearance of longer range anatomical connections is clearly critical to the future validation of DTI-based anatomical networks.

On a final methodological note, the studies described here and elsewhere each proceed with more or less consistent processing steps [52-53, 95]. Further work is necessary to determine the most biologically relevant and robust methods for the analysis of human brain networks derived from neuroimaging data [95].

THE COMPLEX STRUCTURE-FUNCTION RELATIONSHIP

Finally, we cannot leave the discussion of anatomical network architecture without discussing the ramifications for the functional dynamics that occur on top of this substrate. The plethora of cognitive functions necessary to maintain human existence as we know it need to be performed by a single largely hard-wired organ. Granted, some small alterations to this hard-wiring are possible *via* directed training or general activity (for reviews, see [96-97]), but to a first approximation they remain constant. Does a small-world anatomical network constrain the structure of functional connectivity patterns?

While we cannot answer this question directly, it is interesting to note in this context that to date all functional networks studied have displayed small-world properties (for reviews, see [52-53, 95]). A significant body of work has focused on showing some correspondence, both theoretically and experimentally, between the human brain's functional patterns of connectivity at rest and its inherent anatomical connectivity [54, 88-100]. Conceptually, however, the ubiquity of such relationships are necessarily decreased by the inherent variance in resting state connectivity [101]: many resting state functions are possible on a single anatomical/structural form just as many task-related functions are also possible on that same structural form. In the future, it will be interesting to characterize the diversity of functional motifs possible on a single wiring diagram, and which subset of such possible motifs are in fact utilized by the human brain.

CONCLUSION AND FUTURE DIRECTIONS

The brain is a complex system composed of many different components non-trivially interacting with each other over a range of scales of space and time. The analytic tools of both statistical mechanics and graph theory allow the exploration of the topology of these complex networks once they have been abstractly described as a collection of nodes connected by edges. The relative simplicity and generality of this approach seems to be a promising way forward in grasping key organizational principles of brain network organization.

We have summarized some of the convergent evidence from a wide variety of data modalities over a broad range of species for a small-world organization of cortical anatomy. Coarse-grained anatomical brain networks further show a tendency to minimize wiring length and their topologies are dominated by association cortical hubs. Future directions include parsing out the effects of aging, gender, cognitive ability, neuropsychiatric disease, and genetics as well as optimizing analysis pipelines and working to overcome current methodological limitations.

GLOSSARY

Centrality: The centrality of a node is a general term for how important that node is in the network. There are many different types of nodal centrality including degree centrality (*e.g.* hubs), betweenness centrality, eigenvector centrality and closeness centrality; measures for edge centrality have also been proposed [69].

Clustering coefficient: The clustering coefficient, c_i, of a node, n_i, is defined as the ratio of the number of edges connecting its neighbors, k_i, to the number of total possible connections between its neighbors ($k_i (k_i - 1)/2$). The clustering coefficient, C, of a network is equal to the average of c_i over all nodes in the graph and is a good measure of the amount of *local* communication possible in the network [5]. Note: other possible definitions for the clustering coefficient exist [103].

Cost: The cost, κ, of a network is defined as the number of edges present in the network divided by the number of total possible edges (*N(N-1)/2*), where N is the total number of nodes in the network. This term is also often referred to as the sparsity of the network; the tract tracing studies in the macaque and cat suggest that the sparsity of anatomical brain networks at this spatial scale is approximately 0.3 [52].

Degree: The degree, k, of a node is equal to the number of edges emanating from that node. The degree of a node tells you how important that node is in the network in terms of the number of its communication pathways.

Degree distribution: The degree distribution is the probability distribution of nodal degrees, k_i, over all nodes in the network. Degree distributions are usually plotted as cumulative distributions in log-log space. Random graphs have an exponential degree distribution ($P(k) \sim e^{-\alpha k}$) while other complex systems such as the internet and worldwide web have been found to have a power law distribution ($P(k) \sim k^{-\alpha}$) [59]. Power-law distributions are termed "scale-free" and imply a greater probability that nodes with very large degree will exist in the graph [59]. The majority of brain networks as well as transport or infrastructural systems have an exponentially truncated power law distribution of the form $P(k) \sim k^{\alpha-1} e^{k/kc}$ which implies that the probability of highly connected hubs will be greater than in a random graph but smaller than in a "scale-free" network [6].

Edge: An edge, $e_{i,j}$, is a piece of the network that connects two nodes n_i and n_j; it is usually depicted by a line in a graph [3]. In anatomical brain networks, an edge denotes the fact that, for example, two brain regions are connected by white matter tracts.

Efficiency: The efficiency, E, of a network is equal to the inverse of that network's path-length L and measure the global efficiency of a graph [70]. Local efficiency metrics which more closely mimic the clustering coefficient have also been defined [70].

Hierarchy: The hierarchy, β, of a network is given by the slope in log-log space of the clustering coefficient, c_i, *versus* the degree, k_i, of each node in the network [7]. The hierarchy parameter indicates that hubs connect disparate sub-modules which would not otherwise be connected and indicates a structured hierarchical organization of information processing.

Hub: A hub of a network is a node that has a large degree. There are different definitions of hubs which are more or less stringent: *e.g.* a hub must have a degree 1, 2 or 3 standard deviations above the mean degree of the network. Hubs of whole brain functional and anatomical networks have been shown to be located predominantly in association cortex [56,102].

Modularity: the modularity, m, of a network is a measure of the degree to which the network is composed of modules: *e.g.* cohesive communities of nodes that are more connected to each other than to the rest of the network [63,64,105,106]. There is some evidence that modules of the anatomical network underlie functionally coherent sets of brain and nervous system components [50,54].

Minimum Spanning Tree: A minimum spanning tree is a subgraph of the network made up of the smallest subset of edges of the graph where all nodes are still connected together; this subgraph must be a tree meaning that it does not contain any cycles, *e.g.* feedback loops [107]. The minimum spanning tree has been used to create a connectivity "backbone" of an anatomical brain network [79].

Neighbor: A neighbor of node n_i is any node n_j for which there exists an edge $e_{i,j}$; that is, a neighbor of node n_i is any node connected to node n_i.

Node: A node, n, is the smallest part of a network from which an edge emanates and is usually depicted by a circle in a graph [3]. In brain networks, nodes are usually brain regions such as Brodmann areas or voxels.

Path-Length: The path-length, l_i, of a node is defined as the average shortest path between that node and any other node on the graph. The path-length, L, of a network is given by the average of l_i over all nodes in the graph and is a good measure of the amount of *global* communication possible in the network [104].

Small-Worldness: The small-worldness scalar, σ, is the ratio of the clustering coefficient of a network, C, normalized by the clustering coefficient of a random graph, C_r, to the path-length of a network, L, normalized by the path-length of a random graph, L_r: $\sigma = (C/C_r)/(L/L_r) = \gamma/\lambda$ where the normalized clustering coefficient $\gamma = C/C_r$ and the normalized path-length $\lambda = L/L_r$ [5,30]. The small-world property indicates a balance of the possible communication in the network on both a global and local scale: e.g., a balance between integration and segregation of information processing.

REFERENCES

[1]   Karinthy F. Chains. Atheneum Press; 1929.
[2]   de Sola Pool I, Kochen M. Contacts and influence. Social Networks 1978; v1(1).
[3]   Erdos P, Renyi A. On random graphs. Publ Math Debrecen 1959; 6: 290–7.
[4]   Bollabas B. Random Graphs Academic Press, London; 1985.
[5]   Watts DJ, Strogatz SH. Collective dynamics of 'small-world' networks. Nature 1998; 393(6684): 440–2.
[6]   Amaral LAN, Scala A, Barthelemy M, Stanley HE. Classes of small-world networks. Proc Natl Acad Sci USA 2000; 97(21): 11149–52.
[7]   Ravasz E, Barabási, AL. Hierarchical organization in complex networks. Phys Rev E Stat Nonlin Soft Matter Phys 2003; 67(2 Pt 2): 026112.
[8]   Finger S. The origins of neuroscience: A history of explorations into brain function. Oxford University Press; 1994.
[9]   Sporns O, Tononi G, Edelman GM. Connectivity and complexity: the relationship between neuroanatomy and brain dynamics. Neural Networks 2000; 13(8-9): 909–22.
[10]   Sporns O, Tonon G, Edelman G.M. Theoretical neuroanatomy: Relating anatomical and functional connectivity in graphs and cortical connection matrices. Cereb Cortex 2000; 10: 127–41.
[11]   Brodmann K. Vergleichende lokalisationslehre der grosshirnrinde 1909.
[12]   Hubel DH, Wiesel TN. Receptive fields and functional architecture of monkey striate cortex. J Physiol 1968; 195: 215–43.
[13]   Mountcastle VB. Modularity and topographic properties of single neurons of cat's somatic sensory cortex. J Neurophysiol 1957; 20: 408–34.
[14]   da Fontoura Costa L. Diambra L. Topographical maps as complex networks. Phys Rev E 2005; 71(2 Pt 1): 021901.
[15]   Kashtan N, Alon U. Spontaneous evolution of modularity and network motifs. Proc Natl Acad Sci USA 2005; 102(39): 13773–8.
[16]   Wen Q, Chklovskii DB. Segregation of the brain into gray and white matter: A design minimizing conduction delays. PLoS Comput Biol 2005; 1(7): e78.
[17]   Simon H. The architecture of complexity. Proc Amer Philos Soc 1962; 106(6): 467–82.
[18]   Kopell N, Ermentrout GB, Whittington MA, Traub RD. Gamma rhythms and beta rhythms have different synchronization properties. Proc Natl Acad Sci USA 2000; 97: 1867–72.
[19]   Lee K, Williams LM, Breakspear M, Gordon G. Synchronous gamma activity: A review and contribution to an integrative neuroscience model of schizophrenia. Brain Res Rev 2003; 41(1): 57–78.
[20]   Bassett DS, Meyer-Lindenberg A, Achard S, Duke T, Bullmore E. Adaptive reconfiguration of fractal small-world human brain functional networks. Proc Natl Acad Sci USA 2006; 103: 19518–23.
[21]   Bassett DS, Bullmore E, Meyer-Lindenberg A, Apud J, Weinberger DR, Coppola R. Cognitive fitness of cost-efficient brain functional networks. Proc Natl Acad Sci USA 2009; 106(28): 11747–52.
[22]   Lago-Fernandez LF, Huerta R, Corbacho F, Siguenza J.A. Fast response and temporal coding on coherent oscillations in small-world networks. Phys Rev Lett 2000; 84: 2758–61.
[23]   Barahona M, Pecora LM. Synchronization in small-world systems. Phys Rev Lett 2002; 89: 054101.
[24]   Hong H, Choi MY. Synchronization on small-world networks. Phys Rev E 2002; 65: 026139.
[25]   Atay FM, Biyikoğlu T, Jost J. Synchronization of networks with prescribed degree distributions. IEEE Trans Circuits Syst I Regul Pap 2006; 53(1): 92–8.
[26]   Nishikawa T, Motter AE, Lai Y, Hoppensteadt FC. Heterogeneity in oscillator networks: Are smaller worlds easier to synchronize? Phys Rev Lett 2003; 91: 014101.
[27]   Atay FM, Biyikoğlu T. Graph operations and synchronization of complex networks. Phys Rev E 2005; 72: 016217.
[28]   Beggs, J.M, Plenz, D. Neuronal avalanches in neocortical circuits. J Neurosci 2003; 23: 11167–11177.
[29]   Kitzbichler MG, Smith M, Christensen S, Bullmore E. Broadband criticality of human brain network synchronization. PLoS Comput Biol 2009; in press.
[30]   Humphries MD, Gurney K, Prescott TJ. The brainstem reticular formation is a small-world, not scale-free, network. Proc Biol Sci B 2006; 273(1-3): 503–11.
[31]   Kaiser M, Hilgetag CC. Non-optimal component placement, but short processing paths, due to long-distance projections in neural systems. PLoS Comput Biol 2006; 2: e95.
[32]   Chen BL, Hall DH, Chklovskii DB. Wiring optimization can relate neuronal structure and function. Proc Natl Acad Sci USA 2006; 103(12): 4723–8.
[33]   Attwell D, Laughlin SB. An energy budget for signalling in the grey matter of the brain. J Cereb Blood Flow and Metab 2001; 21: 1133–45.

[34]   Ringo JL. Neuronal interconnection as a function of brain size. Brain Behav Evol 1991; 38: 1–6.
[35]   Changizi MA. Principles underlying mammalian neocortical scaling. Biol Cybern 2001; 84(3): 207–15.
[36]   Chklovskii DB, Schikorski T, Stevens CF. Wiring optimization in cortical circuits. Neuron 2002; 34(3): 341–7.
[37]   Stepanyants A, Hof PR, Chklovskii DB. Geometry and structural plasticity of synaptic connectivity. Neuron 2002; 34(2): 275–88.
[38]   Chklovskii DB. Exact solution for the optimal neuronal layout problem. Neural Comput 2004; 16(10): 2067–78.
[39]   Sik A, Penttonen M, Ylinen A, Buzsaki G. Hippocampal CA1 interneurons: An in vivo intracellular labeling study. J Neurosci 1995; 15(10): 6651–65.
[40]   Allman JM. Evolving Brains. Scientific American, New York; 1998.
[41]   Buzsaki G, Geisler C, Henze DA, Wang X.J. Interneuron diversity series: Circuit complexity and axon wiring economy of cortical interneurons. Trends Neurosci 2004; 27(4): 186–93.
[42]   Karbowski J. Optimal wiring principle and plateaus in the degree of separation for cortical neurons. Phys Rev Lett 2001; 86(16): 3674.
[43]   Hilgetag CC, Burns GA, O'Neill MA, Scannell JW, Young MP. Anatomical connectivity defines the organization of clusters of cortical areas in the macaque monkey and the cat. Phil Trans Roy Soc Lon B Biol Sci 2000; 335: 91–110.
[44]   Zhigulin VP. Dynamical motifs: Building blocks of complex dynamics in sparsely connected random networks. Phys Rev Lett 2005; 92: 238701.
[45]   Felleman DJ, Van Essen DC. Distributed hierarchical processing in the primate cerebral cortex. Cereb Cortex 1991; 1: 1–47.
[46]   Young MP. Objective analysis of the topological organization of the primate cortical visual system. Nature 1992; 358(6382): 152–5.
[47]   Young MP. The organization of neural systems in the primate cerebral cortex. Proc R Soc Lond B 1993; 252: 13–18.
[48]   Scannell JW, Blakemore C, Young MP. Analysis of connectivity in the cat cerebral cortex. J Neurosci 1995; 15(2): 1463–83.
[49]   Scannell JW, Burns GAPC, Hilgetag CC, O'Neil MA, Young MP. The connectional organization of the cortico-thalamic system of the cat. Cereb Cortex 1999; 9(3): 277–99.
[50]   Chatterjee N, Sinha S. Understanding the mind of a worm: hierarchical network structure underlying nervous system function in C. elegans. Prog Brain Res 2007; 145–53.
[51]   Sporns O, Zwi J. The small world of the cerebral cortex. Neuroinformatics 2004; 2: 145–62.
[52]   Bassett DS, Bullmore ET. Small-world brain networks. Neuroscientist 2006; 12: 512–23.
[53]   Bullmore ET, Sporns O. Complex brain networks: Graph theoretical analysis of structural and functional systems. Nat Rev Neurosci 2009; 10(3): 186–98.
[54]   Sporns O, Honey CJ, Kotter R. Identification and classification of hubs in brain networks. PLoS One 2007; 2(10): e1049.
[55]   Hagmann P, Kurant M, Gigandet X, et al. Imaging the brain neuronal network with diffusion MRI: A way to understand its global architecture. Proc Intl Soc Mag Reson Med 2006; 14.
[56]   He Y, Chen ZJ, Evans AC. Small-world anatomical networks in the human brain revealed by cortical thickness from MRI. Cereb Cortex 2007; 17: 2407–19.
[57]   Iturria-Medina Y, Sotero RC, Canales-Rodriguez EJ, Aleman-Gomez Y, Melie-Garcia L. Studying the human brain anatomical network via diffusion-weighted MRI and graph theory. Neuroimage 2008; 40(3): 1064–76.
[58]   Gong G, He Y, Concha L, et al. Mapping anatomical connectivity patterns of human cerebral cortex using in vivo diffusion tensor imaging tractography. Cereb Cortex 2009; 19(3): 524–36.
[59]   Albert R, Barabási AL Statistical mechanics of complex networks. Rev Mod Phys 2002; 74: 47–98.
[60]   Achard S, Salvador R, Whitcher B, Suckling J, Bullmore E. A resilient, low-frequency, small-world human brain functional network with highly connected association cortical hubs. J Neurosci 2006; 26(1): 63–72.
[61]   Raichle ME, MacLeod AM, Snyder AZ, Powers WJ, Gusnard DA, Shulman GL. A default mode of brain function. Proc Natl Acad Sci U A 2001; 98(2): 676–82.
[62]   Chen ZJ, He Y, Rosa-Neto P, Germann J, Evans AC. Revealing modular architecture of human brain structural networks by using cortical thickness from MRI. Cereb Cortex 2008; 18(10): 2374–81.
[63]   Blondel VD, Guillaume JL, Lambiotte R, Lefebvre E. Fast unfolding of communities in large networks. J Stat Mech 2008; P10008.
[64]   Leicht EA, Newman, MEJ. Community structure in directed networks. Phys Rev Lett 2008; 100(11): 118703.
[65]   Salvador R, Suckling J, Coleman MR, Pickard JD, Menon D, Bullmore E. Neurophysiological architecture of functional magnetic resonance images of human brain. Cereb Cortex 2005; 15: 1332–42.
[66]   Meunier D, Achard S, Morcom A, Bullmore E. Age-related changes in modular organization of human brain functional networks. NeuroImage 2009; 44: 715–23.
[67]   He Y, Chen ZJ, Evans AC. Structural insights into aberrant topological patterns of large-scale cortical networks in Alzheimer's disease. J Neurosci 2008; 28(18): 4756–66.
[68]   He Y, Dagher A, Chen Z, et al. Impaired small-world efficiency in structural cortical networks in multiple sclerosis associated with white matter lesion load. Brain 2009; Epub ahead of print.
[69]   Freeman LC. A set of measures of centrality based on betweenness. Sociometry 1977; 40: 35–41.
[70]   Latora V, Marchiori M. Economic small-world behavior in weighted networks. Eur Phys J B 2003; 32: 249–63.
[71]   Bassett DS, Bullmore E, Verchinksi BA, Mattay VS, Weinberger, DR, Meyer-Lindenberg A. Hierarchical organization of human cortical networks in health and schizophrenia. J Neurosci 2008; 28: 9239–48.
[72]   Mesulam MM. From sensation to cognition. Brain 1998; 121(Pt 6): 1013–52.
[73]   Wright IC, Sham P, Murray RM, Weinberger DR, Bullmore ET. Genetic contributions to regional variability in human brain structure: methods and preliminary results. Neuroimage 2002; 17(1): 256–71.
[74]   Schmitt JE, Lenroot RK, Wallace GL, et al. Identification of genetically mediated cortical networks: a multivariate study of pediatric twins and siblings. Cereb Cortex 2008; 18(8): 1737–47.
[75]   Smit DJ, Stam CJ, Posthuma D, Boomsma DI, de Geus EJ. Heritability of "small-world" networks in the brain: a graph theoretical analysis of resting-state eeg functional connectivity. Hum Brain Mapp 2008; 29(12): 1368–78.
[76]   Basser P, Mattiello J, LeBihan D. MRI diffusion tensor spectroscopy and imaging. Biophys J 1994; 66: 259–67.
[77]   Mori S, Crain B, Chacko V, van Zijl P. Three-dimensional tracking of axonal projections in the brain by magnetic resonance imaging. Ann Neurol 1999; 45(2): 265–9.
[78]   Iturria-Medina Y, Canales-Rodríguez EJ, Melie-García L, et al. Characterizing brain anatomical connections using diffusion weighted MRI and graph theory. Neuroimage 2007; 36(3): 645–60.
[79]   Hagmann P, Cammoun L, Gigandet X, et al. Mapping the structural core of human cerebral cortex. PLoS Biol 2008; 6(7): e159.
[80]   Hagmann P, Kurant M, Gigandet X, et al. Mapping human whole-brain structural networks with diffusion MRI. PLoS One 2007; 2(7): e597.

[81]   Ahn YY, Jeong H, Kim BJ. Wiring cost in the organization of a biological neuronal network. Physica A 2006; 367: 531–7.
[82]   Kaiser M, Hilgetag CC, van Ooyen A. A simple rule for axon outgrowth and synaptic competition generates realistic connection lengths and filling fractions. Cereb Cortex 2009; Epub ahead of print.
[83]   Wang J, Provan G. Topological analysis of specific spatial complex networks. Adv Complex Syst 2009; 12(1): 45–71.
[84]   Butts CT. Revisiting the foundations of network analysis. Science 2009; 325(5939): 414 – 6.
[85]   Sporns O, Tononi G, Kotter R. The human connectome: A structural description of the human brain. PLoS Comput Biol 2005; 1(4): e42.
[86]   Markram H. The blue brain project. Nat Rev Neurosci 2006; 7: 153–160.
[87]   Stephan KE, Kamper L, Bozkurt A, Burns GAPC, Young MP, K¨otter R. Advanced database methodology for the collation of connectivity data on the macaque brain(CoCoMac). Phil Trans R Soc Lond B 2001; 356: 1159–86.
[88]   White JG, Southgate E, Thomson JN, Brenner S. The structure of the nervous system of the nematode Caenorhabditis elegans. Philos Trans R Soc London B 1986; 314.
[89]   Hall DH, Russel RL. The posterior nervous system of the nematode Caenorhabditis elegans: serial reconstruction of identified neurons and complete pattern of synaptic interactions. J Neurosci 1991; 11: 1–22.
[90]   Wright IC, Sharma T Ellison ZR, *et al.* Supra-regional brain systems and the neuropathology of schizophrenia. Cereb Cortex 1999; 9: 366–78.
[91]   Pezawas L, Meyer-Lindenberg A, Drabant EM, *et al.* 5-HTTLPR polymorphism impacts human cingulate-amygdala interactions: A genetic susceptibility mechanism for depression. Nat Neurosci 2005; 8(6): 828–34.
[92]   Lerch JP, Worsley K, Shaw GP, *et al.* Mapping anatomical correlations across cerebral cortex (MACACC) using cortical thickness from MRI. NeuroImage 2006; 31: 993–1003.
[93]   Dauguet J, Peled S, Berezovskii V, *et al.* Comparison of fiber tracts derived from in-vivo dti tractography with 3D histological neural tract tracer reconstruction on a macaque brain. NeuroImage 2007; 37: 530–8.
[94]   Lewis JD, Theilmann RJ, Sereno MI, Townsend J. The relation between connection length and degree of connectivity in young adults: A DTI analysis. Cereb Cortex 2009; 19(3): 554–62.
[95]   Bassett DS, Bullmore ET. Human brain networks in health and disease. Curr Opin Neurol 1009; 22(4): 340–7.
[96]   Draganski B, May A. Training-induced structural changes in the adult human brain. Behav Brain Res 2008; 192(1): 137–42.
[97]   Butz M, W¨org¨otter F, van Ooyen A. Activity-dependent structural plasticity. Brain Res Rev 2009; 60(2): 287–305.
[98]   Honey CJ, K¨otter R, Breakspear M, Sporns O. Network structure of cerebral cortex shapes functional connectivity on multiple time scales. Proc Natl Acad Sci USA 2007; 104(24): 10240–5.
[99]   Honey C, Sporns O. Dynamical consequences of lesions in cortical networks. Hum Brain Mapp 2008; 29(7): 802–9.
[100]   Honey CJ, Sporns O, Cammoun L, *et al.* Predicting human resting-state functional connectivity from structural connectivity. Proc Natl Acad Sci U S A 2009; 206(6): 2035–40.
[101]   Deuker L, Bullmore ET, Smith M, *et al.* Reproducibility of graph metrics of human brain functional networks. Neuroimage 2009; Epub ahead of print.
[102]   Buckner RL, Sepulcre J, Talukdar T, *et al.* Cortical hubs revealed by intrinsic functional connectivity: mapping, assessment of stability, and relation to alzheimer's disease. J Neurosci 2009; 29(6): 1860–73.
[103]   Schank T, Wagner D. Approximating clustering coefficient and transitivity. J Graph Algorithms Appl 2005; 9(2): 265–275.
[104]   Dijkstra EW. A note on two problems in connexion with graphs. Numerische Mathematik 1959; 1: 269–71.
[105]   Newman MEJ. Modularity and community structure in networks. Proc Natl Acad Sci USA 2006; 103: 8577–85.
[106]   Sales-Pardo M, Guimerà R, Moreira AA Amaral LA. Extracting the hierarchical organization of complex systems. Proc Natl Acad Sci USA 2007; 104(39): 15224–9.
[107]   Graham RL, Hell P. On the history of minimum spanning tree problem. Ann Hist Comput 1985; 7(1): 43–57.
[108]   Lohmann H, Rohrig B. Long-range horizontal connections between supragranular pyramidal cells in the extrastriate visual cortex of the rat. J Comp Neurol 1994; 344: 543–58.

CHAPTER 5

Sleep Physiology Dynamics: Network Analysis and other Quantitative Approaches

Matt T. Bianchi[1,*] and Andrew J. Phillips[2]

[1]*Sleep Division, Neurology Department, 55 Fruit Street, Wang 7, Massachusetts General Hospital, Boston, MA, 02114, USA and* [2]*Division of Sleep Medicine, Brigham & Women's Hospital, Harvard Medical School, 221 Longwood Avenue, Boston, MA 02115, USA*

Abstract: Sleep is a state of altered consciousness accompanied by dynamic changes in metabolic activity and neural activity patterns. As such, research into the mechanisms of sleep and the consequences of sleep related disorders represents a frontier of human physiology in need of increasingly sophisticated analytical tools. Methodologies spanning electroencephalographic, magnetoencephalographic, functional magnetic resonance imaging, and autonomic metrics continue to uncover important details of sleep physiology. In addition, novel approaches to modeling sleep-wake state transitions continue to enhance our understanding of the overall architecture of sleep in healthy and disrupted sleep. Given the importance of sleep for mood, performance, restoration, and plasticity, these approaches hold promise for rapid clinical translation – not only for improved diagnosis and characterization of disrupted sleep across its many contributing etiologies, but also for treatment aimed at harnessing the benefits of consolidated sleep. This chapter reviews recent developments in these domains, and their potential clinical applications.

Keywords: REM sleep, NREM sleep, cerebral metabolism, autonomic, insomnia, slow wave sleep, state transitions.

INTRODUCTION

Multiple endogenous and exogenous factors influence the timing and duration of sleep-wake cycles [1-2]. The mechanisms by which sleep contributes to our sense of alertness and well-being, and to various aspects of metabolism and physiology, remain actively investigated and hotly debated [3-7]. Techniques for assessing human sleep range from highly subjective sleep diaries and questionnaires, to objective rest-activity pattern monitoring *via* actigraphy, clinical laboratory polysomnography (PSG), and modern imaging techniques (such as magnetoencephalography (MEG) or functional magnetic resonance imaging (fMRI)). Each strategy has important advantages and disadvantages, and provides distinct types of information about sleep. Ideally, these diverse techniques will serve complementary roles in our understanding of human sleep physiology. For example, the convenience and capacity for longitudinal monitoring in the home setting are key benefits of wrist actigraphy, which aids in the documentation of circadian phase of sleep-wake patterns. However, limb movement has only modest accuracy in distinguishing sleep from wake, and beyond this binary distinction, no insight is provided into sleep quality, the architecture of sleep stages, or other physiological parameters.

Laboratory PSG is the gold standard for diagnosis of sleep disordered breathing and other types of sleep pathology. In addition, its multi-channel monitoring of physiological signals provides the gold standard for scoring sleep stages, as well as scalp electroencephalography (EEG) "arousals" that may disturb sleep. However, clinical PSG measurements are usually restricted to a single night, and the unfamiliar and potentially disruptive nature of the actual monitoring ensemble may confound interpretation. Thus, laboratory PSG measurements may not accurately reflect home sleep patterns, including features such as night-to-night variability, intrinsic circadian phase, and effects of perturbations (behaviors such as exercise, substances such as caffeine, etc.) that may vary over time. In particular, sleep architecture (arousals, stage transition patterns, sleep efficiency, etc.) may be altered significantly by the testing environment.

Research tools such as high density EEG, electrocorticography (ECoG), MEG, fMRI, and positron emission tomography (PET) imaging continue to provide important insights into brain metabolism and physiology during

*Address correspondence to Matt T. Bianchi: Sleep Division, Neurology Department, 55 Fruit Street, Wang 7, Massachusetts General Hospital, Boston, MA, 02114, USA; Email: mtbianchi@partners.org

both normal and disrupted sleep (for example, experimental disruption *via* caffeine or by acoustic stimulation), and sleep in the setting of neurological or psychiatric disease. However, like the PSG, the implementation of these methods requires an environment that may not be reflective of home sleep.

The literature of applying imaging methodologies to sleep disorders has been reviewed recently [8-9]. Combined with physiological studies, these efforts have led to interesting hypotheses; for example, insomnia has been suggested to be a disorder of hyper-arousal [10]. This idea is supported by several observations in insomnia patients, such as increased beta and gamma frequency EEG activity at sleep onset and during established episodes of NREM sleep [11-12]. Increased metabolism at transitions between sleep and wakefulness has also been reported in patients with insomnia for several brain regions (including the limbic system, thalamus, and cingulate and prefrontal cortices), suggesting that the normal decrease in brain metabolism accompanying the descent into sleep may be impaired [10, 13]. However, other studies have shown the opposite, with reduced cerebral blood flow (CBF) during sleep in cortical and sub-cortical regions of subjects with insomnia [14], which treatment reversed (concurrently with objective improvements in sleep latency). It is possible that the heterogeneity of insomnia as a disorder, combined with the unusual sleep environment in which these metabolic studies are conducted, contribute to the variable findings.

SLOW WAVE OSCILLATIONS IN NREM SLEEP

Slow wave oscillations during sleep have attracted attention in several areas of research [15], including their possible role in synaptic plasticity [16] and their use as a biomarker of the homeostatic sleep drive [17]. The prominent heritability of slow wave oscillations (and other frequency bands) suggests that they may be an important marker of cortical physiology [18]. During NREM sleep (mainly N3 but also N2), cortical neurons transition in a step-like manner between a depolarized 'up' state in which action potential firing can be observed, and a hyperpolarized 'down' state with little or no firing [15, 19-21]. Transitions between up and down states may relate to the ~1 Hz slow waves recorded by scalp EEG during NREM sleep. Linking scalp EEG dynamics to cortical firing patterns, such as the slow wave oscillations to up-down states, provides a mechanistic basis for interpreting non-invasive clinical studies. As further studies solidify these relationships, it is hoped that routine EEG measures will gain increasing utility as biomarkers for underlying cortical function.

Transcranial magnetic stimulation (TMS) has provided an intriguing avenue to test certain hypotheses related to sleep physiology. Massimini *et al.* [22] combined high density (60 channel) EEG with TMS in six healthy subjects, who were recorded during quiet wakefulness (eyes closed) and during NREM sleep (N1-N3). Importantly, subjects reported not being able to identify the timing of TMS pulses, and sleep was not disturbed by TMS. TMS pulses during wakefulness elicited spreading waves of activity that emanated from the stimulation site. During the first ~100 ms, these waves were higher frequency (20-35Hz) than ~100-300ms post-stimulation (8-12 Hz). Upon entry into N1 sleep, the dynamics were immediately distinct, with larger amplitude initial responses (within 50ms), followed by attenuation of the emanating waves of activity within 150-200ms. The initial local response became even larger with progression to N2/N3 sleep, followed by virtually no spreading of activity in subsequent time windows.

The authors interpreted this localized response in NREM sleep compared to wakefulness as evidence of decreased effective connectivity among brain regions associated with sleep. The study contrasts its findings with the well-described increase in coherence between EEG electrodes observed during NREM sleep. Reconciling the mechanisms that could support functional disconnection (non-propagation of TMS stimulation) despite coherent slow wave oscillations may provide insight into normal and pathological sleep-related network activity.

In a follow-up study [23], TMS was shown to trigger slow waves and spindles in healthy subjects during sleep (but not wake) using simultaneous high density EEG recordings. Varying the location and amplitude of TMS stimulation resulted in local versus more global spread of activity. Interestingly, under certain conditions, repeated slow (<1Hz) TMS stimulation caused a global increase in slow wave power, including frequencies above the stimulation range (that is, >1 Hz). Given the possible role of slow wave oscillations in plasticity and/or restorative aspects of sleep, the prospect of non-pharmacological augmentation of this process is intriguing.

Several other studies have continued efforts to draw causal links between waking experience and the manifestation of slow waves of sleep. Local increases in slow wave activity during sleep have been correlated with motor learning in the prior waking period [24], while local decreases in slow wave activity are observed with arm immobilization [25]. Direct current stimulation at the frequency of slow waves during sleep has also been shown to enhance declarative memory [26].

METABOLIC IMAGING IN SLEEP

Before the emergence of fMRI, brain metabolism was known to be altered during sleep compared to wakefulness in healthy subjects, based on PET and SPECT imaging as well as measures of CBF [27]. The overall trends of these studies suggested decreased metabolism and CBF during NREM sleep. In contrast, REM sleep generally exhibited higher activity levels and blood flow, similar to those seen in wakefulness. Moving from light to deeper stages within NREM sleep was generally associated with progressive decreases in metabolism, and was also associated with involvement of additional brain regions in these metabolic changes. During REM sleep, increased metabolism was evident in the pons, limbic system, and visual areas, while parietal regions and the prefrontal cortex showed decreased activity [27].

An early fMRI study employed a special quiet scanning technique to investigate blood oxygen level dependent (BOLD) signal changes during sleep in 5 healthy subjects who were able to achieve both NREM and REM sleep in the scanner over the course of several hours [28]. Simultaneous recording of EEG (6 leads), EOG and EMG was used to identify sleep stages during fMRI acquisition. They found that compared to NREM sleep, REM sleep was associated with decreased frontal and increased occipital BOLD signals. This pattern was consistent with the above mentioned PET and SPECT imaging.

Subsequent studies extended the use of combined EEG and fMRI to investigate sleep, but in these studies only NREM sleep was observed, likely because subjects could not maintain sleep long enough to complete a cycle that included REM sleep. Portas *et al.* [29] and Czisch *et al.* [30] used acoustic stimulation protocols to demonstrate the expected decreased activation in response to auditory stimulation during NREM sleep, compared to wakefulness, in several brain regions. Interestingly, the response to the subject's own name presented in NREM sleep showed relatively greater activation, compared to a beep sound, in the left amygdala and left prefrontal cortex, suggesting that "higher" sensory processing is still occurring to some extent during sleep. Early studies also showed evidence of sensory responsiveness in N1 and N2 sleep during an auditory task, although performance accuracy sharply declined in the latter [31].

In some studies, further details were available such as activity changes specific to N2 compared to other NREM stages, and correlations between hypothalamic and cortical BOLD signal [32]. Spindles recorded by scalp EEG were associated with increased BOLD signal in the thalamus, and the anterior cingulate, insular, and superior temporal cortices [33]. This was the case for both fast (13-15 Hz) and slow (11-13 Hz) spindles. Using an "event-related" design, in which fMRI activity could be linked to discrete EEG slow waves, NREM sleep periods dominated by slow waves (<4 Hz) were shown to exhibit greater BOLD signal compared to lighter NREM sleep (mainly N2 but also N1) [34]. These differences were seen in the inferior frontal, medial prefrontal, precuneus, and posterior cingulate cortices. This finding is interesting because of recent interest in the cortical firing and plasticity potential associated with the oscillations between 'up' and 'down' states [15, 19, 35]. The idea that synaptic downscaling occurs during slow wave sleep to help consolidate waking experiences from the prior day as well as to "make room" for subsequent waking experiences, remains an intriguing possibility that is accumulating evidence [15-16, 19, 36-37].

THE DEFAULT NETWORK IN SLEEP

With the discovery that the "resting" awake brain demonstrates correlated BOLD signal in specific brain regions, which subsequently breaks down with attention to a task, there has been an explosion of studies investigating this so-called "default" brain network. The main regions associated with resting wakefulness are the posterior parietal / precuneus region (PCC), medial prefrontal cortex, and lateral parietal regions [38].

Larson-Prior *et al.* used a combination of 64-lead EEG and fMRI to investigate the BOLD signal patterns associated with sleep in 5 healthy subjects [39]. NREM sleep was obtained for short periods (under 40 minutes) in 5 of 10 subjects attempting to sleep in the scanner. The "light sleep" analyzed in that study was defined as at least 15 minutes of clear N2 sleep; REM was not obtained. Six networks were analyzed from the fMRI data: three primary sensory networks (visual, auditory, and sensory-motor), and three higher networks: the "default" network, the "dorsal attention" network, and the "executive control" network. Given the extensive literature associating the default, attention, and executive networks with various waking (conscious) experiences/tasks, one might expect the descent from wake into sleep to involve alteration or dissolution of these coherent networks, which has been directly suggested by transcranial magnetic stimulation data [22]. Surprisingly however, this study demonstrated the opposite: not only were the sensory networks preserved, but all three higher cognitive networks were unchanged during stage N2 sleep in these subjects. In fact, the attention network actually showed increased BOLD fMRI activity. Like prior studies [40-41], the variance in BOLD signal was greater in NREM sleep compared to wakefulness in all brain regions – although this difference was not statistically significant.

Previous reports had in fact shown persistence of default network activity in light NREM sleep in humans [41]. Interestingly, sensory and default network connectivity has also been shown using fMRI to persist with anesthesia in primates and sedation in humans [42-43]. Possible explanations for this interesting persistence of networks during NREM sleep include one or more of the following: 1) effects on network dynamics were too small to detect with small sample sizes; 2) BOLD activity in these networks is not sufficient itself to provide conscious waking experience; and/or 3) maintaining network correlations during sleep is actually important for memory or other restorative functions. One intriguing alternative relates to the observation that sleep defined by EEG criteria is not always perceived as sleep by subjective report, especially in certain forms of insomnia [44], and sensory processing clearly persists into sleep [31]. Although the authors do not report the subjective sleep perception in these participants, it is possible that light or fragmented sleep in the scanner is perceived as wake or some drowsy intermediate state. If so, could this perception (or in fact misperception) be attributed in part to the persistence of wake-like network correlations amidst otherwise sleep-like EEG patterns?

Patients with epilepsy undergoing invasive monitoring during pre-surgical evaluation offer an important opportunity to measure sleep-related neuronal activity directly – with the obvious caveats of the baseline epilepsy syndrome, the use of anticonvulsant medications, and that the subjects have just undergone neurosurgery. For example, such intracranial recordings facilitated a detailed investigation of the relationship of K-complexes to cortical firing patterns, indicating that this phenomenon represented a cortical down-state [45].

Comparison of ECoG and fMRI were undertaken in five such patients by He *et al.* [46]. fMRI sequences during a visual fixation task were obtained either before or after implantation of ECoG electrodes placed for epilepsy monitoring purposes. These electrodes, which spanned sensory-motor networks, allowed collection of data across all sleep-wake stages (scoring was accomplished *via* ECoG, EOG, and video monitoring). Cortical electrodes overlying epileptic tissue were discarded from the analysis. By comparing correlations in ECoG signals obtained in wake, REM sleep and NREM sleep (N3) with correlations in BOLD fMRI signals obtained during the visual fixation task, they concluded that similar patterns occurred across arousal states. However, as the authors point out, it is important to note that BOLD fMRI fluctuations have been attributed to neuronal as well as non-neuronal factors in the literature [47-50].

FUNCTIONAL CONNECTIVITY NETWORKS IN SLEEP

The landmark 1998 publication by Watts and Strogatz [51] on small world networks sparked an explosion in research documenting the occurrence of this network structure in numerous fields of study. Brain anatomy and physiology proved to be particularly fertile ground for such endeavors (see Chapters 1 and 2). Theoretical work discussed in other chapters supports the general idea that small world network patterns represent an efficient solution to the problem of maintaining local connectivity while allowing long-range communication between portions of the network (see Chapter 2). Network analysis draws from graph theory, and can apply to anatomy (tractography, for example), or physiology ("functional" connectivity between sensors). Comparison is often drawn between small world network architecture and another pervasive connectivity pattern seen in the biological, physical, and social sciences: the scale free network. In the scale free setting, there are relatively few hubs (heavily connected nodes in the network), while there are a large number of nodes with few connections. Network properties such as stability, resilience to perturbation, information transfer speed, and synchronization capacity are influenced by connectivity [52]. It is generally thought that although anatomical connections constrain possible functional dynamics, the functional dynamics can in fact influence anatomical connections through plasticity [53-55].

One recent study used connectivity models based on anatomical data to suggest that the circuitry pattern of the reticular formation resembled a small world, not scale free, network [56]. Although the application of graph theory to sleep physiology remains in its infancy, recent studies have used functional connectivity metrics of surface EEG to compare network dynamics across different arousal states. Ferri *et al.* [57-58] used routine 19 channel surface EEG in 10 healthy adult subjects to record during quiet wakefulness as well as sleep. Like other studies of this type, EEG electrode contact sites are considered nodes in a graphical network. In addition, they investigated possible relationships with the cyclic alternating pattern (CAP), a visual scoring metric applied to NREM sleep [59-60]. NREM sleep can be visually divided into relatively quiescent periods (CAP-B) interrupted by transient events in the 0.5-2.5Hz range. Correlated activity between all possible pairs of electrodes was investigated in different frequency bands, corresponding to delta, theta, alpha, and sigma. The correlated activity demonstrated small world network characteristics during wakefulness, with increase in one small world measure, the clustering coefficient, during sleep. When different frequency bands were analyzed, small world connectivity was seen in bands below 15Hz. Those portions of NREM sleep exhibiting CAP-A (the active component of CAP) showed increased small world character. The interpretation of these changes remains speculative. The prevailing view that sleep is accompanied by breakdown of network correlations [22, 61], and therefore loss of conscious awareness, is difficult to reconcile with the persistence (and indeed strengthening) of small world correlations by Ferri *et al*. In addition, the idea of breakdown of cortical connectivity in sleep contrasts with other studies demonstrating persistence of network activity in sleep and anesthesia, as described above.

Other studies have used correlation metrics based on neuronal firing patterns to understand network dynamics during sleep. Dimitriadis *et al*. [62] studied the correlations in 12-channel surface EEG in 10 healthy young adult males during wakefulness and a full night of sleep (all stages represented). Choosing only segments of at least 8 consecutive minutes of a given stage, their methods allowed connections between nodes to be assigned a weight. Functional clusters within these graphical networks were also defined, which exhibited left-right and anterior-posterior asymmetries in a sleep-wake state-dependent manner. REM sleep showed more prominent coupling anteriorly than posteriorly, while the reverse asymmetry was noted in NREM sleep. REM sleep also showed more coupling in the right hemisphere compared to the left, while coupling in NREM sleep showed the opposite pattern. Again, while the physiological (and pathophysiological) implications of these findings remain uncertain, these measurements of network dynamics may evolve into useful biomarkers for sleep physiology in health and disease as they gain broader application.

EMERGING APPROACHES TO QUANTIFY SLEEP ARCHITECTURE: STATE TRANSITION MODELS

The often observed "disconnect" between objective and subjective data represents an ongoing challenge in clinical sleep medicine: many patients report non-refreshing sleep in the absence of significant obstructive sleep apnea (OSA) or other identifiable causes of sleep disruption (narcolepsy, periodic limb movements), and many patients with severe apnea function quite well during the day. One potential contributor to daytime symptoms involves fragmentation of sleep architecture [63-64]. Metrics of sleep architecture routinely used in a clinical setting include percentage of time in bed that is actually spent sleeping (sleep efficiency) and percentage of sleep time spent in each sleep sub-stage: REM sleep and NREM sleep stages (N1, N2, N3). However, summary percentages are insensitive to fragmentation of sleep architecture, which may be a critical feature of disturbed and/or non-refreshing sleep. For example, consider two patients that exhibit the same total sleep time, and the same 90% sleep efficiency, but one spends 30 minutes falling asleep (then sleeps without interruption), while the other experiences 30 one-minute long waking bouts scattered throughout the night. The two scenarios feature quite different degrees of fragmentation, but this distinction is invisible to sleep efficiency percentage (and potentially even sleep stage percentages). The term "efficiency" may thus be considered something of a misnomer, since a raw assessment of total sleep time arguably provides little insight into sleep continuity. Surrogate measures for fragmentation exist, such as the frequency of arousals and percentage of time spent in light (N1) sleep. Arousals can be sub-divided into "spontaneous" versus those evoked by respiratory events or leg movements, and they are by definition brief (seconds) and thus do not warrant scoring a stage shift to "wake" according to conventional clinical scoring criteria.

To address this potentially important issue, several groups have investigated sleep architecture in terms of stage transitions, thereby incorporating the temporal dynamics rather than simply the percentage of time one spends in any given state. Compelling evidence supporting the critical need for such analysis stems from the work of Swihart *et al*. [65], who investigated the sleep architecture of patients with severe OSA in comparison with matched controls. There were no differences in sleep architecture by routine PSG metrics (total sleep time, sleep efficiency, or percentage of any sub-stage of sleep). However, there were obvious differences in sleep stage transition probability, which captures the fragmentation that clearly accompanies severe OSA. We and others have used the similar approach of survival curve analysis of stage transition statistics to characterize sleep-wake transitions in normal versus sleep apnea patients [66-67], as well as in pain/fatigue syndromes [68-69]. Markov chain models (with either constant or time-varying transition probabilities) have been proposed, as have general transition probability matrix approaches [70-73].

The power of classical Markov modeling, used with great success in describing state transitions at the molecular level [74-76], may be harnessed for quantitative characterization of state transition patterns comprising sleep architecture in health and disease [70-72]. Several statistical properties of sleep-wake transitions, necessary to justify the use of Markov modeling, have already been suggested in the literature. For example, human and rodent sleep-wake behavior demonstrates exponential distribution of sleep bout duration [77-79], with species specific time constants [77]. Whether wake distributions reflect power law (i.e., not a traditional Markov process) or exponential patterns is debated [67, 79-80]. Further assumptions of a Markov state model include mutually exclusive state occupancy. Finally, although Markov processes are memory-less, certain aspects of sleep are clearly history-dependent: the concept of sleep homeostasis is that prior sleep-wake history changes the probability of sleep onset, as well as the architecture of recovery sleep.

The concept of discrete sleep states may be an oversimplification, at least in the sense that transitional or intermediate states may exist, or that sleep itself is a continuum of depths/stages. State space analysis may prove useful in this regard: spectral analysis of the EEG measured in small time windows may reveal additional dynamics compared to standard "epoch" scoring criteria. Although data in this domain are limited, one recent study used a form of state space analysis as a metric for unstable state transitions seen in mice deficient in orexin that are considered a model for narcolepsy [81]. Increased transitions between sleep and wake have been demonstrated in narcolepsy studies, and the state space method may be a marker for sleep-wake state instability. Whether this method reflects more fundamental information about the underlying physiology awaits further study.

EMERGING APPROACHES TO QUANTIFY SLEEP ARCHITECTURE: QUANTITATIVE PHYSIOLOGICAL MODELS

The last decade has seen massive advances in the identification and understanding of the brainstem and hypothalamic nuclei involved in regulating the sleep/wake state of the brain as a whole [82]. During wake, monoaminergic nuclei (including the norepinephrinergic locus coeruleus, the serotonergic dorsal raphé, and the histaminergic tuberomammillary nuclei) are active, promoting cortical activation *via* diffuse ascending projections [83]. During sleep, a hypothalamic region called the ventrolateral preoptic area (VLPO) is active, and GABAergically inhibits the wake-promoting nuclei. Mutual inhibition between these sleep-promoting and wake-promoting regions has been proposed as the basis for switch-like behavior: each group indirectly reinforces its own activity by inhibiting the other, resulting in only one group being active at a time [84].

Alternation between sleep and wake is effected by circadian and homeostatic drives to the sleep-wake switch. The suprachiasmatic nucleus projects a signal to the VLPO, primarily *via* the dorsomedial hypothalamus (DMH) [82]. The physiological basis for the homeostatic drive is less clear, but site-specific accumulation of adenosine in the basal forebrain during wake appears to play an important role, with both direct and indirect effects on the VLPO [83, 85].

Mathematical models of this circuit provide a potentially powerful means of understanding overt behavior in both healthy and pathological phenotypes in terms of the underlying physiology. This may prove critical for improving diagnosis, prognosis, and treatment approaches to human disorders that fragment sleep. In the last few years, several state-space models have been proposed, which can be broadly classified into 2 classes: mean field models, and limit cycle models. Mean field models utilize population state variables by averaging across neuronal properties such as cell body voltages and firing rates, and have been widely used in cortico-thalamic models since the 1970s [86-88]. Mean field models of the sleep-wake switch have reproduced several basic features of wake and sleep in both humans [89-91] and other mammalian species [92]. However, in the absence of noisy input these models are deterministic, and thus do not reproduce the fine timescale of sleep architecture seen in human polysomnography.

Other physiological models have been developed using networks of single neuron limit cycle models, which generate spontaneous oscillations between wake and the stages of sleep [93-94]. These models have been shown to accurately reproduce the raw probabilities of different sleep stages in rodents, but not the power law or exponential statistical distributions for bout lengths [95].

Incorporating the effects of stochastic inputs to both of these model classes will likely improve our understanding of how sleep/wake transition statistics are generated. Using modeling in parallel with state-space analysis of EEG activity during sleep/wake [81] could prove to be a powerful approach. However, it is important to bear in mind that sleep, like many neural phenomena, is a multi-scale process regulated at many levels of the brain, and while mechanisms at the level of the brainstem and hypothalamus are integral to sleep/wake regulation, it is not yet clear what their level of involvement is in very brief arousals. It is possible that different timescale dynamics are hierarchically regulated, with micro-sleeps and micro-arousals being a primarily cortical phenomenon, and feasibly even a local rather than global phenomenon [7, 24]. Integrating models of the higher brain with models of the sleep-wake switch is thus an important future research direction.

EMERGING APPROACHES TO QUANTIFY SLEEP ARCHITECTURE: ECG-DERIVED SPECTROGRAM

Although automated staging has been used, and in some cases is based on minimal biological signal streams [96-101], common clinical and research practice recommends multiple signals (including EEG, EMG, and EOG) as the gold standard for sleep staging. The balance between the time and equipment requirements of laboratory settings and the portability and automation of analysis of home monitors is a consideration relevant for clinical and research endeavors alike. One alternative method of assessing autonomic physiology is through analysis of heart rate variability (HRV). The ease of obtaining a high signal-to-noise ratio makes ECG an ideal candidate for analysis in clinical settings or for extended ambulatory monitoring. HRV may be altered in certain disease states, and certain patterns have been associated with increased risk of cardiovascular mortality [102]. HRV has also been assessed in sleep, and in particular with regard to the impact of aging [103-106].

A related metric that has been proposed as a marker of sleep "stability" involves a novel ECG-derived "cardio-pulmonary coupling" (CPC) metric, using only a single ECG lead [64, 99]. This method uses Fourier analysis to extract the dominant frequencies of fluctuations in R-R interval and QRS amplitudes that occur with respiration. The ECG-spectrogram is based on the physiological principle of cardio-pulmonary coupling, involving two features of the ECG: heart rate variability (reflecting autonomic fluctuations coupling heart rate to respiration), and QRS-wave amplitude fluctuations (due to changes in the distance between the heart and the surface electrode with respiration). The fundamental concept underlying ECG-derived CPC involves state-specific breathing patterns. Because respiration varies with sleep stage, and with sleep apnea, the CPC spectrogram represents a bio-marker for both sleep architecture and sleep disordered breathing. In normal NREM sleep, the spectrogram is dominated by the frequency of normal quiet respiration ("high frequency coupling", HFC; 0.1-0.4 Hz). A subset of NREM sleep (usually N1, portions of N2, and regions of rapid transition between N1, N2 and wake) is considered "unstable" by this metric, which captures the somewhat less regular breathing pattern ("low frequency coupling", LFC; 0.01-0.1 Hz). LFC is observed in healthy individuals without OSA, but the presence of such oscillations is increased in those with OSA (and has been termed elevated low frequency coupling, or eLFC). Wake and REM sleep involve irregular breathing, and are characterized by very low frequency coupling (vLFC; ~0-0.01 Hz). Finally, sleep disordered breathing produces characteristic disruptions in respiration (depending on whether the cause is obstructive, central, or a combination), generating "elevated low frequency coupling" (eLFC, ~0.05 Hz; LFC). Several studies have demonstrated important clinical correlates of the ECG-spectrogram method [64, 99, 107-108]. Two major advantages of this analysis approach are 1) the spectrogram can be calculated from any single lead ECG, such as those obtained for other reasons in various clinical cohorts, and 2) the ECG is relatively easy to measure in the home setting compared to other sleep assessment tools.

AUTONOMIC MEASUREMENTS OF SLEEP PHYSIOLOGY

Recent advances in home sleep monitoring include a device that utilizes the peripheral sympathetic tone in the staging of sleep. The WatchPAT device (Itamar), uses an algorithm that begins with actigraphy measurements to discriminate wake versus sleep, and then, within sleep, uses complex feature analysis algorithms to distinguish REM, light NREM (N1 and N2) and deep NREM (N3) sleep [109-112]. This device is considered a Type IV device according to the Center for Medicare and Medicaid Services guidelines for clinical sleep studies. The sleep staging algorithm does have certain limitations as described in the literature, including a bias against brief transitions, and a bias towards REM detection during certain time intervals (for example, the algorithm does not consider REM sleep as a possibility within the first 60 minutes of sleep onset). Finally, the measurements of autonomic tone and heart rate variability may be compromised in populations with impaired autonomic nervous system function, such as those with peripheral neuropathy, peripheral vascular disease, atrial fibrillation, or diabetes, for example. Also, the impact of medications active on the autonomic nervous system may confound evaluation of sleep by this device.

COMPUTATIONAL APPROACHES TO ACTIGRAPHY DATA

Actigraphy is typically used to track rest-activity patterns to investigate circadian rhythm disorders [113-115], or to verify activity in the days before a multiple sleep latency test is conducted to investigate narcolepsy (because circadian phase delay can potentially result in falsely "positive" sleep-onset REM periods in morning naps). Actigraphy involves wearing a watch-like device, usually on the wrist (but it can be worn on the leg to track leg movements associated with restless legs syndrome or periodic limb movements of sleep). The device contains an accelerometer that detects movements, and may also contain a light meter and an event button. There are several algorithms employed to analyze the resulting data, including zero-crossings, thresholds, and integrals of (typically 1-minute duration) binned activity measurements. Studies on the clinical use of actigraphy have been reviewed elsewhere [113].

A more sophisticated analytical approach was recently proposed for actigraphy data, which focuses on the variability in the data over different time scales. The technique, called de-trended fluctuation analysis (DFA) [116-117], was applied to mouse and human activity measures, with the goal of understanding correlations over different time scales in the variance or fluctuations in the data. Briefly, the technique involves a sequence of analytical steps designed to 1) remove the global mean, 2) "de-trend" the data in time windows of various lengths (through polynomial fitting), and 3) measuring the root mean square variance in the residual values after this subtraction and de-trending. This analysis distinguishes external variations in activity (such as those arising from social scheduling) from inherent or intrinsic sources of variation (such as might arise from central regulation nodes such as the suprachiasmatic nucleus (SCN)). External stimulation or activities are presumed to have only local effects from a temporal standpoint – there is no reason to think that, say, riding a bike would introduce correlations with activity hours before or after the event. Short-term correlations would therefore predominate, and would not manifest on longer time scales. In contrast, inherent fluctuations in behavioral control (potentially of central origin or influence, such as from the SCN) are presumed to emanate from brain circuit behavior, which may be expected to demonstrate correlations over diverse time scales.

Hu *et al.* [118-120] showed that fluctuations in activity levels exhibited scale free (or scale invariant) correlations, and that the correlations were independent of light-dark cycle, absolute differences in activity levels, scheduled activities, or naps. The correlations spanned a wide range of time scales, from minutes to 24 hours, consistent with the idea of scale-invariance. The scaling exponent, interestingly, was similar between rats and humans. This led the investigators to test the hypothesis that the SCN was important in the control of activity fluctuations (not simply activity levels). Rats harboring SCN lesions had abolished correlations on time scales greater than 4 hours.

This technique was then applied to analyzing actigraphy data obtained from patients with Alzheimer's disease (AD). Compared to matched controls, dementia was associated with alterations in the scale-free correlations obtained from DFA of the actigraphy data. Independent of differences in baseline activity levels between individuals and between clinical groups, the authors found a significant "breakdown" of scale-free correlations in activity, as indicated by a decrease in the scaling exponent of the power law function used to fit such scale-free processes. Thus, a single parameter, the scaling exponent, was significantly altered in patients with dementia. Importantly, this effect can be seen at the level of the individual patient (as well as the combined group data). The breakdown in correlations was intermediate compared to the total loss of correlated activity seen in complete lesions of the SCN in rats. This suggests that changes in the scaling exponent may reflect the degree of degeneration of the SCN associated with degenerative diseases such as AD [121-122].

DFA of actigraphy data is a promising approach to clinical disorders for several reasons, including that actigraphy is non-invasive, can be used in patients with cognitive impairment (it requires minimal user interaction), and measurements reflect the natural activity fluctuations over time whether in the home or in a facility setting. In addition to providing standard information about sleep-wake patterns and circadian dysregulation, DFA of actigraphy fluctuations may provide an important objective biomarker with diagnostic or prognostic utility in disorders of brain function. As a potential marker of SCN integrity, it may be useful for individualizing therapy designed to optimize circadian rhythms. Interestingly, disruption of rest-activity cycles preceded cognitive impairments in a mouse model of Huntington's Disease, and correction of this irregularity with pharmacologically enforced rhythms delays the onset of neurological dysfunction [123].

CLINICAL IMPLICATIONS

In addition to the value of improving our understanding of normal sleep physiology, studies of sleep physiology and staging architecture has specific relevance to patient care as tools to improve phenotyping of sleep pathology in a diversity of clinical circumstances. For example, risk stratification, prognosis, and medication responses can potentially be improved through more objective and detailed diagnostic descriptions. As has been found in other fields, understanding individual differences or sub-populations (such as genetic markers of chemotherapeutic sensitivity in cancer) can greatly enhance personalized management decisions. It is possible, for example, that heterogeneity within populations of insomnia patients may dilute clinical associations and/or medication effects in research studies. The seemingly complex and variable manifestations of "fragmented" sleep architecture that accompany disease states such as sleep disordered breathing may in fact possess underlying patterns of architecture, which may correlate with clinically relevant endpoints (hypertension, sleepiness, cognitive impairment). Phenotyping also holds promise for rapid clinical translation as small wearable technologies improve the capacity to measure sleep in the home setting, over time, with minimal disruption to the patient. In many neurological diseases, fluctuations in symptoms or daytime function may be linked to fluctuations in sleep quality and/or quantity. PSG offers little utility for evaluating such "real life" fluctuations since it is typically recorded on only one night in laboratory conditions.

Longitudinal data acquisition will thus help address important deficits in our understanding of variability of sleep quality, quantity and timing in health and disease (outside of the controlled settings of research laboratory settings). For example, subjective and objective measures of sleep may be altered by fluctuations in pain or mood, each of which may vary in a given patient over time and with treatment or relapses. Understanding sleep in the habitual routine of a given patient is currently cumbersome (often involving sleep diaries) and is vulnerable to the phenomenon of sleep-state misperception in which patients typically underestimate sleep and overestimate wakefulness when self-reporting their sleep complaints [124]. The discrepancies between subjective and objective assessments of sleep may itself contain important clinical information [125].

METHODOLOGICAL AND PRACTICAL CONSIDERATIONS

Anecdotal reports by many patients undergoing diagnostic PSG in the laboratory suggest that the act of recording sleep in this setting may in fact be disruptive of sleep (or at least its subjective perception by the individual). Whether "normal" sleep can be obtained during similarly (or even more) un-natural conditions such as recordings requiring special scanners, head or body restraint, and/or extensive scalp sensors, is therefore a major concern. Even if laboratory sleep is found to be similar to home sleep under certain conditions, many of these methods are limited to only one or a few nights of sleep per individual (due to cost, comfort, or other practical issues). Given the numerous intrinsic, behavioral, and extrinsic factors influencing sleep that fluctuate from night to night, evidence from laboratory studies should be interpreted with caution. The major tool for longitudinal home sleep monitoring is wrist actigraphy [113], which estimates sleep versus wake based on limb movement and therefore provides no explicit information about individual sleep stages. The distinction between sleep and wake by actigraphy has variable accuracy, and depends on the patient population and analysis algorithm [113]. Despite widespread research use, these limitations may restrict clinical utility to studies of circadian rhythm disorders (which are often fairly evident by history alone, but may need to be confirmed objectively).

The relationship of neural activity to the BOLD fMRI signal continues to be debated, although much progress is being made in this arena [126]. At the most basic level, there are several steps separating neuronal activity from hemoglobin oxygenation. In neurology and psychiatry, it may be particularly important to consider factors that alter neurovascular coupling, such as atherosclerosis of cervical and/or intracranial vessels, medications, age, and/or the underlying disease process. Also, the baseline partial pressure of oxygen in the blood may impact the degree to which a given level of neuronal activity is predicted to alter the hemoglobin oxygenation percentage. The classic hemoglobin-oxygen sigmoidal curve is quite flat at "healthy" levels of oxygen partial pressure, and thus it is possible that subjects with higher baseline oxygen partial pressures would require more neuronal activity to produce a measurable decrease in hemoglobin oxygen saturation. Cardiopulmonary dynamics change in sleep (and within sleep, differently in REM versus NREM stages), raising a further possibility that oxyhemoglobin saturation as a measure of changes in neural activity may differ with arousal state. Studies involving an intervention such as transcranial magnetic stimulation (see Chapter 8) during sleep to strengthen or disrupt certain networks hold promise for raising these otherwise correlation-based studies to the level of causation.

CONCLUSIONS

Human sleep represents an important yet challenging frontier for both research and clinical investigations. Sleep disruption can be the cause or the result (and possibly both in a vicious cycle) of various diseases spanning neurology, psychiatry, and general medicine. The very act of measuring sleep may itself induce disruption, especially in the individual who already reports poor sleep. Despite these caveats, sleep represents a field rich with multi-channel physiology, and it is hoped that advanced analytical tools will provide insight into normal and pathological sleep by integrating information across multiple physiological arenas spanning EEG, autonomic fluctuations, arousals, circadian rhythms, and sleep homeostasis.

REFERENCES

[1] Fuller PM, Gooley JJ, Saper CB. Neurobiology of the sleep-wake cycle: sleep architecture, circadian regulation, and regulatory feedback. J Biol Rhythms 2006; 21(6): 482-93.
[2] Espana RA, Scammell TE. Sleep neurobiology for the clinician. Sleep 2004; 27(4): 811-20.
[3] Tononi G, Cirelli C. Sleep and synaptic homeostasis: a hypothesis. Brain Res Bull 2003; 62(2): 143-50.
[4] Siegel JM. Sleep viewed as a state of adaptive inactivity. Nat Rev Neurosci 2009 10(10): 747-53.
[5] Kolokotrones T, Van S, Deeds EJ, Fontana W. Curvature in metabolic scaling. Nature 2010; 464(7289): 753-6.
[6] Ohayon MM. From wakefulness to excessive sleepiness: what we know and still need to know. Sleep Med Rev 2008; 12(2): 129-41.
[7] Vassalli A, Dijk DJ. Sleep function: current questions and new approaches. Eur J Neurosci 2009; 29(9): 1830-41.
[8] Dang-Vu TT, Desseilles M, Petit D, Mazza S, Montplaisir J, Maquet P. Neuroimaging in sleep medicine. Sleep Med 2007; 8(4): 349-72.
[9] Desseilles M, Dang-Vu T, Schabus M, Sterpenich V, Maquet P, Schwartz S. Neuroimaging insights into the pathophysiology of sleep disorders. Sleep 2008; 31(6): 777-94.
[10] Bonnet MH, Arand DL. Hyperarousal and insomnia. Sleep Med Rev 1997; 1(2): 97-108.
[11] Perlis ML, Merica H, Smith MT, Giles DE. Beta EEG activity and insomnia. Sleep Med Rev 2001; 5(5): 363-74.
[12] Perlis ML, Smith MT, Andrews PJ, Orff H, Giles DE. Beta/Gamma EEG activity in patients with primary and secondary insomnia and good sleeper controls. Sleep 2001; 24(1): 110-7.
[13] Nofzinger EA, Buysse DJ, Germain A, Price JC, Miewald JM, Kupfer DJ. Functional neuroimaging evidence for hyperarousal in insomnia. Am J Psychiatry 2004; 161(11): 2126-8.
[14] Smith MT, Perlis ML, Chengazi VU, et al. Neuroimaging of NREM sleep in primary insomnia: a Tc-99-HMPAO single photon emission computed tomography study. Sleep 2002; 25(3): 325-35.
[15] Tononi G. Slow wave homeostasis and synaptic plasticity. J Clin Sleep Med 2009; 5(2 Suppl): S16-9.
[16] Tononi G, Cirelli C. Sleep function and synaptic homeostasis. Sleep Med Rev 2006; 10(1): 49-62.
[17] Achermann P, Borbely AA. Mathematical models of sleep regulation. Front Biosci 2003; 8: s683-93.
[18] Linkowski P, Spiegel K, Kerkhofs M, et al. Genetic and environmental influences on prolactin secretion during wake and during sleep. Am J Physiol 1998; 274(5 Pt 1): E909-19.
[19] Vyazovskiy VV, Olcese U, Lazimy YM, et al. Cortical firing and sleep homeostasis. Neuron 2009; 63(6): 865-78.
[20] Destexhe A, Hughes SW, Rudolph M, Crunelli V. Are corticothalamic 'up' states fragments of wakefulness? Trends Neurosci 2007; 30(7): 334-42.
[21] Holcman D, Tsodyks M. The emergence of Up and Down states in cortical networks. PLoS Comput Biol 2006; 2(3): e23.
[22] Massimini M, Ferrarelli F, Huber R, Esser SK, Singh H, Tononi G. Breakdown of cortical effective connectivity during sleep. Science 2005; 309(5744): 2228-32.
[23] Massimini M, Ferrarelli F, Esser SK, et al. Triggering sleep slow waves by transcranial magnetic stimulation. Proc Natl Acad Sci USA 2007; 104(20): 8496-501.
[24] Huber R, Ghilardi MF, Massimini M, Tononi G. Local sleep and learning. Nature 2004; 430(6995): 78-81.
[25] Huber R, Ghilardi MF, Massimini M, et al. Arm immobilization causes cortical plastic changes and locally decreases sleep slow wave activity. Nat Neurosci 2006; 9(9): 1169-76.
[26] Marshall L, Helgadottir H, Molle M, Born J. Boosting slow oscillations during sleep potentiates memory. Nature 2006; 444(7119): 610-3.
[27] Maquet P. Functional neuroimaging of normal human sleep by positron emission tomography. J Sleep Res 2000; 9(3): 207-31.
[28] Lovblad KO, Thomas R, Jakob PM, et al. Silent functional magnetic resonance imaging demonstrates focal activation in rapid eye movement sleep. Neurology 1999; 53(9): 2193-5.
[29] Portas CM, Krakow K, Allen P, Josephs O, Armony JL, Frith CD. Auditory processing across the sleep-wake cycle: simultaneous EEG and fMRI monitoring in humans. Neuron 2000; 28(3): 991-9.
[30] Czisch M, Wetter TC, Kaufmann C, Pollmacher T, Holsboer F, Auer DP. Altered processing of acoustic stimuli during sleep: reduced auditory activation and visual deactivation detected by a combined fMRI/EEG study. Neuroimage 2002; 16(1): 251-8.
[31] Ogilvie RD, Wilkinson RT. The detection of sleep onset: behavioral and physiological convergence. Psychophysiology 1984; 21(5): 510-20.
[32] Kaufmann C, Wehrle R, Wetter TC, et al. Brain activation and hypothalamic functional connectivity during human non-rapid eye movement sleep: an EEG/fMRI study. Brain 2006; 129(Pt 3): 655-67.

[33]   Schabus M, Dang-Vu TT, Albouy G, *et al.* Hemodynamic cerebral correlates of sleep spindles during human non-rapid eye movement sleep. Proc Natl Acad Sci USA 2007; 104(32): 13164-9.

[34]   Dang-Vu TT, Schabus M, Desseilles M, *et al.* Spontaneous neural activity during human slow wave sleep. Proc Natl Acad Sci USA 2008; 105(39): 15160-5.

[35]   Massimini M, Tononi G, Huber R. Slow waves, synaptic plasticity and information processing: insights from transcranial magnetic stimulation and high-density EEG experiments. Eur J Neurosci 2009; 29(9): 1761-70.

[36]   Liu ZW, Faraguna U, Cirelli C, Tononi G, Gao XB. Direct evidence for wake-related increases and sleep-related decreases in synaptic strength in rodent cortex. J Neurosci 2010; 30(25): 8671-5.

[37]   Gilestro GF, Tononi G, Cirelli C. Widespread changes in synaptic markers as a function of sleep and wakefulness in Drosophila. Science 2009; 324(5923): 109-12.

[38]   Buckner RL, Andrews-Hanna JR, Schacter DL. The brain's default network: anatomy, function, and relevance to disease. Ann N Y Acad Sci 2008; 1124: 1-38.

[39]   Larson-Prior LJ, Zempel JM, Nolan TS, Prior FW, Snyder AZ, Raichle ME. Cortical network functional connectivity in the descent to sleep. Proc Natl Acad Sci USA 2009; 106(11): 4489-94.

[40]   Fukunaga M, Horovitz SG, van Gelderen P, *et al.* Large-amplitude, spatially correlated fluctuations in BOLD fMRI signals during extended rest and early sleep stages. Magn Reson Imaging 2006; 24(8): 979-92.

[41]   Horovitz SG, Fukunaga M, de Zwart JA, *et al.* Low frequency BOLD fluctuations during resting wakefulness and light sleep: a simultaneous EEG-fMRI study. Hum Brain Mapp 2008; 29(6): 671-82.

[42]   Greicius MD, Kiviniemi V, Tervonen O, *et al.* Persistent default-mode network connectivity during light sedation. Hum Brain Mapp 2008; 29(7): 839-47.

[43]   Vincent JL, Patel GH, Fox MD, *et al.* Intrinsic functional architecture in the anaesthetized monkey brain. Nature 2007; 447(7140): 83-6.

[44]   Edinger JD, Krystal AD. Subtyping primary insomnia: is sleep state misperception a distinct clinical entity? Sleep Med Rev 2003; 7(3): 203-14.

[45]   Cash SS, Halgren E, Dehghani N, *et al.* The human K-complex represents an isolated cortical down-state. Science 2009; 324(5930): 1084-7.

[46]   He BJ, Snyder AZ, Zempel JM, Smyth MD, Raichle ME. Electrophysiological correlates of the brain's intrinsic large-scale functional architecture. Proc Natl Acad Sci USA 2008; 105(41): 16039-44.

[47]   Shmueli K, van Gelderen P, de Zwart JA, *et al.* Low-frequency fluctuations in the cardiac rate as a source of variance in the resting-state fMRI BOLD signal. Neuroimage 2007; 38(2): 306-20.

[48]   Birn RM, Diamond JB, Smith MA, Bandettini PA. Separating respiratory-variation-related fluctuations from neuronal-activity-related fluctuations in fMRI. Neuroimage 2006; 31(4): 1536-48.

[49]   Wise RG, Ide K, Poulin MJ, Tracey I. Resting fluctuations in arterial carbon dioxide induce significant low frequency variations in BOLD signal. Neuroimage 2004; 21(4): 1652-64.

[50]   Kleinfeld D, Mitra PP, Helmchen F, Denk W. Fluctuations and stimulus-induced changes in blood flow observed in individual capillaries in layers 2 through 4 of rat neocortex. Proc Natl Acad Sci USA 1998; 95(26): 15741-6.

[51]   Watts DJ, Strogatz SH. Collective dynamics of 'small-world' networks. Nature 1998; 393(6684): 440-2.

[52]   Li C, Chen G. Stability of a neural network model with small-world connections. Phys Rev E Stat Nonlin Soft Matter Phys 2003; 68(5 Pt 1): 052901.

[53]   Honey CJ, Thivierge JP, Sporns O. Can structure predict function in the human brain? Neuroimage 2010 Jan 29.

[54]   Honey CJ, Sporns O, Cammoun L, *et al.* Predicting human resting-state functional connectivity from structural connectivity. Proc Natl Acad Sci USA 2009; 106(6): 2035-40.

[55]   Honey CJ, Kotter R, Breakspear M, Sporns O. Network structure of cerebral cortex shapes functional connectivity on multiple time scales. Proc Natl Acad Sci USA 2007; 104(24): 10240-5.

[56]   Humphries MD, Gurney K, Prescott TJ. The brainstem reticular formation is a small-world, not scale-free, network. Proc Biol Sci 2006; 273(1585): 503-11.

[57]   Ferri R, Rundo F, Bruni O, Terzano MG, Stam CJ. The functional connectivity of different EEG bands moves towards small-world network organization during sleep. Clin Neurophysiol 2008; 119(9): 2026-36.

[58]   Ferri R, Rundo F, Bruni O, Terzano MG, Stam CJ. Small-world network organization of functional connectivity of EEG slow-wave activity during sleep. Clin Neurophysiol 2007; 118(2): 449-56.

[59]   Gilmartin GS, Thomas RJ. Mechanisms of arousal from sleep and their consequences. Curr Opin Pulm Med 2004; 10(6): 468-74.

[60]   Terzano MG, Parrino L. Origin and Significance of the Cyclic Alternating Pattern (CAP). REVIEW ARTICLE. Sleep Med Rev 2000; 4(1): 101-23.

[61]   Ferrarelli F, Massimini M, Sarasso S, *et al.* Breakdown in cortical effective connectivity during midazolam-induced loss of consciousness. Proc Natl Acad Sci USA 2010; 107(6): 2681-6.

[62]   Dimitriadis SI, Laskaris NA, Del Rio-Portilla Y, Koudounis G. Characterizing dynamic functional connectivity across sleep stages from EEG. Brain Topogr 2009; 22(2): 119-33.

[63]   Bonnet MH, Arand DL. Clinical effects of sleep fragmentation versus sleep deprivation. Sleep Med Rev 2003; 7(4): 297-310.

[64]   Thomas RJ. Sleep fragmentation and arousals from sleep-time scales, associations, and implications. Clin Neurophysiol 2006; 117(4): 707-11.

[65] Swihart BJ, Caffo B, Bandeen-Roche K, Punjabi NM. Characterizing sleep structure using the hypnogram. J Clin Sleep Med 2008; 4(4): 349-55.

[66] Norman RG, Scott MA, Ayappa I, Walsleben JA, Rapoport DM. Sleep continuity measured by survival curve analysis. Sleep 2006; 29(12): 1625-31.

[67] Bianchi MT, Cash SS, Mietus J, Peng CK, Thomas R. Obstructive sleep apnea alters sleep stage transition dynamics. PLoS One 2010; 5(6): e11356.

[68] Togo F, Natelson BH, Cherniack NS, FitzGibbons J, Garcon C, Rapoport DM. Sleep structure and sleepiness in chronic fatigue syndrome with or without coexisting fibromyalgia. Arthritis Res Ther 2008; 10(3): R56.

[69] Kishi A, Struzik ZR, Natelson BH, Togo F, Yamamoto Y. Dynamics of sleep stage transitions in healthy humans and patients with chronic fatigue syndrome. Am J Physiol Regul Integr Comp Physiol 2008; 294(6): R1980-7.

[70] Kemp B, Kamphuisen HA. Simulation of human hypnograms using a Markov chain model. Sleep 1986; 9(3): 405-14.

[71] Kim JW, Lee JS, Robinson PA, Jeong DU. Markov analysis of sleep dynamics. Phys Rev Lett. 2009; 102(17): 178104.

[72] Yang MC, Hursch CJ. The use of a semi-Markov model for describing sleep patterns. Biometrics 1973; 29(4): 667-76.

[73] Bianchi MT, Eiseman N, Cash S, Mietus J, Peng CK, Thomas RJ. Markov models of sleep architecture with and without sleep apnea. European Journal of Neuroscience 2010; under review.

[74] Cannon RC, D'Alessandro G. The ion channel inverse problem: neuroinformatics meets biophysics. PLoS Comput Biol 2006; 2(8): e91.

[75] McManus OB, Spivak CE, Blatz AL, Weiss DS, Magleby KL. Fractal models, Markov models, and channel kinetics. Biophys J 1989; 55(2): 383-5.

[76] VanDongen AM. Idealization and simulation of single ion channel data. Methods Enzymol 2004; 383: 229-44.

[77] Lo CC, Chou T, Penzel T, et al. Common scale-invariant patterns of sleep-wake transitions across mammalian species. Proc Natl Acad Sci USA 2004; 101(50): 17545-8.

[78] Blumberg MS, Seelke AM, Lowen SB, Karlsson KA. Dynamics of sleep-wake cyclicity in developing rats. Proc Natl Acad Sci USA 2005; 102(41): 14860-4.

[79] Joho RH, Marks GA, Espinosa F. Kv3 potassium channels control the duration of different arousal states by distinct stochastic and clock-like mechanisms. Eur J Neurosci 2006; 23(6): 1567-74.

[80] Chu-Shore J, Westover MB, Bianchi MT. Power law versus exponential state transition dynamics: Application to sleep-wake architecture. PLoS One 2010; under revision.

[81] Diniz Behn CG, Klerman EB, Mochizuki T, Lin SC, Scammell TE. Abnormal sleep/wake dynamics in orexin knockout mice. Sleep 2010; 33(3): 297-306.

[82] Saper CB, Scammell TE, Lu J. Hypothalamic regulation of sleep and circadian rhythms. Nature 2005; 437(7063): 1257-63.

[83] Pace-Schott EF, Hobson JA. The neurobiology of sleep: genetics, cellular physiology and subcortical networks. Nat Rev Neurosci 2002; 3(8): 591-605.

[84] Saper CB, Chou TC, Scammell TE. The sleep switch: hypothalamic control of sleep and wakefulness. Trends Neurosci 2001; 24(12): 726-31.

[85] Porkka-Heiskanen T, Alanko L, Kalinchuk A, Stenberg D. Adenosine and sleep. Sleep Med Rev 2002; 6(4): 321-32.

[86] Wilson HR, Cowan JD. A mathematical theory of the functional dynamics of cortical and thalamic nervous tissue. Kybernetik 1973; 13(2): 55-80.

[87] Liley DTJ, Cadusch PJ, Wright JJ. A continuum theory of electro-cortical activity. Neurocomputing. [doi: DOI: 10.1016/S0925-2312(98)00149-0] 1999; 26-27: 795-800.

[88] Rennie CJ, Robinson PA, Wright JJ. Unified neurophysical model of EEG spectra and evoked potentials. Biol Cybern 2002; 86(6): 457-71.

[89] Tamakawa Y, Karashima A, Koyama Y, Katayama N, Nakao M. A quartet neural system model orchestrating sleep and wakefulness mechanisms. J Neurophysiol 2006; 95(4): 2055-69.

[90] Phillips AJ, Robinson PA. A quantitative model of sleep-wake dynamics based on the physiology of the brainstem ascending arousal system. J Biol Rhythms 2007; 22(2): 167-79.

[91] Fulcher BD, Phillips AJ, Robinson PA. Quantitative physiologically based modeling of subjective fatigue during sleep deprivation. J Theor Biol 2010; 264(2): 407-19.

[92] Phillips AJ, Robinson PA, Kedziora DJ, Abeysuriya RG. Mammalian sleep dynamics: how diverse features arise from a common physiological framework. PLoS Comput Biol 2010; 6(6): e1000826.

[93] Behn CG, Brown EN, Scammell TE, Kopell NJ. Mathematical model of network dynamics governing mouse sleep-wake behavior. J Neurophysiol 2007; 97(6): 3828-40.

[94] Rempe MJ, Best J, Terman D. A mathematical model of the sleep/wake cycle. J Math Biol 2010; 60(5): 615-44.

[95] Diniz Behn CG, Kopell N, Brown EN, Mochizuki T, Scammell TE. Delayed orexin signaling consolidates wakefulness and sleep: physiology and modeling. J Neurophysiol 2008; 99(6): 3090-103.

[96] Chua CP, Garvey J, Redmond S, Heneghan C, McNicholas WT. Towards automated sleep state estimation using a Holter-oximeter. Conf Proc IEEE Eng Med Biol Soc 2007; 2007: 3998-4001.

[97] Caffarel J, Gibson GJ, Harrison JP, Griffiths CJ, Drinnan MJ. Comparison of manual sleep staging with automated neural network-based analysis in clinical practice. Med Biol Eng Comput 2006; 44(1-2): 105-10.

[98]   Flexer A, Gruber G, Dorffner G. A reliable probabilistic sleep stager based on a single EEG signal. Artif Intell Med 2005; 33(3): 199-207.

[99]   Thomas RJ, Mietus JE, Peng CK, Goldberger AL. An electrocardiogram-based technique to assess cardiopulmonary coupling during sleep. Sleep 2005; 28(9): 1151-61.

[100]   Agarwal R, Gotman J. Computer-assisted sleep staging. IEEE Trans Biomed Eng 2001; 48(12): 1412-23.

[101]   Penzel T, Conradt R. Computer based sleep recording and analysis. Sleep Med Rev 2000; 4(2): 131-48.

[102]   Havlin S, Buldyrev SV, Goldberger AL, *et al.* Fractals in biology and medicine. Chaos Solitons Fractals 1995; 6: 171-201.

[103]   Goldberger AL, Amaral LA, Hausdorff JM, Ivanov P, Peng CK, Stanley HE. Fractal dynamics in physiology: alterations with disease and aging. Proc Natl Acad Sci USA 2002; 99(Suppl 1): 2466-72.

[104]   Peng CK, Buldyrev SV, Hausdorff JM, *et al.* Non-equilibrium dynamics as an indispensable characteristic of a healthy biological system. Integr Physiol Behav Sci 1994; 29(3): 283-93.

[105]   Seely AJ, Macklem PT. Complex systems and the technology of variability analysis. Crit Care 2004; 8(6): R367-84.

[106]   Hu K, Scheer FA, Buijs RM, Shea SA. The circadian pacemaker generates similar circadian rhythms in the fractal structure of heart rate in humans and rats. Cardiovasc Res 2008; 80(1): 62-8.

[107]   Thomas RJ, Mietus JE, Peng CK, *et al.* Differentiating obstructive from central and complex sleep apnea using an automated electrocardiogram-based method. Sleep 2007; 30(12): 1756-69.

[108]   Thomas RJ, Weiss MD, Mietus JE, Peng CK, Goldberger AL, Gottlieb DJ. Prevalent hypertension and stroke in the Sleep Heart Health Study: association with an ECG-derived spectrographic marker of cardiopulmonary coupling. Sleep 2009; 32(7): 897-904.

[109]   Pang KP, Gourin CG, Terris DJ. A comparison of polysomnography and the WatchPAT in the diagnosis of obstructive sleep apnea. Otolaryngol Head Neck Surg 2007; 137(4): 665-8.

[110]   Schnall RP, Shlitner A, Sheffy J, Kedar R, Lavie P. Periodic, profound peripheral vasoconstriction--a new marker of obstructive sleep apnea. Sleep 1999; 22(7): 939-46.

[111]   Herscovici S, Pe'er A, Papyan S, Lavie P. Detecting REM sleep from the finger: an automatic REM sleep algorithm based on peripheral arterial tone (PAT) and actigraphy. Physiol Meas 2007; 28(2): 129-40.

[112]   Bar A, Pillar G, Dvir I, Sheffy J, Schnall RP, Lavie P. Evaluation of a portable device based on peripheral arterial tone for unattended home sleep studies. Chest 2003; 123(3): 695-703.

[113]   Ancoli-Israel S, Cole R, Alessi C, Chambers M, Moorcroft W, Pollak CP. The role of actigraphy in the study of sleep and circadian rhythms. Sleep 2003; 26(3): 342-92.

[114]   Morgenthaler TI, Lee-Chiong T, Alessi C, *et al.* Practice parameters for the clinical evaluation and treatment of circadian rhythm sleep disorders. An American Academy of Sleep Medicine report. Sleep 2007; 30(11): 1445-59.

[115]   Sack RL, Auckley D, Auger RR, *et al.* Circadian rhythm sleep disorders: part II, advanced sleep phase disorder, delayed sleep phase disorder, free-running disorder, and irregular sleep-wake rhythm. An American Academy of Sleep Medicine review. Sleep 2007; 30(11): 1484-501.

[116]   Peng CK, Mietus JE, Liu Y, *et al.* Quantifying fractal dynamics of human respiration: age and gender effects. Ann Biomed Eng 2002; 30(5): 683-92.

[117]   Stanley HE, Amaral LA, Goldberger AL, Havlin S, Ivanov P, Peng CK. Statistical physics and physiology: monofractal and multifractal approaches. Physica A 1999; 270(1-2): 309-24.

[118]   Hu K, Ivanov P, Chen Z, Hilton MF, Stanley HE, Shea SA. Non-random fluctuations and multi-scale dynamics regulation of human activity. Physica A 2004; 337(1-2): 307-18.

[119]   Hu K, Scheer FA, Ivanov P, Buijs RM, Shea SA. The suprachiasmatic nucleus functions beyond circadian rhythm generation. Neuroscience 2007; 149(3): 508-17.

[120]   Hu K, Van Someren EJ, Shea SA, Scheer FA. Reduction of scale invariance of activity fluctuations with aging and Alzheimer's disease: Involvement of the circadian pacemaker. Proc Natl Acad Sci USA 2009; 106(8): 2490-4.

[121]   Swaab DF, Fliers E, Partiman TS. The suprachiasmatic nucleus of the human brain in relation to sex, age and senile dementia. Brain Res 1985; 342(1): 37-44.

[122]   Hoogendijk WJ, van Someren EJ, Mirmiran M, *et al.* Circadian rhythm-related behavioral disturbances and structural hypothalamic changes in Alzheimer's disease. Int Psychogeriatr 1996; 8(Suppl 3): 245-52; discussion 69-72.

[123]   Pallier PN, Morton AJ. Management of sleep/wake cycles improves cognitive function in a transgenic mouse model of Huntington's disease. Brain Res 2009; 1279: 90-8.

[124]   Edinger JD, Fins AI, Glenn DM, *et al.* Insomnia and the eye of the beholder: are there clinical markers of objective sleep disturbances among adults with and without insomnia complaints? J Consult Clin Psychol 2000; 68(4): 586-93.

[125]   Edinger JD, Bonnet MH, Bootzin RR, *et al.* Derivation of research diagnostic criteria for insomnia: report of an American Academy of Sleep Medicine Work Group. Sleep 2004; 27(8): 1567-96.

[126]   Lee JH, Durand R, Gradinaru V, *et al.* Global and local fMRI signals driven by neurons defined optogenetically by type and wiring. Nature 2010; 465(7299): 788-92.

CHAPTER 6

Multimodal Imaging in Epilepsy: Combining EEG and fMRI

Helmut Laufs[*]

Department of Neurology and Brain Imaging Center, Goethe-University Frankfurt am Main, Theodor-Stern-Kai 2-16, 60590 Frankfurt am Main, Germany

Abstract: This chapter introduces a multimodal imaging approach to "epileptic networks". It is explained why electroencephalography (EEG) in combination with functional magnetic resonance imaging (fMRI) is an ideal tool to study spontaneous brain activity such as spontaneously occurring interictal epileptic discharges, typical sleep graphoelements, or characteristic EEG oscillations. This is closely related to resting state brain activity in healthy subjects and has been studied *via* analysis of spontaneous neuronal oscillations and their fMRI correlates. The application of EEG/fMRI to disease, with epilepsy as the primary example, is reviewed. It starts from the original goal, the identification of the region of the brain in which interictal epileptic activity arises, moves on to studies not in line with this idea but introducing the new concept that fMRI maps may reflect entire epileptic networks, and finally to the clinical applicability of EEG/fMRI patient studies and publications suggesting the method may provide insight into the neurobiology of epilepsy. The chapter concludes with a look into the future: intracranial EEG/fMRI.

Keywords: Resting network, epilepsy, inter-ictal, temporal lobe, methodology, conscious states, epileptogenic zone.

THE RELATIONSHIP OF NETWORKS AND BRAIN STATES

Brain states in the strict sense of the word do not exist, as the living brain hosts dynamic processes. Similarly, the frequently [ab]used term "network" is vague. In line with the previous chapters of this e-Book, a brain state should be understood as a temporally and spatially stable set of brain regions the activity of which is (non-)linearly related and that together subserve or cause a common observable function or measurable effect. A state hence describes the configuration of a temporally stable (sub-)set of networks. For example, at the macroscopic level, a subject can be observed in the "awake" or the "asleep" state, implying the associated state of the brain as a whole to be "awake" or "asleep". More fine-grained observation or measurement will define more detailed brain states within the awake and asleep macro-states. For example, sleep by visual or more precisely basic electroencephalogram (EEG) observation can be subdivided into states of light sleep, deep sleep, arousal and rapid eye movement (REM) sleep, each of which may be further subdivided.

STUDYING "ACTION VERSUS REST" VERSUS STUDYING "REST"

Classically in neuroimaging experiments, paradigms are designed and used to induce brain activity thought to be specific to a task of interest ("activation study"), and paradigm-related analysis methods are chosen to detect the brain regions subserving the task-specific function [1]. In recent years, paradigm-less experiments have moved into the focus of research investigating the brain "at rest", which shall be understood as endogenous brain activity that is not intentionally externally induced or voluntarily generated by the subject, i.e. ongoing brain activity at rest [2-3]. At least three scenarios exist that make the study of the brain at rest an advantageous approach: (a) subjects are in a condition when they cannot engage in a paradigm, for example during sleep [4], coma [5] or an epileptic seizure [6] and especially if that condition itself is the object of interest; other examples include studies of infants [7] or (untrained) animals [8]. (b) Spontaneously occurring phenomena shall be examined, for example epileptic spikes [9-10], sleep spindles, vertex sharp waves, K-complexes, or resting EEG oscillations [11-13]. (c) The activity of networks the function of which was previously described in "activation studies" shall be characterized at rest and compared between healthy subjects and patient groups, and differences may serve as biomarkers [14]. Last but not least, early disease stages may be studied when malfunctioning of the brain due to compensatory mechanisms or strategies cannot yet be observed in behavioural changes, but may be caught using multi modal imaging techniques [11].

From a basic science perspective, neural processes can be perceived as mainly intrinsic - weighting, gating and subsequently integrating new and external information into the brain - as opposed to a rather absolute resting state contrasting momentary activity driven by external demands [3]. This view further motivates that the brain be studied at rest.

*****Address correspondence to Helmut Laufs:** Department of Neurology and Brain Imaging Center, Goethe-University Frankfurt am Main, Theodor-Stern-Kai 2-16, 60590 Frankfurt am Main, Germany; E-mail: *h.laufs@em.uni-frankfurt.de*

Matt T. Bianchi, Verne S. Caviness and Sydney S. Cash (Eds.)

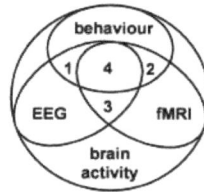

Fig. (6.1). An analytical perspective on the integration of electrophysiological and hemodynamic data. A fraction of all neural processes is reflected by EEG, fMRI and behavior. Some neural processes manifest in EEG and behavior ("1"), or fMRI and behavior ("2"). Of the neural processes reflected in both EEG and fMRI there may also be measurable behavioral manifestations ("4") or not ("3"). In both cases, "3" and "4", however, the correlation between EEG and fMRI is direct in that there is a common substrate of neural activity. If behaviors related to neural processes that also manifest in EEG ("1") and fMRI ("2") independently, yet without being the identical processes at the source of EEG and fMRI effects, this situation can still result in an indirect but meaningful correlation between fMRI and EEG. Simultaneous multi-modal experiments benefit from situations where common neural processes are at the origin of EEG and fMRI signals but the most benefit is derived when these neural processes cannot be monitored by or recalibrated to behavior ("3"), such as endogenous brain activity. (Figure taken from Neuroimage 40, Laufs et al., Recent advances in recording electrophysiological data simultaneously with magnetic resonance imaging, 515-28, 2008, with permission from Elsevier).

METHODS TO STUDY THE BRAIN AT REST

It is difficult to study the brain 'at rest' with the approach generally pursued in science when external manipulation (independent variable) is used to obtain informative measurements (dependent variable) about the object of interest, because it may suspend the resting state: as soon as the previously resting subject is confronted with a task, he or she will no longer be at (unbiased) rest. Multimodal imaging, i.e. the application of two experimental imaging techniques in parallel, allows studying the brain's activity from two angles. One modality can be chosen to be interpreted as the independent variable and the other one as the dependent variable, as described below.

MULTIMODAL IMAGING EXAMPLES IN DISEASES

Eidelberg reviewed how voxel-based network modeling algorithms can be applied to metabolic imaging data (e.g. positron emission tomography (PET) and single photon emission tomography (SPECT)) to study changes in brain function in neurodegenerative disease (Alzheimer's dementia, AD; Parkinson's disease, PD) (15). Consistent disease-related network abnormalities reflect stereotyped changes in the functional interactions of discrete sets of brain regions in these disorders. These specific spatial patterns can be quantified and upon their validation eventually be used as biomarkers of disease progression and treatment effects at the systems level [15]. Damoiseaux and Greicius review multimodal imaging studies including diffusion tractography imaging (DTI) combined fMRI and volumetry-correlated DTI concluding that multimodal imaging of resting state connectivity will enhance diagnostic as well as prognostic scope in diseases like AD, multiple sclerosis (MS) and stroke [16]. However, the potential of these diagnostic developments to be exploited at the single subject level remains to be established[14]. In epilepsy, multimodal imaging by means of EEG-combined fMRI in some patients adds valuable diagnostic information while other observations are the result of group studies and not yet exploitable at the individual subject level [10, 17-20].

Without external manipulation, within-subject state changes in endogenous brain activity can be observed across different stages of vigilance in healthy subjects. In certain patients, pathologic activity can occur intrinsically, as in the case of epileptic activity. Both types of changes can be detected and characterized using EEG, the gold standard of determining sleep stages [21] and non-invasively detecting epileptiform activity [22]. Although blood oxygen level-dependent (BOLD) fMRI is a more indirect measure of neuronal activity than EEG both in terms of the temporal scale and the signal source, MRI's spatial resolution complements the relative blindness of surface EEG to deep and subcortical sources [23]. These regions are especially relevant in the mentioned application fields of sleep and epilepsy. Hence this chapter will focus on EEG-combined BOLD-fMRI (EEG/fMRI) as a particularly exciting multimodal imaging approach.

THE COMBINATION OF EEG AND fMRI

When studying spontaneous neuronal activity without external manipulation using EEG/fMRI, the EEG data describes endogenous modulations of vigilance or spontaneous events (sleep spindles, epileptic discharges) and can be treated as the independent variable, forming a regressor to interrogate the fMRI data (dependent variable). The opposite regression is also possible; and data fusion attempts are being made using all data both as dependent and independent variables [23-26].

THE PHYSIOLOGY OF THE SIGNALS AND THEIR CONCEPTUAL LINK

BOLD-fMRI measures the haemodynamic correlate of neuronal activity, probably local field potentials (LFP) and – to a lesser degree – multi unit activity [27]. Accordingly, BOLD signal decreases are related to neuronal activity decreases [28], however the reference system (i.e. the so-called "baseline") needs to be considered [3]. The BOLD signal may reflect also sub-threshold activity, simultaneous inhibition with excitation and the result of modulating afferent input of remote neurons [29]. Of note, astrocytic processes contribute to the BOLD response [30] and may be involved in epileptogenesis [31] but evade surface EEG.

Scalp EEG measures neuronal activity in the form of postsynaptic excitatory and inhibitory potentials (EPSP and IPSP) of pyramidal cells aligned perpendicular to the cortical surface. The overlap between EPSP and LFP remains unknown, and fMRI and EEG are measurements not of identical neuronal processes, providing valuable complementary information. Because of this, the relationship between simultaneously acquired EEG and fMRI data needs further consideration (see Fig. **6.1**) [11].

MOTIVATION AND FEASIBILITY OF COMBINING EEG AND fMRI

The development of EEG recording during fMRI (Fig. **6.2**) was initially clinically motivated by the wish to localize electrical sources of neuronal activity, in particular epileptic discharges [32]. This intention led epilepsy researchers to develop both acquisition hardware and artifact reduction algorithms (Fig. **6.3**), such that the methodology today is sufficiently developed to implement a wide variety of experiments as reviewed elsewhere [9, 33-35].

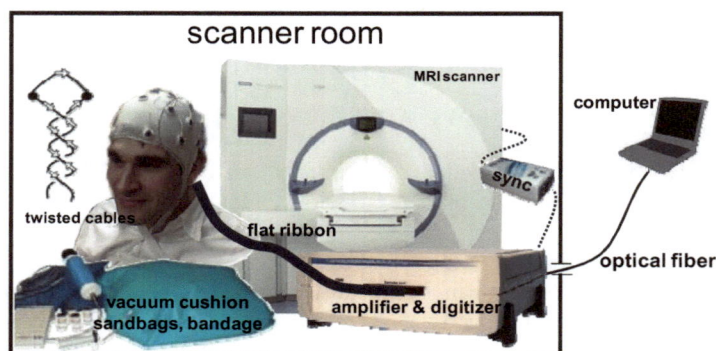

Fig. (**6.2**). A schematic of an example EEG/fMRI experimental setup. EEG ring electrodes with current limiting safety resistors are woven into a cap. Their bundled wires converge into a flat ribbon cable which connects to the battery-driven amplifier and digitizer, which is usually positioned at the head end of the scanner bore (a second amplifier and digitizer, e.g. for EMG recordings, may be positioned near the subject's lower extremities). The digitizer is connected to the MRI scanner clock *via* a synchronization device (frequency divider). A fiber-optical cable transmits the digitized electrophysiological signals through the wave guide to a recording computer outside the scanner room. Vacuum cushions serve subject comfort and can reduce subject motion. Twisting of wires has also been proposed and may be useful in bipolar recordings. (Figure taken from Neuroimage 40, Laufs et al., Recent advances in recording electrophysiological data simultaneously with magnetic resonance imaging, 515-28, 2008, with permission from Elsevier).

When studying rest with fMRI alone, mainly data driven analysis approaches (functional connectivity, principal, or independent component analysis) have been used, and about a dozen consistent resting state networks have been identified [36]. The so called "default mode" network (DMN) is a set of brain regions that are active when an individual is not focused on the outside world and the brain is at wakeful rest as opposed to the individual being asleep or engaged in a task [37]. The DMN is a special one of several resting state networks (RSN) described in the literature. As historically being among the first to be described [38], the DMN seeded the concept of RSN in general [3]. These are sets of brain regions known to be active during typical (classes of) tasks exhibiting coherent activity fluctuations also at rest. Deviations from "normal" resting state network behavior are in the focus of current research hypothesizing that they reflect disease-specific pathology [39].

However, the interpretation of their functional significance remains difficult when assessed unimodally and – necessarily – in the absence of a task or context. Objective assessment of each subject's state during data acquisition (e.g. external observation or *via* a post hoc questionnaire) has to remain indirect and potentially inaccurate, especially in situations of reduced vigilance. A second perspective on, *via* a second measure of, brain activity at rest can be obtained by measuring EEG. It can give information on the subject's "state of mind". Of course, the benefit from EEG when interpreting fMRI maps is limited by how well resting state EEG phenomena and their functional meaning have been studied alone [40], or on the strength of prior hypotheses [41]. Still, its combination with fMRI in the study of the resting state is of great value. In a complementary sense, EEG/fMRI can help to elucidate the physiology and brain processes that underlie specific EEG phenomena [12-13].

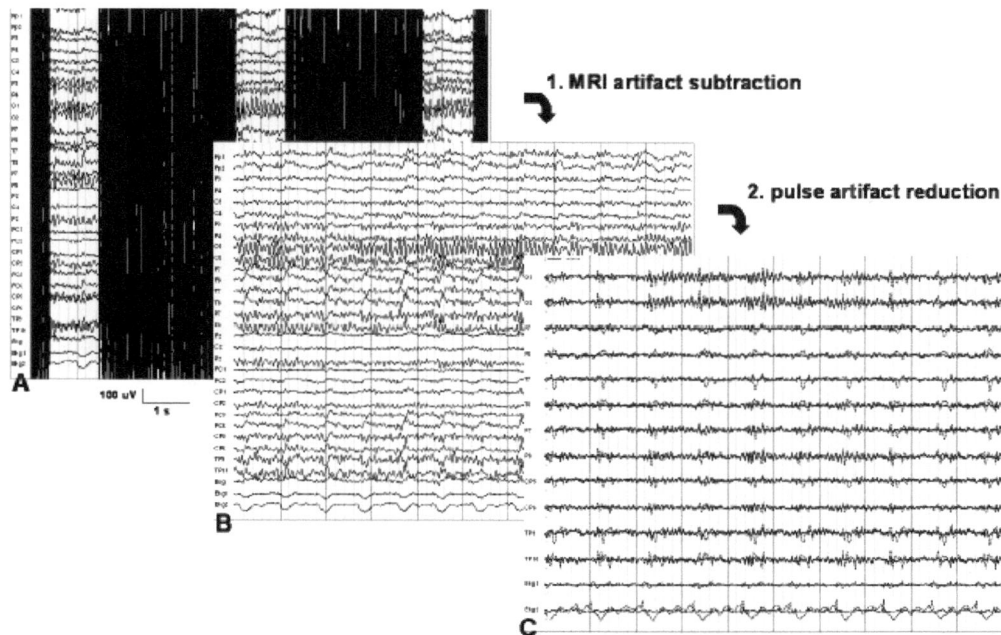

Fig. (6.3). A schematic of preprocessing stages of MRI and pulse artifact affected EEG. Panel (A) shows a segment (10 seconds) of a 32 channel electrophysiological recording during "interleaved" fMRI acquisition at 1.5 Tesla (T) with about 3 seconds of imaging per acquired volume followed by a gap in scanning of about 1 second in duration. In panel (B), we see the same segment after channel-wise subtraction of a template MRI artifact obtained by averaging. The identical segment (dotted lines) is shown in panel (C) after channel-wise pulse artifact reduction (solid line) *via* subtraction of an EKG-locked sliding average. (Figure taken from Neuroimage 40, Laufs et al., Recent advances in recording electrophysiological data simultaneously with magnetic resonance imaging, 515-28, 2008, with permission from Elsevier.

ENDOGENOUS NEURONAL OSCILLATIONS IN HEALTHY VOLUNTEERS AT REST

EEG/fMRI of Ongoing Neuronal Oscillations in the Awake State

While neuronal oscillations in different EEG frequency bands and associated topographies have been identified in the context of different types of active mental activity, endogenous brain activity during relaxed wakefulness ("awake rest") inherently has been less well characterized, despite being recorded in day-to-day clinical practice and having been the first condition that was ever reported to have been assessed with EEG [42]. Hans Berger named the posterior 8-12 Hz oscillations "alpha rhythm", the most prominent EEG rhythm during the awake resting state. He noticed its desynchronization with ceasing vigilance on the one hand and with engagement in attention-demanding tasks on the other [42].

Unsurprisingly, the first EEG/fMRI investigations studying healthy volunteers at rest were concerned with the BOLD correlates of this very prominent EEG feature. In line with electrophysiological animal studies, Goldman *et al.*, Moosmann *et al.* and – similarly – later Mantini *et al.* identified thalamic BOLD activity to be positively and occipital-parietal areas to be inversely correlated with alpha oscillations on scalp EEG, this in turn reflecting their scalp topography [43-45]. In a larger cohort of 35 subjects studied at 4T, diFrancesco reported a posterior alpha power-associated spatial BOLD pattern including positive thalamic and negative fusiform and visual association and dorsolateral prefrontal cortices, in line with the previous studies [46].

Laufs *et al.* – and, similarly again, Mantini *et al.* - found a frontal-parietal network to be associated with alpha desynchronization [45, 47]. In line with Berger's observations, they claimed to have visualized endogenously waxing and waning attention *via* alpha desynchronization-associated activity changes in a frontal-parietal network, previously and independently established as an attentional system [47-48]. The group of König *et al.* found evidence for the "dorsal attentional" system to be an fMRI correlate of 8.5 to 10.5 Hz alpha activity in the form of global field synchronization, i.e. a quantification of alpha phase synchronization across the entire scalp [49]. In line with the work by Mantini *et al.*, Jann *et al.* found an overlap of alpha phase-associated fMRI maps and independently identified resting state networks [49]. In the context of resting state fMRI signal fluctuations, DiFrancesco highlighted similar temporal characteristics of alpha magnitude variations (period of 10 s) [46], as had Laufs *et al.* [40].

Laufs *et al.* had described fMRI signal alterations in regions of the 'default mode' network (see below), a prominent resting state network, to be positively correlated with 17-23 Hz beta band power [48], similar to Mantini *et al.* [45], who demonstrated that multiple frequency bands are correlated simultaneously with fMRI activity fluctuations. This fact was further highlighted by deMunck and colleagues, who argued that, in addition to inter-subject variability [50], high between-EEG band power correlation could be responsible for discrepant spatial findings across studies [51].

Taking a more methodological perspective, Tyvaert and colleagues tested the hypothesis that BOLD correlates of neuronal background rhythm oscillations may confound fMRI results in general. Their results were based on data sets obtained from a cohort of epilepsy patients with background (inter-ictal) EEG activity that was considered comparable to that of healthy volunteers. Tyvaert *et al.* studied alpha, higher beta, theta and delta band power derived from posterior (for individual alpha frequencies) and more anterior EEG channels (for the other bands), respectively. They found that in around 7% of gray matter voxels BOLD signal variations at the order of 5% could be explained by spontaneous ongoing EEG oscillations [52]. While this study was performed during task-free rest, it should not be forgotten that in activation studies EEG oscillations may be induced by (and hence correlated with) the task and as such cannot necessarily be seen as a pure confound especially where EEG- and task-associated activations overlap. Tyvaert's findings at the group level found alpha power-associated positive signal changes in the thalamus (and putamen) and a negative response in widespread and symmetrical cortical regions, which in principle is in line with the topographies discussed above. Group analysis of the other frequency bands, spontaneous beta, theta and delta (during awake and sleep) oscillations, failed to identify significant BOLD clusters [52]. Pushing technical limits, Mullinger and colleagues studied (driven) EEG alpha correlates at 7T and found related activations in visual cortex [53].

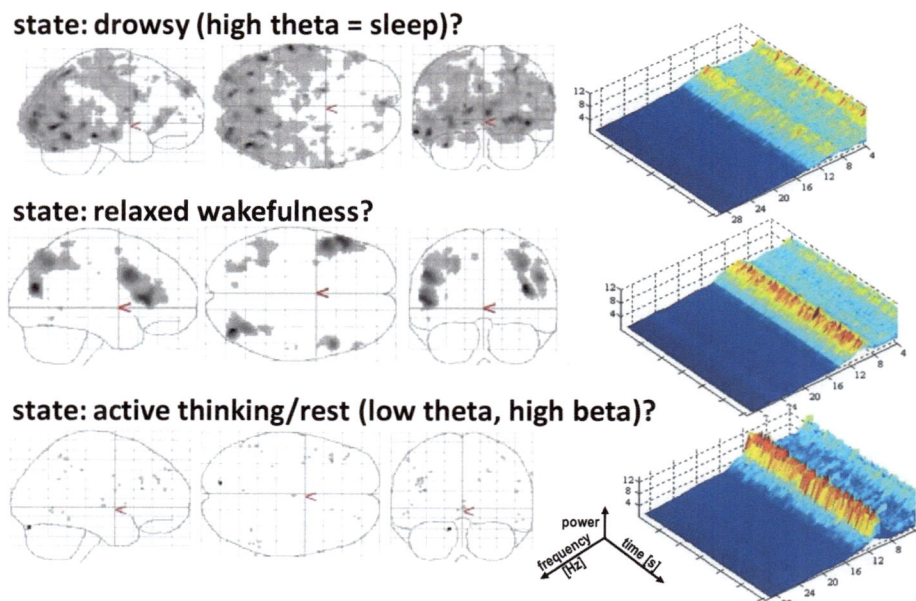

Fig. (6.4). illustrates the hemodynamic signatures of human posterior alpha activity. Analysis of fMRI correlates of EEG 8-12 Hz alpha power resulted in three different average fMRI maps and spectral patterns. Laufs *et al.* hypothesized that the state of vigilance reflected in the EEG also underlies the different fMRI patterns. (Figure taken from Neuroimage 31, Laufs et al., Where the BOLD signal goes when alpha EEG leaves, 1408-18, 2006, with permission from Elsevier.

Critically, apart from the thalamic activation associated with increased alpha power [43-46, 52, 54], none of the mentioned studies in the stricter sense revealed coherent [cortical] correlates of scalp EEG alpha oscillations; instead, by identifying inverse relationships, they identified brain regions that increase their activity in the absence of marked alpha activity [40]. In congruence with Hans Berger's observations, Laufs *et al.* found the occipitally pronounced, inversely alpha-associated pattern to occur in association with a decline in vigilance (Fig. **6.4**). This was supported by a corresponding enhanced spectral density in the theta (4-7 Hz) band, usually observed in drowsiness. Furthermore, activation in occipital brain regions during light sleep compared to wakefulness had been shown with positron emission tomography (PET) [55]. The failure across studies to identify an average cortical BOLD signal pattern that is positively correlated with alpha power may be explained by non-uniform brain activity at the population level during periods of prominent alpha oscillations such that fMRI group analysis must fail to detect [40].

A frequency-independent perspective on resting state EEG activity was introduced by Lehmann: EEG microstates. These relate to functional states of the brain each characterized uniquely by a fixed spatial distribution of active neuronal generators with time varying intensity (i.e. EEG amplitude topography maps around local peaks of global field power). Brain electrical activity is modeled as being composed of a time sequence of non-overlapping microstates with variable duration [56-58]. A reproducible set of a limited number of EEG microstates was identified to characterize resting state brain activity. Musso, Britz, and colleagues examined fMRI correlates of EEG microstates and found more or less spatial similarity to previously identified generic fMRI RSN [59-60]. Future work in this area may be able to establish a "microstate alphabet" of resting state brain activity including across different vigilance states. The much higher temporal resolution of the EEG microstate sequence compared to BOLD signal fluctuations should help study in detail the interaction and temporal relationship of different RSN with respect to one another [61].

EEG/fMRI of Endogenous Neuronal Oscillations During Sleep and Reduced Consciousness

Sleep by polysomnographic criteria is generally subdivided into dream sleep ("rapid eye movement" [REM] sleep), light sleep (non-REM [NREM] "stages N1 and N2") and deep sleep (NREM "stage N3"). These stages are mainly defined by characteristic EEG oscillations (e.g. in the alpha, theta, delta frequency band) and grapho-elements (e.g. vertex sharp waves, K-complexes, sleep spindles) [21, 62]. Significant insights into the neuroanatomy of sleep were gained based on studies with positron emission tomography (PET) in combination with EEG [63]. In general, the simultaneously recorded EEG was used to define sleep stages that were then analyzed in a so-called block design, e.g. comparing stages between one another or to awake rest. For methodological reasons detailed elsewhere, such an analysis approach is not possible with BOLD-fMRI data [12]. In short, due to hardware constraints, the BOLD signal undergoes a scanner- and sequence-specific slow drift that will bias the comparison of epochs (blocks) that are temporally distant to one another. High pass filtering will remove the drift, but potentially also the signal changes of interest. An alternative approach to be used when comparing temporally distant epochs is arterial spin labeling that is sensitive to perfusion changes and drift resistant because pairs of images are acquired containing an individual reference [64].

Similarly, in early fMRI studies, the EEG was used to define sleep depth - but not as an analysis parameter itself – for example to indicate when to perform sensory stimulation during specific sleep stages [65-66]. In their study on acoustic stimulus-induced BOLD signal decreases, Czisch and colleagues correlated the number of K-complexes and the amount of delta power occurring during NREM sleep with the extent and amplitude of the fMRI signal changes [67]. The same group later were the first to study "sleep itself" with EEG/fMRI in a way analogous to the earlier PET sleep studies [68]. Such an approach needs to be appreciated with caution since resting state BOLD-fMRI data does not serve well the analysis of longer epochs in a block design fashion, as above. In contrast, it is ideally suited to analyze brief EEG-defined events and to correlate ongoing EEG oscillations with the BOLD time course [64, 69]. Laufs et al. demonstrated exactly this in a single case studied with EEG/fMRI during sleep: they correlated the power of EEG oscillations typically occurring during NREM sleep stages with the BOLD data and found a wide overlap of the detected regions with those previously reported as a 'default mode' network by Raichle and colleagues, the activity of which had previously been reported to be higher during resting wakefulness compared to both sleep and also active perception and action. Laufs et al. speculated that their findings indicated that this set of brain areas is still dynamically active during sleep - possibly at a lower activity level compared to wakefulness [12]. On a much larger data set, Horovitz et al. made a parallel observation using functional connectivity analysis, which showed disintegration and reintegration of the default mode during light and deep sleep [70-71]. Functionally, examining patients with different degrees of impaired consciousness it was recently generalized that default mode network connectivity correlates with the level of consciousness [72].

Olbrich and colleagues extended work by Picchioni [73] by examining vigilance states from relaxed wakefulness to sleep onset. The EEG-defined vigilance stages served as regressors for the analysis of simultaneously acquired fMRI data. Results showed increased BOLD signal in the occipital cortex, the anterior cingulate cortex, the frontal cortex, the parietal cortices and the temporal cortices, and decreasing BOLD signals in the thalamus and the frontal cortex for declining vigilance stages compared to the fully awake stage. One important implication of these findings was for cognitive fMRI-research that presumably task-related results may be biased by vigilance switches [74]. Using (event-related) factorial designs and performing group analysis will help to protect against both false positives and negatives [75]. Based on findings in an epilepsy study, Moehring *et al.* proposed a more fundamental effect of vigilance in that it may influence the net neuronal excitability [76].

Laufs et al. in the mentioned case study analyzed EEG grapho-elements characteristic for stage N2 sleep, namely K-complexes (KC) and sleep spindles (Sp), which unsurprisingly often occurred in close temporal association. Sp- and KC-associated BOLD signal changes were observed in the thalamus, frontal and central, temporal and, to a lesser degree, occipital cortices. They proposed this reflected synchronized activity of primary (sensory-motor, visual, auditory) cortices and thalamus. Signal changes were opposite in direction—KC were related to deactivation while Sp were correlated with activation that was seen, in agreement with studies at the cellular level and the observation in rats that KC mark the transition from 'down-to-up' states, whilst Sp activity typically occurs in the subsequent upstate. BOLD signal changes observed in bilateral superior and middle temporal gyri, cortices implied in memory formation, were argued to support the hypothesis of synchronized activity serving memory consolidation, and BOLD changes in sensorimotor, auditory and visual cortices to reflect the involved replay of behavioral experience [12].

Highlighting the increasing interest in studying sleep with EEG/fMRI, recent methodological work has focused on optimizing pulse (ballistocardiographic) artifact reduction for EEG acquired during light and deep sleep [77-78]. Good pulse artifact reduction is especially important when EEG oscillations (e.g. spectral power analysis) or grapho-elements (e.g. amplitude) are quantified for analysis.

Endogenous Neuronal Activity in Epilepsy

The literature on EEG/fMRI in epilepsy has meanwhile become extensive, and it is beyond the scope of this chapter to review all studies in detail. The following shall create an understanding of the past, current and future direction of this type of research while mainly listing supportive studies. Several review articles, each with a different perspective, are available discussing these studies in more detail [9-10, 18-20, 35, 79-83].

Technical Remarks

For the current typical clinical settings (1.5T or 3T MRI scanners) the main technical and safety challenges [84] of recording EEG during fMRI can be addressed. Simultaneous and continuous EEG/fMRI acquisition readily allows the identification of epileptic activity on surface EEG while obtaining hemodynamic measurements. More technical details have been reviewed elsewhere [34, 85-86]. Advantages and disadvantages of EEG/fMRI originate from each technique's characteristics: surface EEG lacks non-ambiguous and high spatial resolution and is blind to sources not projecting to the scalp [87], which is of particular relevance in frontal lobe epilepsies. Despite fMRI's ability to cover the whole brain including subcortical and mesio-temporal structures, its temporal resolution is limited, currently at the order of seconds (versus milliseconds for EEG) due to physical constraints and biologically because of the time taken for a BOLD signal change to occur consequent to a change in neuronal activation. While in cognitive fMRI studies an effectively higher temporal resolution can be achieved by optimising the stimulus presentation (fast event-related designs), this cannot be done in fMRI studies of interictal epileptic activity (IEA) that are dependent on spontaneously occurring IEA.

MR sequences need to be tailored to imaging certain brain areas, in order that the BOLD-fMRI signal will not be too compromised in certain parts of the brain (e.g. susceptibility artifacts, partial volume effects), such as the temporal lobe [88]. TLE is of particular interest in clinical epilepsy practice because of its high prevalence in the adult population and the occurrence of drug-resistant TLE that may be amenable to surgical treatment [89].

THE PAST AND FUTURE ROUTE OF EEG/FMRI RESEARCH IN EPILEPSY

Feasibility

Early EEG/fMRI research in the field of epilepsy included several feasibility studies and has been summarized previously [9, 80-83, 90]. Later, large patient cohorts were subjected to the study of IEA-correlated focal [91-94] and generalized epileptic discharges [95-96] exploring both the usefulness and limitations of EEG/fMRI in epilepsy. The general analysis approach pursued was to model IEA in an event-related fashion within the framework of a general linear model, where the occurrence of IEA in time served as an event that was then convolved with a hemodynamic response function like the one observed in healthy subjects arising with a delay of around 2 to 6 seconds after an induced neuronal event.

Initial Aim: Mapping the Origin of Epileptic Activity

The initial research was motivated by the vision to use EEG/fMRI as a diagnostic tool to non-invasively identify the irritative zone (where IEA are generated) or ideally the epileptogenic zone, i.e. that brain region the surgical removal of which makes a subject seizure free [97]. Subsequently, case series were broken down based on the spatial location of IEA [98-99] or pathology findings [100-103]. The more data became available the more it was obvious that the initial vision was tinted by findings not easily interpretable [10], such as both positive and negative IEA-associated BOLD signal changes [9], and widespread as well as distant activity changes relative to the presumed (determined by other diagnostic means) origin of epileptic activity [18]. Consequently, another wave of methodologically oriented studies followed.

Inconclusive Results: Methodological Refinement

On the fMRI side, studies probed different hemodynamic models in response to IEA [104-116] and attempted improved modelling of artifacts [91, 117-118]. On the EEG side, apart from attempts to improve (pulse) artifact reduction [119-120] more sophisticated and automated IEA detection and classification were explored [49, 91, 116, 121-125] and the influence of vigilance and of EEG oscillations accompanying IEA were tested [52, 76, 126]. Finally, methods that had meanwhile become established in "classical" neuroimaging studies, i.e. in cognitive neuroscience, were also applied to EEG/fMRI studies of epilepsy. Such methods include independent component analysis [127-128] and other methods with and without the integration of the available EEG information [129-132].

Ictal and Interictal Activity: Analysing Epileptic Networks

Advanced methodology proved useful also in the analysis of fMRI data acquired during epileptic seizure activity that can easily be compromised by subject motion and related artefacts [6, 79, 128, 132-142]. The widespread ictal and interictal signal changes often observed nourished the concept that BOLD maps might reflect the spread of epileptic activity collapsed in a static image [128, 133, 143-146], a reasonable assumption given typical fMRI repetition times of several seconds and (inter)ictal EEG spreading occurring at a similar temporal scale [147].

Effective connectivity analysis is one method that, in the BOLD-fMRI domain, allows the assessment of what in the EEG domain would be IEA propagation. Put another way, it allows the study of which brain region drives the activity of another. Hamandi and colleagues using EEG-dependent dynamic causal modelling (DCM) and diffusion tensor imaging tractography in a patient with refractory temporal lobe epilepsy found supporting evidence for propagation of neural activity from the temporal focus to an area of occipital fMRI activation [144]. They showed that temporal lobe activity drove the activity in the occipital region of interest. In a slightly different context, Vaudano applied DCM to assess effective connectivity between regions commonly exhibiting BOLD activity changes in association with generalized spike and wave discharges [148].

Clinical Implications: Validation Studies

After two decades of EEG/fMRI epilepsy research, its clinical usefulness is increasingly apparent. The obvious clinical potential is that of an additional non-invasive tool to localize epileptic activity as part of the pre-surgical evaluation of patients with focal epilepsy [9, 80, 91-92]. It is important, therefore, to understand the sensitivity and specificity of EEG/fMRI data, and these will help to determine the reliability of the results. Few reports exist in which the reliability has been determined against intracranial EEG recordings. One study demonstrated that EEG/fMRI activation maxima on average were 6 cm away from the dipolar sources of surface EEG spikes [106]. This is not unexpected since the BOLD signal originates mainly in draining veins and is only an indirect measure of the activity of some synapses, not all of which is detected by the EEG [27-28]. The BOLD signal arises from changes in blood oxygenation within the capillaries where the oxygenation change occurs, as well as within downstream draining veins. Neuronal activation thus alters susceptibility signal in the blood of the active capillaries and veins, leading to a change in the magnetic field within active vessels that correlates with the activity. Because it is believed that the most relevant cortical activations detected through BOLD contrast are those which are tied to the microvasculature, where the blood oxygenation change occurs, many attempts have been made (especially relevant at higher field strengths) to reduce the contributions from the macrovasculature, or large draining veins, to the BOLD-computed cortical activations [149]. Nevertheless, the important clinical question is how the scalp IEA-correlated hemodynamic changes benefit the individual with epilepsy, i.e. the better localization of the irritative and seizure onset zones [97]. Of primary interest to interpreting EEG/fMRI results clinically is the knowledge of how they relate to ictal and interictal intracranial electrophysiology recordings.

While the simultaneous acquisition of intracranial EEG and fMRI is on its way [150-151], the comparison of non-invasive EEG/fMRI with invasive electrophysiology data on individual patients has suggested that there is generally good concordance of some but not all scalp IEA-correlated fMRI changes with ictal and interictal invasive EEG findings [92, 152-156]. From a relatively large cohort of patients, the concordance between EEG/fMRI signal changes and stereotactic EEG was investigated in 5 patients. Bénar and colleagues showed that if intracranial EEG was sampled from near a region of BOLD activation or deactivation, then usually at least one contact was "active" [157]. Ziljmans and colleagues showed that in four of 29 patients EEG/fMRI results motivated the reconsideration of patients previously considered not eligible for epilepsy surgery. In two of them intracranial EEG confirmed epileptic activity in the region of BOLD activation [116].

Another validation approach is to compare the location of IEA-related BOLD signal changes obtained preoperatively with the region actually resected and subsequent postoperative outcome. In a patient series analysed by Thornton and colleagues, seven of ten patients showing epileptic activity-related BOLD signal changes were seizure free following surgery and the area of maximal BOLD signal change was concordant with the resected area in six of seven cases. In the remaining 3 patients with reduced seizure frequency post-surgically, areas of significant IEA-correlated BOLD signal change lay outside the resection area [158]. Hence, EEG/fMRI may add to preoperative evaluation when patients have frequent IED on routine EEG by supporting localization theories suggested by complementary diagnostic tests (e.g. EEG, structural imaging) or proposing regions particularly when other tests do not indicate a clear-cut epileptogenic focus. Thus, EEG/fMRI potentially can be of predictive value for surgical outcome in focal epilepsy.

Controversial Findings: Possible Explainations

As discussed in the preceding paragraphs, the cumulative body of EEG/fMRI studies in epilepsy made it clear that the convolution of scalp EEG-marked IEA with a fixed hemodynamic response function as used in standard fMRI analyses of healthy volunteers does not unambiguously reveal the "irritative zone" [110]. Instead, data support the likely possibility that scalp EEG changes reflect only a part of the assumed "epileptogenic network" activity that is at least spatially more comprehensively captured by fMRI. Reasons for this include that EEG and fMRI measure different biological processes as discussed above. Furthermore, among those neuronal processes that scalp EEG indeed is known to be capable in principle of registering, surface recordings may not reflect neuronal discharges of certain spatial configurations or locations. It is hence unsurprising that hemodynamic changes have been found to precede or outlast scalp EEG changes [105, 111, 138], reflecting evolution as well as propagation of epileptiform activity [159]. That alone would suffice to explain the often difficult to interpret results of routine analysis. Additionally, whether the neurovascular coupling in brain regions affected by epilepsy is disturbed [110] or not [160-163] remains uncertain. In other words, IEA-associated hemodynamic changes derived from surface EEG will reflect different aspects of the epileptogenic processes depending on the underlying pathology: in some circumstances (as demonstrated) the IEA-related BOLD response indeed will reflect the irritative zone, while in others it may reflect propagated activity, or in some instances, the resulting associated cognitive state of the individual. The latter may relate to what clinically is referred to as "semiology", which will be discussed in the following paragraph. Assessment of the clinical applicability or yield of EEG/fMRI [10, 91, 158, 164] will become more meaningful in the future as they consider which part of the epileptogenic process is being measured.

A Different Application: Insights into the Neurobiology of Epilepsy?

Some aspects of the IEA-correlated EEG/fMRI results were clearer when groups of patients with particular epilepsy syndromes were considered compared to when individual subjects were analyzed. While such group studies do not benefit individual patients, they contribute to the understanding of the neurobiology of the epilepsies. In the context of the above, they relate to the average epileptogenic process time-linked to the EEG phenomena on which the analyses are based.

Accordingly, they identified the temporally related subpart of the epileptic network (brain regions that change their activity in association with IEA without necessarily being their actual electrical source) in temporal lobe [98-99] and generalized epilepsies [96, 165-166]. In generalized epilepsy, both at the individual subject [166-169] and the group level [96, 165], fMRI activations in response to generalized spike and wave activity (GSW) were found in the thalamus along with cortical deactivations – similar to electrophysiological data obtained in animal studies suggesting a cortico-thalamic loop of excitatory and inhibitory synaptic activity [170]. The particular patterns of cortical deactivation may specifically be related to the semiology of typical absences: 'default mode' areas of the brain exhibit reduced activity during GSW [165, 167, 169]. The precuneus and bilateral frontal and parietal cortices are usually more active during relaxed wakefulness than either goal directed behaviour or states of reduced consciousness, such as sleep and anaesthesia [37]. Reduced consciousness during absences parallels that during reduced vigilance both phenomenologically and in the in cortical areas hemodynamically. It may be that because of the analysis strategy (fMRI block design), only the common relay station, the thalamus, and the lower activity in default mode brain regions are detected [48] and the BOLD correlates of the sources of the generalized EEG discharges are not identified.

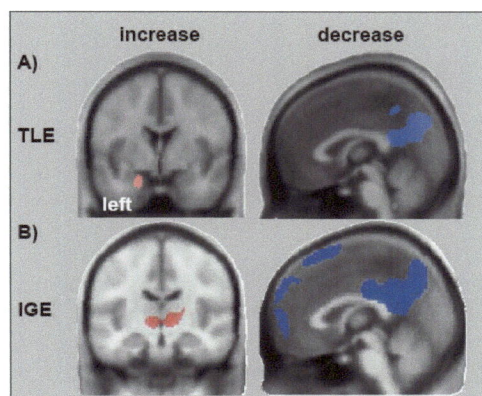

Fig. (6.5). shows brain regions typically involved in temporal lobe and idiopathic generalized epilepsies. EEG/fMRI in epilepsy had initially been used attempting to map the area of cortical tissue that generates interictal epileptic discharges. Panel (A) shows the common BOLD signal increases in response to frequent focal interictal spikes in a group of patients with left temporal lobe epilepsy (TLE). Despite heterogeneous EEG features and histopathology, the hippocampus, known to play a crucial role in TLE, was activated. BOLD signal decreases were commonly observed in the retrosplenium and precuneus, brain areas typically active during conscious rest, suggesting that focal interictal discharges affect ongoing brain function even when a seizure cannot be observed. Panel (B) shows that, in idiopathic generalized epilepsies with absence seizures, similar brain regions exhibit generalized spike and wave-associated BOLD signal decreases. BOLD signal increases typically occur bilaterally in the thalamus. Figure taken from Laufs, Duncan, Electroencephalography/functional MRI in human epilepsy: what it currently can and cannot do, Curr Opin Neurol 2007, 20:4, 417-23 with permission from Wolters Kluwer Health.

Interestingly, an analogous pattern of sub-neocortical activation and neocortical deactivation was found in a group analysis of patients with heterogeneous temporal lobe epilepsy syndromes with frequent IEA. There was common ipsilateral IEA-correlated hippocampal activation and cortical deactivation of default mode brain regions, which included areas distant to the temporal lobe [99]. Remote intra- and extra-temporal activations and deactivations, including the contralateral temporal lobe, have also been associated with temporal lobe spikes [98].

It was suggested that the hippocampus might act as a common relay station in temporal lobe epilepsy, with some analogy to the thalamus in generalized epilepsies [99]. The activity decrease of consciousness-subserving default mode areas, in association with *inter*ictal epileptic activity, may explain the phenomenon of transient cognitive impairment [99, 171][1]. Contrasting this interpretation, activity patterns in the precuneus may facilitate the occurrence of the epileptic process [148]. The widespread deactivations in default mode brain regions during both focal and generalized epileptiform

---

[1] "Epileptiform discharges not accompanied by obvious clinical events are generally regarded as subclinical or interictal. However, in many patients sensitive methods of observation, notably continuous psychological testing, show brief episodes of impaired cognitive function during such discharges. This phenomenon of transitory cognitive impairment (TCI) is found in about 50% of patients who show discharges during testing. TCI is not simple inattention. The effects are material and site specific: lateralised discharges are associated with deficits of functions mediated by the hemisphere in which the discharges occur. Conversely, specific tasks can activate or suppress focal discharges over the brain regions that mediate the cognitive activity in question. TCI clearly contributes to the cognitive problems of some people with epilepsy and may cause deficits that pass unrecognised" (171.
Binnie CD. Cognitive impairment during epileptiform discharges: is it ever justifiable to treat the EEG? Lancet Neurol 2003; 2(12): 725-30).

discharges suggest that the term '*inter*ictal epileptic activity' may need to be understood with caution: a distinction between ictal and interictal epileptiform activity may be difficult to make (Fig. **6.5**).

THE FUTURE

EEG/fMRI will not replace intracranial EEG studies in the near future because of the discussed problem that the former cannot specifically distinguish between the irritative zone, the epileptogenic zone as well as prodromal and propagation effects. More recently developed analysis strategies such as effective connectivity studies of the EEG as well as the fMRI data however may open new avenues.

In some epilepsy surgery centres, EEG/fMRI in certain cases is used as an additional non-invasive diagnostic tool. Its future clinical role will crucially depend on comparative studies of intracranial EEG and interictal as well as ictal EEG/fMRI studies but which is complicated by the different spatial coverage of these investigations. Given current technical developments and safety evaluations of simultaneous intracranial EEG recordings during fMRI [151, 172], this next important milestone in the field is about to be at hand.

EEG/FMRI STUDIES IN CHILDREN

Paralleling the mentioned development of EEG/fMRI studies mainly performed in adults, a growing number of studies have been performed in the paediatric population [109, 112, 114-115, 126, 153, 173-182]. They have enhanced the conceptual understanding of EEG/fMRI studies in epilepsy and have been discussed alongside the adult population studies above.

In addition to this, in children, the role of EEG/fMRI as a non-invasive pre-surgical diagnostic tool is of particular interest: early surgical treatment of medically refractory epilepsy should be sought [183], and because the threshold to perform invasive investigations is often higher than in adults, this non-invasive investigation would be of great benefit. Longitudinal EEG/fMRI studies of epilepsy syndromes in paediatric populations should help to better understand disease progression revealing starting points for new treatment strategies before the epilepsy syndromes reach their adult forms, which can be potentially more resistant to treatment.

SUMMARY AND FUTURE DIRECTIONS

This chapter has reviewed simultaneous EEG/fMRI studies of healthy subjects across different vigilance states and of patients with epilepsy. The acquisition techniques have reached a level of sophistication that does not currently impose relevant constraints. The analysis and interpretation levels however suffer from the fact that as much as the relationship between neuronal activity and the BOLD signal is not yet fully understood, even more complex is the combination of EEG with BOLD-fMRI. While in studies of healthy subjects meaningful inferences can be made after careful intellectual conceptualization (compare Fig. **6.1**), this is hardly possible in patient populations: firstly, it is unclear whether neurovascualer coupling can be treated as normal allowing the same methodologies and interpretations to be applied as in studies of healthy individuals. Secondly, it is unknown which part of the underlying epileptic processes are reflected in the (scalp) EEG to which the observed fMRI changes are linked.

The way forward might partly lie in the thorough detailed methodological refinements at the individual study level, and by the further development of data fusion methods in the wider sense. These advances can incorporate the entirety of the acquired EEG and fMRI data as well as focus on phenomena of particular interest. This should allow the better appreciation of observed effects in the broader context of the experiment. Nevertheless, the joint interpretation of EEG and fMRI whole brain data remains an ill-posed problem due to the modalities' physical (temporal and spatial sampling), physiological (signal substrate) and technical (noise sources and characteristics) disjunction. Invasive electrophysiological recordings, which are limited by their spatial coverage, in combination with high resolution fMRI represent the obvious next step resulting in interpretation models for this type of multimodal imaging data at least within circumscribed brain regions.

ACKNOWLEDGEMENT

"Helmut Laufs is funded by the Bundesministerium für Bildung und Forschung (Germany), BMBF 01 EV 0703 and this work in part by LOEWE Neuronale Koordination Forschungsschwerpunkt Frankfurt (NeFF)".

REFERENCES

[1]   Friston KJ. Statistical parametric mapping: the analysis of functional brain images. Amsterdam ; London: Elsevier/Academic Press; 2007.

[2]   Buckner RL, Vincent JL. Unrest at rest: default activity and spontaneous network correlations. Neuroimage 2007; 37(4): 1091-6; discussion 7-9.

[3]   Raichle ME, Snyder AZ. A default mode of brain function: a brief history of an evolving idea. Neuroimage 2007; 7(4): 1083-90; discussion 97-9.

[4]   Dang-Vu TT, Schabus M, Desseilles M, *et al.* Spontaneous neural activity during human slow wave sleep. Proc Natl Acad Sci USA 2008.

[5]   Owen AM, Schiff ND, Laureys S. A new era of coma and consciousness science. Prog Brain Res 2009; 177: 399-411.

[6]   Tyvaert L, Hawco C, Kobayashi E, Levan P, Dubeau F, Gotman J. Different structures involved during ictal and interictal epileptic activity in malformations of cortical development: an EEG-fMRI study. Brain 2008; 131(Pt 8): 2042-60.

[7]   Ment LR, Hirtz D, Huppi PS. Imaging biomarkers of outcome in the developing preterm brain. Lancet Neurol 2009; 8(11): 1042-55.

[8]   Vincent JL, Patel GH, Fox MD, *et al.* Intrinsic functional architecture in the anaesthetized monkey brain. Nature 2007; 447(7140): 83-6.

[9]   Gotman J, Kobayashi E, Bagshaw AP, Benar CG, Dubeau F. Combining EEG and fMRI: a multimodal tool for epilepsy research. J Magn Reson Imaging 2006; 23(6): 906-20.

[10]   Laufs H, Duncan JS. Electroencephalography/functional MRI in human epilepsy: what it currently can and cannot do. Curr Opin Neurol 2007; 20(4): 417-23.

[11]   Laufs H. Endogenous brain oscillations and related networks detected by surface EEG-combined fMRI. Hum Brain Mapp 2008; 29(7): 762-9.

[12]   Laufs H, Walker MC, Lund TE. "Brain activation and hypothalamic functional connectivity during human non-rapid eye movement sleep: an EEG/fMRI study" - its limitations and an alternative approach. Brain 2007; 130(Pt 7): e75.

[13]   Schabus M, Dang-Vu TT, Albouy G, *et al.* Hemodynamic cerebral correlates of sleep spindles during human non-rapid eye movement sleep. Proc Natl Acad Sci USA 2007; 104(32): 13164-9.

[14]   Greicius M. Resting-state functional connectivity in neuropsychiatric disorders. Curr Opin Neurol 2008; 21(4): 424-30.

[15]   Eidelberg D. Metabolic brain networks in neurodegenerative disorders: a functional imaging approach. Trends Neurosci 2009 ; 32(10): 548-57.

[16]   Damoiseaux JS, Greicius MD. Greater than the sum of its parts: a review of studies combining structural connectivity and resting-state functional connectivity. Brain Struct Funct 2009; 213(6): 525-33.

[17]   Moeller F, Tyvaert L, Nguyen DK, *et al.* EEG-fMRI: adding to standard evaluations of patients with nonlesional frontal lobe epilepsy. Neurology 2009; 73(23): 2023-30.

[18]   Gotman J. Epileptic networks studied with EEG-fMRI. Epilepsia 2008; 49 Suppl 3: 42-51.

[19]   Krakow K. Imaging epileptic activity using functional MRI. Neurodegener Dis 2008; 5(5): 286-95.

[20]   Cunningham CJ, Zaamout Mel F, Goodyear B, Federico P. Simultaneous EEG-fMRI in human epilepsy. Can J Neurol Sci 2008; 35(4): 420-35.

[21]   Rechtschaffen A, Kales AA. A manual of standardized terminology, techniques and scoring system for sleep stages of human subjects. Washington, D.C.: Government Printing Office; 1968.

[22]   Gibbs FA, Davis H, Lennox WG. The electro-encephalogram in epilepsy and in conditions of impaired consciousness. Arch Neurol Psych 1935(34): 1133.

[23]   Laufs H, Daunizeau J, Carmichael DW, Kleinschmidt A. Recent advances in recording electrophysiological data simultaneously with magnetic resonance imaging. Neuroimage 2008; 40(2): 515-28.

[24]   Daunizeau J, Vaudano AE, Lemieux L. Bayesian multi-modal model comparison: a case study on the generators of the spike and the wave in generalized spike-wave complexes. Neuroimage 2010; 49(1): 656-67.

[25]   Daunizeau J, Grova C, Marrelec G, *et al.* Symmetrical event-related EEG/fMRI information fusion in a variational Bayesian framework. Neuroimage 2007; 36(1): 69-87.

[26]   Valdes-Sosa PA, Sanchez-Bornot JM, Sotero RC, *et al.* Model driven EEG/fMRI fusion of brain oscillations. Hum Brain Mapp 2009; 30(9): 2701-21.

[27]   Logothetis NK, Pauls J, Augath M, Trinath T, Oeltermann A. Neurophysiological investigation of the basis of the fMRI signal. Nature 2001; 412(6843): 150-7.

[28]   Shmuel A, Augath M, Oeltermann A, Logothetis NK. Negative functional MRI response correlates with reases in neuronal activity in monkey visual area V1. Nat Neurosci 2006; 9(4): 569-77.

[29]   Nunez PL, Silberstein RB. On the relationship of synaptic activity to macroscopic measurements: does co-registration of EEG with fMRI make sense? Brain Topogr 2000; 13(2): 79-96.

[30]   Takano T, Tian GF, Peng W, *et al.* Astrocyte-mediated control of cerebral blood flow. Nat Neurosci 2006; 9(2): 260-7.

[31]   Tian GF, Azmi H, Takano T, *et al.* An astrocytic basis of epilepsy. Nat Med 2005; 11(9): 973-81.

[32]   Ives JR, Warach S, Schmitt F, Edelman RR, Schomer DL. Monitoring the patient's EEG during echo planar MRI. Electroencephalogr Clin Neurophysiol 1993; 87(6): 417-20.

[33]   Laufs H, Daunizeau J, Carmichael D, Kleinschmidt AK. Recent advances in recording electrophysiological data simultaneously with magnetic resonance imaging. Neuroimage 2007: in press.

[34]   Ritter P, Villringer A. Simultaneous EEG-fMRI. Neurosci Biobehav Rev 2006; 30(6): 823-38.

[35]   Richardson M. Current themes in neuroimaging of epilepsy: Brain networks, dynamic phenomena, and clinical relevance. Clin Neurophysiol 2010.

[36]   Fox MD, Raichle ME. Spontaneous fluctuations in brain activity observed with functional magnetic resonance imaging. Nat Rev Neurosci 2007; 8(9): 700-11.

[37]   Raichle ME, MacLeod AM, Snyder AZ, Powers WJ, Gusnard DA, Shulman GL. A default mode of brain function. Proc Natl Acad Sci USA 2001; 98(2): 676-82.

[38]   Mazoyer B, Zago L, Mellet E, et al. Cortical networks for working memory and executive functions sustain the conscious resting state in man. Brain Res Bull 2001; 54(3): 287-98.

[39]   Broyd SJ, Demanuele C, Debener S, Helps SK, James CJ, Sonuga-Barke EJ. Default-mode brain dysfunction in mental disorders: a systematic review. Neurosci Biobehav Rev 2009; 33(3): 279-96.

[40]   Laufs H, Holt JL, Elfont R, et al. Where the BOLD signal goes when alpha EEG leaves. Neuroimage 2006; 31(4): 1408-18.

[41]   Giraud AL, Kleinschmidt AK, Poeppel D, Lund TE, Frackowiak R, Laufs H. Endogenous cortical rhythms determine cerebral specialisation for speech perception and production. Neuron 2007; In Press, Accepted Manuscript.

[42]   Berger H. Über das Elektrenkephalogramm des Menschen. Archiv für Psychiatrie und Nervenkrankheiten 1929; 87: 527-70.

[43]   Moosmann M, Ritter P, Krastel I, et al. Correlates of alpha rhythm in functional magnetic resonance imaging and near infrared spectroscopy. Neuroimage 2003; 20(1): 145-58.

[44]   Goldman RI, Stern JM, Engel J, Jr., Cohen MS. Tomographic mapping of alpha rhythm using simultaneous EEG/fMRI. NeuroImage 2001. p. S1291.

[45]   Mantini D, Perrucci MG, Del Gratta C, Romani GL, Corbetta M. Electrophysiological signatures of resting state networks in the human brain. Proc Natl Acad Sci USA 2007; 104(32): 13170-5.

[46]   Difrancesco MW, Holland SK, Szaflarski JP. Simultaneous EEG/functional magnetic resonance imaging at 4 Tesla: correlates of brain activity to spontaneous alpha rhythm during relaxation. J Clin Neurophysiol 2008; 25(5): 255-64.

[47]   Laufs H, Kleinschmidt A, Beyerle A, et al. EEG-correlated fMRI of human alpha activity. Neuroimage 2003; 19(4): 1463-76.

[48]   Laufs H, Krakow K, Sterzer P, et al. Electroencephalographic signatures of attentional and cognitive default modes in spontaneous brain activity fluctuations at rest. Proc Natl Acad Sci USA 2003; 100(19): 11053-8.

[49]   Jann K, Wiest R, Hauf M, et al. BOLD correlates of continuously fluctuating epileptic activity isolated by independent component analysis. Neuroimage 2008; 42(2): 635-48.

[50]   Goncalves SI, de Munck JC, Pouwels PJ, et al. Correlating the alpha rhythm to BOLD using simultaneous EEG/fMRI: Inter-subject variability. Neuroimage 2006; 30(1): 203-13.

[51]   de Munck JC, Goncalves SI, Mammoliti R, Heethaar RM, Lopes da Silva FH. Interactions between different EEG frequency bands and their effect on alpha-fMRI correlations. Neuroimage 2009; 47(1): 69-76.

[52]   Tyvaert L, Levan P, Grova C, Dubeau F, Gotman J. Effects of fluctuating physiological rhythms during prolonged EEG-fMRI studies. Clin Neurophysiol 2008; 119(12): 2762-74.

[53]   Mullinger K, Brookes M, Stevenson C, Morgan P, Bowtell R. Exploring the feasibility of simultaneous electroencephalography/functional magnetic resonance imaging at 7 T. Magn Reson Imaging 2008; 26(7): 968-77.

[54]   Feige B, Scheffler K, Esposito F, Di Salle F, Hennig J, Seifritz E. Cortical and subcortical correlates of electroencephalographic alpha rhythm modulation. J Neurophysiol 2005; 93(5): 2864-72.

[55]   Kjaer TW, Law I, Wiltschiotz G, Paulson OB, Madsen PL. Regional cerebral blood flow during light sleep--a H(2)(15)O-PET study. J Sleep Res 2002; 11(3): 201-7.

[56]   Lehmann D, Ozaki H, Pal I. EEG alpha map series: brain micro-states by space-oriented adaptive segmentation. Electroencephalogr Clin Neurophysiol 1987; 67(3): 271-88.

[57]   Lehmann D, Skrandies W. Reference-free identification of components of checkerboard-evoked multichannel potential fields. Electroencephalogr Clin Neurophysiol 1980; 48(6): 609-21.

[58]   Pascual-Marqui RD, Michel CM, Lehmann D. Segmentation of brain electrical activity into microstates: model estimation and validation. IEEE Trans Biomed Eng 1995; 42(7): 658-65.

[59]   Britz J, Van De Ville D, Michel CM. BOLD correlates of EEG topography reveal rapid resting-state network dynamics. Neuroimage 2010.

[60]   Musso F, Brinkmeyer J, Mobascher A, Warbrick T, Winterer G. Spontaneous brain activity and EEG microstates. A novel EEG/fMRI analysis approach to explore resting-state networks. Neuroimage 2010.

[61]   Laufs H. Multimodal analysis of resting state cortical activity: What does EEG add to our knowledge of resting state BOLD networks? Neuroimage 2010.

[62]   Iber C, Ancoli-Israel S, Chesson A, Quan S, Medicine. ftAAoS, editors. The AASM Manual for the Scoring of Sleep and Associated Events: Rules, Terminology and Technical Specification. Westchester: American Academy of Sleep Medicine; 2007.

[63]   Maquet P. Functional neuroimaging of normal human sleep by positron emission tomography. J Sleep Res 2000; 9(3): 207-31.

[64]   Lund TE, Madsen KH, Sidaros K, Luo WL, Nichols TE. Non-white noise in fMRI: does modelling have an impact? Neuroimage 2006; 29(1): 54-66.

[65]   Czisch M, Wetter TC, Kaufmann C, Pollmacher T, Holsboer F, Auer DP. Altered processing of acoustic stimuli during sleep: reduced auditory activation and visual deactivation detected by a combined fMRI/EEG study. Neuroimage 2002; 16(1): 251-8.

[66]   Born AP, Law I, Lund TE, *et al.* Cortical deactivation induced by visual stimulation in human slow-wave sleep. Neuroimage 2002; 17(3): 1325-35.

[67]   Czisch M, Wehrle R, Kaufmann C, *et al.* Functional MRI during sleep: BOLD signal reases and their electrophysiological correlates. Eur J Neurosci 2004; 20(2): 566-74.

[68]   Kaufmann C, Wehrle R, Wetter TC, *et al.* Brain activation and hypothalamic functional connectivity during human non-rapid eye movement sleep: an EEG/fMRI study. Brain 2006; 129(Pt 3): 655-67.

[69]   Laufs H, Walker MC, Lund TE. 'Brain activation and hypothalamic functional connectivity during human non-rapid eye movement sleep: an EEG/fMRI study'--its limitations and an alternative approach. Brain 2007; 130(Pt 7): e75; author reply e6.

[70]   Horovitz SG, Fukunaga M, de Zwart JA, *et al.* Low frequency BOLD fluctuations during resting wakefulness and light sleep: a simultaneous EEG-fMRI study. Hum Brain Mapp 2008; 29(6): 671-82.

[71]   Horovitz SG, Braun AR, Carr WS, *et al.* oupling of the brain's default mode network during deep sleep. Proc Natl Acad Sci USA 2009; 106(27): 11376-81.

[72]   Vanhaudenhuyse A, Noirhomme Q, Tshibanda LJ, *et al.* Default network connectivity reflects the level of consciousness in non-communicative brain-damaged patients. Brain 2010; 133(Pt 1): 161-71.

[73]   Picchioni D, Fukunaga M, Carr WS, *et al.* fMRI differences between early and late stage-1 sleep. Neurosci Lett 2008; 441(1): 81-5.

[74]   Olbrich S, Mulert C, Karch S, *et al.* EEG-vigilance and BOLD effect during simultaneous EEG/fMRI measurement. Neuroimage 2009; 45(2): 319-32.

[75]   Josephs O, Henson RN. Event-related functional magnetic resonance imaging: modelling, inference and optimization. Philos Trans R Soc Lond B Biol Sci 1999; 354(1387): 1215-28.

[76]   Moehring J, Moeller F, Jacobs J, *et al.* Non-REM sleep influences results of fMRI studies in epilepsy. Neurosci Lett 2008; 443(2): 61-6.

[77]   Leclercq Y, Balteau E, Dang-Vu T, *et al.* Rejection of pulse related artefact (PRA) from continuous electroencephalographic (EEG) time series recorded during functional magnetic resonance imaging (fMRI) using constraint independent component analysis (cICA). Neuroimage 2009; 44(3): 679-91.

[78]   Lee JH, Oh S, Jolesz FA, Park H, Yoo SS. Application of independent component analysis for the data mining of simultaneous Eeg-fMRI: preliminary experience on sleep onset. Int J Neurosci 2009; 119(8): 1118-36.

[79]   Hamandi K, Duncan JS. FMRI in the Evaluation of the Ictal Onset Zone. In: Lüders HO, editor. Textbook of Epilepsy Surgery: informa healthcare; 2008. p. Chapter 80.

[80]   Hamandi K, Salek-Haddadi A, Fish DR, Lemieux L. EEG/functional MRI in epilepsy: The Queen Square Experience. J Clin Neurophysiol 2004; 21(4): 241-8.

[81]   Salek-Haddadi A, Friston KJ, Lemieux L, Fish DR. Studying spontaneous EEG activity with fMRI. Brain Res Brain Res Rev 2003; 43(1): 110-33.

[82]   Stern JM. Simultaneous electroencephalography and functional magnetic resonance imaging applied to epilepsy. Epilepsy Behav 2006; 8(4): 683-92.

[83]   Yu AH, Li KC, Piao CF, Li HL. Application of functional MRI in epilepsy. Chin Med J (Engl) 2005; 118(12): 1022-7.

[84]   Lemieux L, Allen PJ, Franconi F, Symms MR, Fish DR. Recording of EEG during fMRI experiments: patient safety. Magn Reson Med 1997; 38(6): 943-52.

[85]   Laufs H, Daunizeau J, Kleinschmidt AK. Recent advances in recording electrophysiological data simultaneously with magnetic resonance imaging. Current Medical Imaging Reviews 2007.

[86]   Gotman J, Benar CG, Dubeau F. Combining EEG and FMRI in epilepsy: methodological challenges and clinical results. J Clin Neurophysiol 2004; 21(4): 229-40.

[87]   Nunez PL, Srinivasan R. Electric fields of the brain : the neurophysics of EEG. 2nd ed. Oxford: Oxford University Press; 2006.

[88]   Bagshaw AP, Torab L, Kobayashi E, *et al.* EEG-fMRI using z-shimming in patients with temporal lobe epilepsy. J Magn Reson Imaging 2006; 24(5): 1025-32.

[89]   Wiebe S, Blume WT, Girvin JP, Eliasziw M. A randomized, controlled trial of surgery for temporal-lobe epilepsy. N Engl J Med 2001; 345(5): 311-8.

[90]   Lemieux L. Electroencephalography-correlated functional MR imaging studies of epileptic activity. Neuroimaging Clin N Am 2004; 14(3): 487-506.

[91]   Salek-Haddadi A, Diehl B, Hamandi K, *et al.* Hemodynamic correlates of epileptiform discharges: an EEG-fMRI study of 63 patients with focal epilepsy. Brain Res 2006; 1088(1): 148-66.

[92]   Al-Asmi A, Benar CG, Gross DW, *et al.* fMRI activation in continuous and spike-triggered EEG-fMRI studies of epileptic spikes. Epilepsia 2003; 44(10): 1328-39.

[93]   Patel MR, Blum A, Pearlman JD, *et al.* Echo-planar functional MR imaging of epilepsy with concurrent EEG monitoring. AJNR Am J Neuroradiol 1999; 20(10): 1916-9.

[94]   Krakow K, Woermann FG, Symms MR, *et al.* EEG-triggered functional MRI of interictal epileptiform activity in patients with partial seizures. Brain 1999; 122 (Pt 9): 1679-88.

[95]   Aghakhani Y, Bagshaw AP, Benar CG, *et al.* fMRI activation during spike and wave discharges in idiopathic generalized epilepsy. Brain. 2004; 127(Pt 5): 1127-44.

[96]   Hamandi K, Salek-Haddadi A, Laufs H, *et al.* EEG-fMRI of idiopathic and secondarily generalized epilepsies. Neuroimage 2006; 31(4): 1700-10.

[97]   Rosenow F, Luders H. Presurgical evaluation of epilepsy. Brain 2001; 124(Pt 9): 1683-700.

[98]   Kobayashi E, Bagshaw AP, Benar CG, *et al.* Temporal and extratemporal BOLD responses to temporal lobe interictal spikes. Epilepsia 2006; 47(2): 343-54.

[99]   Laufs H, Hamandi K, Salek-Haddadi A, Kleinschmidt AK, Duncan JS, Lemieux L. Temporal lobe interictal epileptic discharges affect cerebral activity in "default mode" brain regions. Hum Brain Mapp 2006; 28(10): 1923-32.

[100]   Federico P, Archer JS, Abbott DF, Jackson GD. Cortical/subcortical BOLD changes associated with epileptic discharges: an EEG-fMRI study at 3 T. Neurology 2005; 64(7): 1125-30.

[101]   Kobayashi E, Bagshaw AP, Gotman J, Dubeau F. Metabolic correlates of epileptic spikes in cerebral cavernous angiomas. Epilepsy Res 2007; 73(1): 98-103.

[102]   Kobayashi E, Bagshaw AP, Grova C, Gotman J, Dubeau F. Grey matter heterotopia: what EEG-fMRI can tell us about epileptogenicity of neuronal migration disorders. Brain 2006; 129(Pt 2): 366-74.

[103]   Kobayashi E, Bagshaw AP, Jansen A, *et al.* Intrinsic epileptogenicity in polymicrogyric cortex suggested by EEG-fMRI BOLD responses. Neurology 2005; 64(7): 1263-6.

[104]   Lemieux L, Laufs H, Carmichael D, Paul JS, Walker MC, Duncan JS. Noncanonical spike-related BOLD responses in focal epilepsy. Hum Brain Mapp 2007; doi: 10.1002/hbm.20389.

[105]   Hawco CS, Bagshaw AP, Lu Y, Dubeau F, Gotman J. BOLD changes occur prior to epileptic spikes seen on scalp EEG. Neuroimage 2007; 35(4): 1450-8.

[106]   Bagshaw AP, Kobayashi E, Dubeau F, Pike GB, Gotman J. Correspondence between EEG-fMRI and EEG dipole localisation of interictal discharges in focal epilepsy. Neuroimage 2006; 30(2):417-25.

[107]   Lu Y, Grova C, Kobayashi E, Dubeau F, Gotman J. Using voxel-specific hemodynamic response function in EEG-fMRI data analysis: An estimation and detection model. Neuroimage 2007; 34(1): 195-203.

[108]   Lu Y, Bagshaw AP, Grova C, Kobayashi E, Dubeau F, Gotman J. Using voxel-specific hemodynamic response function in EEG-fMRI data analysis. Neuroimage 2006; 32(1): 238-47.

[109]   Masterton RA, Harvey AS, Archer JS, *et al.* Focal epileptiform spikes do not show a canonical BOLD response in patients with benign rolandic epilepsy (BECTS). Neuroimage 2010.

[110]   Grouiller F, Vercueil L, Krainik A, Segebarth C, Kahane P, David O. Characterization of the hemodynamic modes associated with interictal epileptic activity using a deformable model-based analysis of combined EEG and functional MRI recordings. Hum Brain Mapp 2010.

[111]   Moeller F, Siebner HR, Wolff S, *et al.* Changes in activity of striato-thalamo-cortical network precede generalized spike wave discharges. Neuroimage 2008; 39(4): 1839-49.

[112]   Moeller F, Siebner HR, Wolff S, *et al.* Simultaneous EEG-fMRI in drug-naive children with newly diagnosed absence epilepsy. Epilepsia 2008; 49(9): 1510-9.

[113]   Kang JK, Benar C, Al-Asmi A, *et al.* Using patient-specific hemodynamic response functions in combined EEG-fMRI studies in epilepsy. Neuroimage 2003; 20(2): 1162-70.

[114]   Jacobs J, Hawco C, Kobayashi E, *et al.* Variability of the hemodynamic response as a function of age and frequency of epileptic discharge in children with epilepsy. Neuroimage 2008; 40(2): 601-14.

[115]   Jacobs J, Kobayashi E, Boor R, *et al.* Hemodynamic responses to interictal epileptiform discharges in children with symptomatic epilepsy. Epilepsia 2007; 48(11): 2068-78.

[116]   Zijlmans M, Huiskamp G, Hersevoort M, Seppenwoolde JH, van Huffelen AC, Leijten FS. EEG-fMRI in the preoperative work-up for epilepsy surgery. Brain 2007; 130(Pt 9): 2343-53.

[117]   Lemieux L, Salek-Haddadi A, Lund TE, Laufs H, Carmichael D. Modelling large motion events in fMRI studies of patients with epilepsy. Magn Reson Imaging 2007; 25(6): 894-901.

[118]   Liston AD, Lund TE, Salek-Haddadi A, Hamandi K, Friston KJ, Lemieux L. Modelling cardiac signal as a confound in EEG-fMRI and its application in focal epilepsy studies. Neuroimage 2006; 30(3): 827-34.

[119]   Siniatchkin M, Moeller F, Jacobs J, *et al.* Spatial filters and automated spike detection based on brain topographies improve sensitivity of EEG-fMRI studies in focal epilepsy. Neuroimage 2007; 37(3): 834-43.

[120]   Huiskamp GJ. Reduction of the Ballistocardiogram Artifact in Simultaneous EEG-fMRI using ICA. Conf Proc IEEE Eng Med Biol Soc 2005; 4: 3691-4.

[121]   Flanagan D, Abbott DF, Jackson GD. How wrong can we be? The effect of inaccurate mark-up of EEG/fMRI studies in epilepsy. Clin Neurophysiol 2009; 120(9): 1637-47.

[122]   Liston AD, De Munck JC, Hamandi K, *et al.* Analysis of EEG-fMRI data in focal epilepsy based on automated spike classification and Signal Space Projection. Neuroimage 2006; 31(3): 1015-24.

[123]   Marques JP, Rebola J, Figueiredo P, Pinto A, Sales F, Castelo-Branco M. ICA omposition of EEG signal for fMRI processing in epilepsy. Hum Brain Mapp 2009; 30(9): 2986-96.

[124]   Bagshaw AP, Hawco C, Benar CG, *et al.* Analysis of the EEG-fMRI response to prolonged bursts of interictal epileptiform activity. Neuroimage 2005; 24(4): 1099-112.

[125]   Vulliemoz S, Rodionov R, Carmichael DW, *et al*. Continuous EEG source imaging enhances analysis of EEG-fMRI in focal epilepsy. Neuroimage 2010; 49(4): 3219-29.

[126]   Siniatchkin M, van Baalen A, Jacobs J, *et al*. Different Neuronal Networks Are Associated with Spikes and Slow Activity in Hypsarrhythmia. Epilepsia 2007; doi:10.1111/j.1528-1167.2007.01195.x.

[127]   Rodionov R, De Martino F, Laufs H, *et al*. Independent component analysis of interictal fMRI in focal epilepsy: comparison with general linear model-based EEG-correlated fMRI. Neuroimage 2007; 38(3): 488-500.

[128]   LeVan P, Tyvaert L, Moeller F, Gotman J. Independent component analysis reveals dynamic ictal BOLD responses in EEG-fMRI data from focal epilepsy patients. Neuroimage 2010; 49(1): 366-78.

[129]   Hamandi K, Salek Haddadi A, Liston A, Laufs H, Fish DR, Lemieux L. fMRI temporal clustering analysis in patients with frequent interictal epileptiform discharges: comparison with EEG-driven analysis. Neuroimage 2005; 26(1): 309-16.

[130]   Morgan VL, Price RR, Arain A, Modur P, Abou-Khalil B. Resting functional MRI with temporal clustering analysis for localization of epileptic activity without EEG. Neuroimage 2004; 21(1): 473-81.

[131]   Morgan VL, Gore JC, Abou-Khalil B. Cluster analysis detection of functional MRI activity in temporal lobe epilepsy. Epilepsy Res 2007; 76(1): 22-33.

[132]   Donaire A, Falcon C, Carreno M, *et al*. Sequential analysis of fMRI images: A new approach to study human epileptic networks. Epilepsia 2009; 50(12): 2526-37.

[133]   Salek-Haddadi A, Merschhemke M, Lemieux L, Fish DR. Simultaneous EEG-Correlated Ictal fMRI. Neuroimage 2002; 16(1): 32-40.

[134]   Detre JA, Alsop DC, Aguirre GK, Sperling MR. Coupling of cortical and thalamic ictal activity in human partial epilepsy: demonstration by functional magnetic resonance imaging. Epilepsia 1996; 37(7): 657-61.

[135]   Auer T, Veto K, Doczi T, *et al*. Identifying seizure-onset zone and visualizing seizure spread by fMRI: a case report. Epileptic Disord 2008; 10(2): 93-100.

[136]   Bonaventura CD, Vaudano AE, Carni M, *et al*. EEG/fMRI Study of Ictal and Interictal Epileptic Activity: Methodological Issues and Future Perspectives in Clinical Practice. Epilepsia 2006; 47 Suppl 5: 52-8.

[137]   Di Bonaventura C, Carnfi M, Vaudano AE, *et al*. Ictal hemodynamic changes in late-onset rasmussen encephalitis. Ann Neurol 2006; 59(2): 432-3.

[138]   Federico P, Abbott DF, Briellmann RS, Harvey AS, Jackson GD. Functional MRI of the pre-ictal state. Brain 2005; 128(Pt 8): 1811-7.

[139]   Kobayashi E, Hawco CS, Grova C, Dubeau F, Gotman J. Widespread and intense BOLD changes during brief focal electrographic seizures. Neurology 2006; 66(7): 1049-55.

[140]   Liu Y, Yang T, Liao W, *et al*. EEG-fMRI study of the ictal and interictal epileptic activity in patients with eyelid myoclonia with absences. Epilepsia 2008; 49(12): 2078-86.

[141]   Marrosu F, Barberini L, Puligheddu M, *et al*. Combined EEG/fMRI recording in musicogenic epilepsy. Epilepsy Res 2009; 84(1): 77-81.

[142]   Salek Haddadi A, er T, Hamandi K, *et al*. Imaging seizure activity: a combined EEG/EMG-fMRI study in reading epilepsy. Epilepsia 2008; DOI: 10.1111/j.1528-1167.2008.01737.x(Epub ahead of print).

[143]   Vulliemoz S, Thornton R, Rodionov R, *et al*. The spatio-temporal mapping of epileptic networks: combination of EEG-fMRI and EEG source imaging. Neuroimage 2009; 46(3): 834-43.

[144]   Hamandi K, Powell HW, Laufs H, *et al*. Combined EEG-fMRI and tractography to visualise propagation of epileptic activity. J Neurol Neurosurg Psychiatry 2008; 79(5): 594-7.

[145]   De Tiege X, Harrison S, Laufs H, *et al*. Impact of interictal epileptic activity on normal brain function in epileptic encephalopathy: an electroencephalography-functional magnetic resonance imaging study. Epilepsy Behav 2007; 11(3): 460-5.

[146]   Tyvaert L, Chassagnon S, Sadikot A, LeVan P, Dubeau F, Gotman J. Thalamic nuclei activity in idiopathic generalized epilepsy: an EEG-fMRI study. Neurology 2009; 73(23): 2018-22.

[147]   Gotz-Trabert K, Hauck C, Wagner K, Fauser S, Schulze-Bonhage A. Spread of ictal activity in focal epilepsy. Epilepsia 2008; 49(9): 1594-601.

[148]   Vaudano AE, Carmichael DW, Thornton R, *et al*. Dynamic causal modelling of fMRI data suggests a balanced cortico-subcortical loop influenced by the precuneal state during generalized spike-wave discharges. Epilepsia 2007; 48(s6): 157.

[149]   Nencka AS, Rowe DB. Reducing the unwanted draining vein BOLD contribution in fMRI with statistical post-processing methods. Neuroimage 2007; 37(1): 177-88.

[150]   Carmichael DW, Thornton JS, Rodionov R, *et al*. Safety of localizing epilepsy monitoring intracranial electroencephalograph electrodes using MRI: radiofrequency-induced heating. J Magn Reson Imaging 2008; 28(5): 1233-44.

[151]   Carmichael DW, Thornton JS, Rodionov R, *et al*. Feasibility of simultaneous intracranial EEG-fMRI in humans: a safety study. Neuroimage 2010; 49(1): 379-90.

[152]   Laufs H, Hamandi K, Walker MC, *et al*. EEG-fMRI mapping of asymmetrical delta activity in a patient with refractory epilepsy is concordant with the epileptogenic region determined by intracranial EEG. Magn Reson Imaging 2006; 24(4): 367-71.

[153]   De Tiege X, Laufs H, Boyd SG, *et al*. EEG-fMRI in children with pharmacoresistant focal epilepsy. Epilepsia 2007; 48(2): 385-9.

[154]   Seeck M, Lazeyras F, Michel CM, *et al*. Non-invasive epileptic focus localization using EEG-triggered functional MRI and electromagnetic tomography. Electroencephalogr Clin Neurophysiol 1998; 106(6): 508-12.

[155] Lazeyras F, Zimine I, Blanke O, Perrig SH, Seeck M. Functional MRI with simultaneous EEG recording: feasibility and application to motor and visual activation. J Magn Reson Imaging 2001; 13(6): 943-8.

[156] Bagshaw AP, Aghakhani Y, Benar CG, et al. EEG-fMRI of focal epileptic spikes: analysis with multiple haemodynamic functions and comparison with gadolinium-enhanced MR angiograms. Hum Brain Mapp 2004; 22(3): 179-92.

[157] Benar CG, Grova C, Kobayashi E, et al. EEG-fMRI of epileptic spikes: concordance with EEG source localization and intracranial EEG. Neuroimage 2006; 30(4): 1161-70.

[158] Thornton R, Laufs H, Rodionov R, et al. EEG-correlated fMRI and Post-Operative Outcome in Focal Epilepsy. JNNP 2010; in press.

[159] Vulliemoz S, Lemieux L, Daunizeau J, Michel CM, Duncan JS. The combination of EEG Source Imaging and EEG-correlated functional MRI to map epileptic networks. Epilepsia 2009.

[160] Lemieux L, Laufs H, Carmichael D, Paul JS, Walker MC, Duncan JS. Noncanonical spike-related BOLD responses in focal epilepsy. Hum Brain Mapp 2008; 29(3): 329-45.

[161] Hamandi K, Laufs H, Noth U, Carmichael DW, Duncan JS, Lemieux L. BOLD and perfusion changes during epileptic generalised spike wave activity. Neuroimage 2008; 39(2): 608-18.

[162] Carmichael DW, Hamandi K, Laufs H, Duncan JS, Thomas DL, Lemieux L. An investigation of the relationship between BOLD and perfusion signal changes during epileptic generalised spike wave activity. Magn Reson Imaging 2008; 26(7): 870-3.

[163] Stefanovic B, Warnking JM, Kobayashi E, et al. Hemodynamic and metabolic responses to activation, deactivation and epileptic discharges. Neuroimage 2005; 28(1): 205-15.

[164] Rosenkranz K, Lemieux L. Present and future of simultaneous EEG-fMRI. MAGMA 2010.

[165] Gotman J, Grova C, Bagshaw A, Kobayashi E, Aghakhani Y, Dubeau F. Generalized epileptic discharges show thalamocortical activation and suspension of the default state of the brain. Proc Natl Acad Sci USA 2005.

[166] Archer JS, Abbott DF, Waites AB, Jackson GD. fMRI "deactivation" of the posterior cingulate during generalized spike and wave. Neuroimage 2003; 20(4): 1915-22.

[167] Laufs H, Lengler U, Hamandi K, Kleinschmidt A, Krakow K. Linking generalized spike-and-wave discharges and resting state brain activity by using EEG/fMRI in a patient with absence seizures. Epilepsia 2006; 47(2): 444-8.

[168] Salek-Haddadi A, Lemieux L, Merschhemke M, Friston KJ, Duncan JS, Fish DR. Functional magnetic resonance imaging of human absence seizures. Ann Neurol 2003; 53(5): 663-7.

[169] De Tiege X, Harrison S, Laufs H, et al. Impact of interictal secondary-generalized activity on brain function in epileptic encephalopathy: an EEG-fMRI study. submitted to Epilepsy and Behavior; in press.

[170] Steriade M. Neuronal substrates of spike-wave seizures and hypsarrhythmia in corticothalamic systems. Adv Neurol 2006; 97: 149-54.

[171] Binnie CD. Cognitive impairment during epileptiform discharges: is it ever justifiable to treat the EEG? Lancet Neurol 2003; 2(12): 725-30.

[172] Carmichael DW, Pinto S, Limousin-Dowsey P, et al. Functional MRI with active, fully implanted, deep brain stimulation systems: Safety and experimental confounds. Neuroimage 2007; 37(2): 508-17.

[173] Lengler U, Kafadar I, Neubauer BA, Krakow K. fMRI correlates of interictal epileptic activity in patients with idiopathic benign focal epilepsy of childhood. A simultaneous EEG-functional MRI study. Epilepsy Res 2007; 75(1): 29-38.

[174] Jacobs J, Rohr A, Moeller F, et al. Evaluation of epileptogenic networks in children with tuberous sclerosis complex using EEG-fMRI. Epilepsia 2008; 49(5): 816-25.

[175] Groening K, Brodbeck V, Moeller F, et al. Combination of EEG-fMRI and EEG source analysis improves interpretation of spike-associated activation networks in paediatric pharmacoresistant focal epilepsies. Neuroimage 2009; 46(3): 827-33.

[176] Li Q, Luo C, Yang T, et al. EEG-fMRI study on the interictal and ictal generalized spike-wave discharges in patients with childhood absence epilepsy. Epilepsy Res 2009; 87(2-3): 160-8.

[177] De Tiege X, Goldman S, Van Bogaert P. Insights into the pathophysiology of psychomotor regression in CSWS syndromes from FDG-PET and EEG-fMRI. Epilepsia 2009; 50 Suppl 7: 47-50.

[178] Boor S, Vucurevic G, Pfleiderer C, Stoeter P, Kutschke G, Boor R. EEG-related functional MRI in benign childhood epilepsy with centrotemporal spikes. Epilepsia 2003; 44(5): 688-92.

[179] Boor R, Jacobs J, Hinzmann A, et al. Combined spike-related functional MRI and multiple source analysis in the non-invasive spike localization of benign rolandic epilepsy. Clin Neurophysiol 2007; 118(4): 901-9.

[180] Archer JS, Briellman RS, Abbott DF, Syngeniotis A, Wellard RM, Jackson GD. Benign epilepsy with centro-temporal spikes: spike triggered fMRI shows somato-sensory cortex activity. Epilepsia 2003; 44(2): 200-4.

[181] Labate A, Briellmann RS, Abbott DF, Waites AB, Jackson GD. Typical childhood absence seizures are associated with thalamic activation. Epileptic Disord 2005; 7(4): 373-7.

[182] Leal A, Dias A, Vieira JP, Secca M, Jordao C. The BOLD effect of interictal spike activity in childhood occipital lobe epilepsy. Epilepsia 2006; 47(9): 1536-42.

[183] Cross JH. Epilepsy surgery in childhood. Epilepsia 2002; 43 Suppl 3: 65-70.

CHAPTER 7

Abnormal Synchrony and Oscillations in Neuropsychiatric Disorders

Peter J. Uhlhaas[1,2,*] and Wolf Singer[1,3]

[1]*Department of Neurophysiology, Max Planck Institute for Brain Research, Deutschordenstrasse 46 Frankfurt am Main, 60528, Germany,* [2]*Laboratory for Neurophysiology and Neuroimaging, Department of Psychiatry, Johann Wolfgang Goethe University, Heinrich-Hoffmann-Strasse 10, Frankfurt am Main, 60528, Germany and* [3]*Frankfurt Institute for Advanced Studies, Johann Wolfgang Goethe University, Max-von-Laue-Strasse 1, Frankfurt am Main, 60438, Germany*

Abstract: Following the discovery of context-dependent synchronization of oscillatory neuronal responses in the visual system, novel methods of time series analysis have been developed for the examination of task- and performance-related oscillatory activity and its synchronization. Studies employing these advanced techniques revealed that synchronization of oscillatory responses in the β- and γ-band is involved in a variety of cognitive functions, such as perceptual grouping, attention-dependent stimulus selection, routing of signals across distributed cortical networks, sensory-motor integration, working memory, and perceptual awareness. Here, we review evidence that certain brain disorders, such as schizophrenia, epilepsy, autism, Alzheimer's disease, and Parkinson's are associated with abnormal neural synchronization. The data suggest close correlations between abnormalities in neuronal synchronization and cognitive dysfunctions, emphasizing the importance of temporal coordination. Thus, a focused search for abnormalities in temporal patterning may be of considerable clinical relevance.

Keywords: EEG, time series, binding, synchrony, schizophrenia, autism, epilepsy, Alzheimer's, Parkinson's.

INTRODUCTION

Most of the brain's cognitive functions are based on the coordinated interactions of large numbers of neurons that are distributed within and across different specialized brain areas. A fundamental, yet unresolved, problem of modern neuroscience is how this coordination is achieved. Integration and segregation of neural activity needs to occur at various spatial and temporal scales, and these scales must be dynamically adjusted depending on the nature of the respective cognitive tasks. In contrast to the large number of studies that investigated the role of synchrony in a wide range of cognitive and executive processes during normal brain functioning, relatively few investigations have examined the possible relevance of neural synchrony in pathological brain states, such as schizophrenia, epilepsy, autism, and Alzheimer's disease (AD). Therefore, we focus this review on studies that specifically investigated neural synchrony in association with circumscribed impairments in cognition in schizophrenia, epilepsy, autism, and AD. Furthermore, we review recent data on the relation between abnormal synchronization and motor deficits in Parkinson's disease (PD). In addition to the obvious medical relevance of this research, further insights into the underlying pathophysiological mechanisms are also likely to enhance our understanding of normal brain functions. Specifically, we hope that these correlations between neural synchrony and pathological brain states will shed some new light on the respective pathophysiological mechanisms and the role of synchrony in normal brain functions.

DISTRIBUTED PROCESSING AND NEURONAL SYNCHRONIZATION

The brain is a highly distributed system in which numerous operations are executed in parallel and that lacks a single coordinating center. This raises the questions of i) how the computations occurring simultaneously in spatially segregated processing areas are coordinated and bound together to give rise to coherent percepts and actions, ii) how signals are selected and routed from sensory to executive structures without being confounded, and finally, iii) how information about the relatedness of contents is encoded. One of the coordinating mechanisms appears to be the synchronization of neuronal activity by phase locking of self-generated network oscillations.

An important link between oscillations and cortical computations was the discovery of the role of oscillatory rhythms in the beta (β) / gamma (γ) range (20-80 Hz) in establishing precise synchronization of distributed neural responses. Gray and colleagues [1] showed that action potentials generated by cortical cells align with the oscillatory rhythm in the

*Address correspondence to Peter J. Uhlhaas: Department of Neurophysiology, Max Planck Institute for Brain Research, Deutschordenstrasse 46 and Laboratory for Neurophysiology and Neuroimaging, Department of Psychiatry, Johann Wolfgang Goethe University, Heinrich-Hoffmann-Strasse 10, Frankfurt am Main, 60528, Germany; Email: uhlhaas@mpih-frankfurt.mpg.de

Matt T. Bianchi, Verne S. Caviness and Sydney S. Cash (Eds.)

β and γ range, which has the consequence that neurons participating in the same oscillatory rhythm synchronize their discharges with high precision. Thus, it is a central role of cortical oscillations in the β/γ range to enable neuronal synchronization and by virtue of establishing systematic phase lags, i.e. shifts between the cycles of two oscillations, to define precise temporal relations between the discharges of distributed neurons [2-3], whereas lower frequencies preferentially establish synchronization over longer distances [4]. These temporal correlations are functionally relevant as there is abundant evidence for a close relationship between the occurrence of oscillations and cognitive and behavioral responses, such as perceptual grouping, attention-dependent stimulus selection, working memory, and consciousness (Table **7.1**) (for a recent review see reference [5]).

Table 7.1 Summarizes Types of Neuronal Oscillations

	Theta (4-7 Hz)	Alpha (8-12 Hz)	Beta (13-30 Hz)	Gamma (30-200 Hz)
Anatomy	Hippocampus, Prefrontal Corted, Sensory Cortex	Thalamus, Hippocampus, Reticular Formation, Sensory Cortex, Motor Cortex	All Cortical Structures, Subthalamic, Nucleus, Hippocampus, Basal Ganglia, Olfactory Bulb	All Brain Strcture, Retina, Olfactory Bulb
Neurotransmitters	GABA, Glutamate, Acetycholine	Glutamate, Acetycholine, Serotonin	Glutamate, GABA, Dopamine	GABA, Glutamate, Acetycholine
Function	Memory, Synaptic Plasticity, Top-Down Control, Long-Range Synchronization	Inhibition, Attention, Consciousness, Top-Down Control, Long-Range Synchronization	Sensory Gating, Attention Perception, Motor Control, Long-Range Syncchronization	Perception, Attention, Memory, Consciousness, Synaptic Plasticity, Motor Control

More recent evidence indicates that these oscillations are not only instrumental for the synchronization of neuronal discharges, but can also support other consistent temporal relations by establishing systematic phase lags between the discharges of distributed neurons. *In vitro* studies [6] and multi-site recordings in the visual cortex of cats [7] provided evidence that the oscillatory patterning of neuronal activity is an efficient mechanism to adjust the precise timing of spikes and is potentially a versatile mechanism to convert rate coded input to cells into a temporal code defined by the time of occurrence of spikes relative to the oscillation cycle (see also reference [2]).

Following the initial descriptions of context dependent synchronization in the visual cortex, numerous studies have been initiated in order to investigate the functional role of this phenomenon. These have demonstrated that response synchronization is a ubiquitous phenomenon in cortical networks and likely to serve a variety of different functions in addition to feature binding at early levels of sensory processing.

Studies in the motion sensitive area MT of the visual cortex of awake monkeys [8], the optic tectum of pigeons [9], other cortical areas in the cat [10], and the retina [11] provided evidence that the oscillatory patterning of neuronal responses and the synchronization of these oscillations is highly sensitive to perceptual context. Multi-site recordings also provided evidence that synchronization occurs between widely distributed structures, such as the primary visual cortex, the optic tectum and the suprasylvian cortex [12], and that it plays a role in the coordination of widely distributed functions as is required, for example, in sensory-motor processing [13]. This latter study indicated further that synchronized oscillatory activity is not only stimulus driven but also generated in anticipation of a visual discrimination task requiring fast motor responses. This observation led to the hypothesis that self-generated oscillatory activity in the β and γ frequency range could be a correlate of focused attention and serve both modality specific selection of stimuli and the coordination of sensory and executive subsystems required for the execution of the anticipated task. A close relation between synchronization and input selection has also been found in experiments on binocular rivalry [14], a phenomenon in which perception alternates between different images presented to each eye.

The notion of an involvement of synchronized β and γ oscillations in attention dependent processes agrees also with the evidence that there is a close relation between arousal, activated cortical states and the occurrence of high frequency oscillations. γ oscillations occur only with activated cortical states and require for their expression activation of muscarinic receptors in the cortex [15-16].

Taken together, the results suggested that synchronization enhances the saliency of the synchronized responses which can in turn be used for a variety of different operations. Joint increases of saliency favor joint selection and processing of signals which can in principle support attention dependent stimulus selection and feature binding. The notion that the saliency of responses can be enhanced in a complementary way either by increases of discharge rate or by synchronization has later received direct support from experiments on apparent brightness perception [17].

STUDIES IN HUMAN SUBJECTS

Non invasive electrophysiological methods such as electroencephalography (EEG) and magnetoencephalography (MEG) recordings register preferentially if not exclusively synchronized neuronal activity because they average over large populations of neurons. Thus, non-synchronized sources of activity tend to cancel out and synchronized signals are enhanced. This, together with the ease to perform demanding psychophysical experiments, is one of the reasons why investigations on synchronized oscillations and their putative function have been particularly rewarding in human subjects. These studies provided rapidly growing evidence for a close relation between synchronous oscillatory activity in the β and γ frequency range and a variety of cognitive functions such as perceptual grouping, focused attention, maintenance of contents in short term memory, poly-sensory integration, formation of associative memories and sensory motor coordination (for review see reference [5]).

MEASURES OF OSCILLATORY ACTIVITY AND SYNCHRONY

Recording methods that assess the activity of large populations of neurons, such as microelectrode recordings of local field potentials (LFPs) or EEG- and MEG-registrations, can only detect neuronal activity if it exhibits some degree of synchrony. Entirely uncoordinated activity would not be detectable because the currents of synaptic events, which are the major source of the measured signals [18], would cancel out.

In most cases, the signals recorded from neuron populations consist of oscillations that cover a broad frequency spectrum and are usually quantified by computing the relative power in distinct frequency bands. Until a decade ago, the most frequently applied technique for this spectral decomposition was the Fourier analysis. This classical method has recently been complemented by wavelet-based techniques [19] and multitaper analyses [20], which are better adapted for the spectral decomposition of nonstationary time series. All these methods have in common that they estimate the amplitude of oscillatory activity.

In addition to analyzing the frequency spectrum of spontaneous oscillations, it is of interest to determine the time course of stimulus- or task-related oscillations. Two forms of stimulus-related oscillatory activity need to be distinguished: (1) evoked and (2) induced oscillations [21]. Evoked oscillations are strictly phase-locked to the onset of a stimulus and, therefore, can be measured by stimulus-triggered averaging of responses. Although these evoked oscillations are related to early, stimulus-driven encoding processes, they are state-dependent and can be modulated by top-down processes such as attention [22]. In contrast, induced oscillations appear in association with stimulus-triggered cognitive processes, but reflect self-paced temporal coordination of neuronal responses. They are not phase-locked with external events, and are therefore abolished by averaging.

Although the amplitude of LFP, EEG, or MEG signals correlates with the degree of synchrony of neuronal responses, there are numerous confounding variables that make it difficult to draw firm conclusions on synchrony by considering only amplitude measures. Among these are the size and the alignment of the dipole fields of the contributing neurons, the fraction of synchronously active neurons in the population of cells contributing to the signal, and, above all, the degree of precision with which the neuronal discharges are synchronized. The latter variable is particularly critical when neurons engage in high-frequency oscillatory activity. In this case, the precision of synchrony needs to be in the millisecond range in order to permit effective summation of synaptic currents and to yield a measurable signal. Therefore, methods have been developed which permit assessment of synchrony independently of amplitude [23]. In essence, they determine separately for different frequency bands the precision and inter-trial variance of phase relations between signals recorded simultaneously from different sites (phase locking). These measures need to be distinguished from measures of "coherence," which determine the covariance of the amplitude of oscillations recorded from different sites for the various frequency bands [24].

In addition to measures that examine the amplitude and synchrony of oscillatory activity at the scalp level, new methods have been developed that improve the spatial resolution of EEG and MEG recordings. Measurement of synchronized, oscillatory activity in scalp EEG and MEG data is contaminated by volume conduction and muscle artifacts that can mimic neural synchrony. One solution is the transformation of EEG and MEG data into source space. Besides more precise estimation of synchronous, oscillatory activity, this technique has the additional advantage of substantially improving the spatial resolution of EEG and MEG measurements. Several techniques have been developed to achieve this goal. They allow the measurement of synchronization between sources, yielding new insights into the relationship between synchronous, oscillatory activity and cognitive processes [25].

Finally, measures for large-scale coordination of neuronal activity have also been derived from covariations of the amplitudes and latencies of hemodynamic signals in different brain regions [26]. Although this method has very low temporal resolution and cannot assess the synchrony of evoked and induced oscillatory activity, it provides indications on functional connectivity and can contribute to the identification of the distributed networks supporting particular cognitive processes. Because clinical studies using measurements of phase synchronization to determine deficiencies in temporal coordination are still sparse, we also included in this review selected studies that applied coherence analysis to EEG and MEG signals and discuss functional magnetic resonance imaging (fMRI) data on functional connectivity.

ANATOMICAL SUBSTRATES, TRANSMITTER-SYSTEMS AND THE GENERATION OF NEURAL SYNCHRONY

Studies involving lesions [27] and developmental manipulations [28] indicate that neural synchronization in the high-frequency range (β- and γ-band) is mainly mediated by cortico-cortical connections that reciprocally link cells situated in the same cortical area, but also cells distributed across different areas and even across the two hemispheres. Accordingly, synchronization probability between neurons reflects the anatomical layout of excitatory cortico-cortical connections [29-30]. Direct evidence for the synchronizing function of reciprocal cortico-cortical connections comes from the finding that sectioning the corpus callosum abolishes synchronization of induced oscillatory responses between neurons located in different hemispheres [27]. These and related studies indicate that cortical mechanisms dominate in the generation and precise synchronization of high-frequency oscillatory activity in the β- and γ-frequency bands. In contrast, subcortical structures, and especially the thalamus, appear to dominate in the generation and synchronization of oscillatory activity in the lower frequency bands (alpha (α), θ, delta (Δ), and below)[1]. However, more research is needed to clarify how exactly cortical and subcortical mechanisms cooperate in the generation and synchronization of rhythmic activity in the various frequency bands.

The discovery of synchronized oscillations has motivated a large number of *in vitro* studies searching for the mechanisms that would generate these oscillations and this led to a re-evaluation of the functional role of inhibitory inter-neurons. Classically, the network of inhibitory inter-neurons has been considered as a mechanism for gain control and improvement of signal to noise ratios. *In vitro* investigations of oscillating networks led to the conclusion that it is the network of inhibitory interneurons that is responsible for the rhythmic pacing of neuronal activity. Thus, inhibitory interneurons appear to play a crucial role not only in controlling response amplitudes but also in adjusting the precise timing of discharges of excitatory neurons. Through the latter effect they assume a pivotal function in the temporal structuring and coordination of neuronal responses (for a review see reference [31]).

Furthermore, recent evidence indicates that cholinergic modulation plays a crucial role in the fast, state-dependent facilitation of high-frequency oscillations and the associated response synchronization [32]. In addition to chemical synaptic transmission, direct electrotonic coupling through gap junctions between inhibitory neurons also contributes to the temporal patterning of population activity and, in particular, to the precise synchronization of oscillatory activity [33].

NEURAL SYNCHRONY IN SCHIZOPHRENIA

Schizophrenia is a severe mental disorder with an estimated life-time prevalence of 1%. The disorder is characterized by psychotic symptoms (delusions, hallucinations), negative symptoms (flattening of affect, apathy), and disorganization of thought and behavior. Cognitive dysfunctions are prominent throughout the course of schizophrenia and have been shown to be a better predictor for outcome than psychotic or negative symptoms, suggesting that cognitive deficits represent a core pathology of the disorder [34]. The pathophysiological mechanisms leading to the overt symptoms and deficits in cognition are, however, largely unknown.

---

[1]Steriade M. Cellular substrates of brain rhythms. In: E. Niedermeyer and F. Lopes Da Silva, Editors, *Electroencephalography: Basic Principles, Clinical Applications, And Related Fields* (Fifth Edition), Lippincott Williams and Wilkins, Philadelphia, 505–621, 2005.

Current theories of schizophrenia [35] emphasize that core aspects of the pathophysiology are due to deficits in the coordination of distributed processes that both involve multiple cortical areas and are associated with specific cognitive deficits. Some of the deficits concern functions, such as working memory, attention, and perceptual organization, that have been proposed to involve synchronization of oscillatory activity in the high-frequency band (β and γ) [35].

Evidence for impairment in neural synchrony has been observed with Steady-State evoked potentials (SSEP). SSEPs represent a basic neural response to a temporally modulated stimulus to which it is synchronized in frequency and phase. Thus, steady-state paradigms are ideally suited to probe the ability of neuronal networks to generate and maintain oscillatory activity in different frequency bands. Patients with schizophrenia are characterized by impaired auditory SSEPs, especially to click-trains presented at γ-frequency [36]. However, deficits in SSEPs in response to stimulus presentation in lower frequency bands have also been shown [37]. Deficits have also been reported for visual SSEPs, in particular to stimuli in the β-frequency range [38].

Consistent with the evidence that early sensory processes are impaired in schizophrenia, several studies have demonstrated abnormalities in the stimulus-locked activity that occurs within 50-150 ms after a stimulus is presented (Fig. **7.1**). For example, reductions in the amplitude and phase-locking of evoked oscillations have been shown during the processing of visual information [39-40], suggesting an impaired ability to precisely align oscillatory activity with incoming sensory information. Correlations between behavioral performance and the degree to which evoked γ-band oscillations are reduced in patients with schizophrenia suggests that this phenomenon is related to perceptual dysfunctions [41]. The data for deficits in evoked activity in the auditory domain is less consistent. Several studies have shown that patients with schizophrenia are characterized by reduced amplitude and phase-locking of evoked β- and γ-band oscillations [42-43], but a recent study [40] did not confirm this finding.

Reductions in evoked γ-band oscillations have also been demonstrated in frontal regions, an area that has been a traditional focus of schizophrenia research, through measurement of EEG responses following the application of transcranial magnetic stimulation (TMS) to the premotor cortex [44]. Relative to healthy controls, schizophrenia patients had a marked decrease in γ oscillations within the first 100 ms after TMS, particularly in a cluster of electrodes located in a fronto-central region. Source-analyses revealed that in schizophrenia patients γ-band oscillations triggered by TMS did not propagate beyond the area of stimulation whereas in controls activity was found in several motor and sensorimotor areas.

The finding that there are intrinsic deficits in neural oscillations in frontal circuits in schizophrenia is compatible with EEG studies that have tested frontal γ- and theta (θ)-oscillations during executive and working memory tasks. Patients with schizophrenia were characterized by a reduced amplitude of γ- and θ-oscillations in frontal regions [45-46] and an impaired stimulus-induced phase-resetting of ongoing oscillations at low and high frequencies [47].

Panel (**A**) shows auditory steady-state responses in schizophrenia patients. The left panel shows the average electroencephalographic frequency over a midline frontal electrode site (Fz) in controls (n = 15) and patients with schizophrenia (n = 15) during presentation of a train of clicks at 40 Hz, 30 Hz and 20 Hz. Y-axis shows the mean power in microvolts squared of oscillations at different frequencies (x axis) for each stimulus rate. Schizophrenia patients show decreased power in the 40 Hz band at 40-Hz stimulation compared with control subjects, but no difference at lower frequencies of stimulation. (This panel is adapted from reference [23]).

Reductions in the amplitude of neural oscillations during cognitive tasks are accompanied by reduced phase-synchronization of induced oscillatory activity. Phase-synchronization has been proposed to provide an effective mechanism for the integration of neural responses in distributed neural responses in local cortical networks [48]. Several studies have shown that schizophrenia patients have reduced phase-synchronization of oscillations in the β- and γ- frequency-band during perceptual organization and auditory processing [39, 49]. These findings suggest that impaired synchronization of β- and γ-band oscillations underlie the hypothesized functional dysconnectivity of cortical networks in schizophrenia [35]. It is currently unclear, however, to what extent impairments in local circuits contribute to long-range synchronization impairments or whether these represent two independent phenomena.

Recent evidence indicates that dysfunctional neural oscillations represent an endophenotype of the disorder. Work in healthy twins has demonstrated that the power and temporal correlations of oscillations during the resting state are highly heritable [50], indicating that neural oscillations can be exploited in the search for genetic contributions to schizophrenia. Indeed, a recent study [51] has provided important evidence for the relationship between impaired neural oscillations and genetic predisposition to schizophrenia.

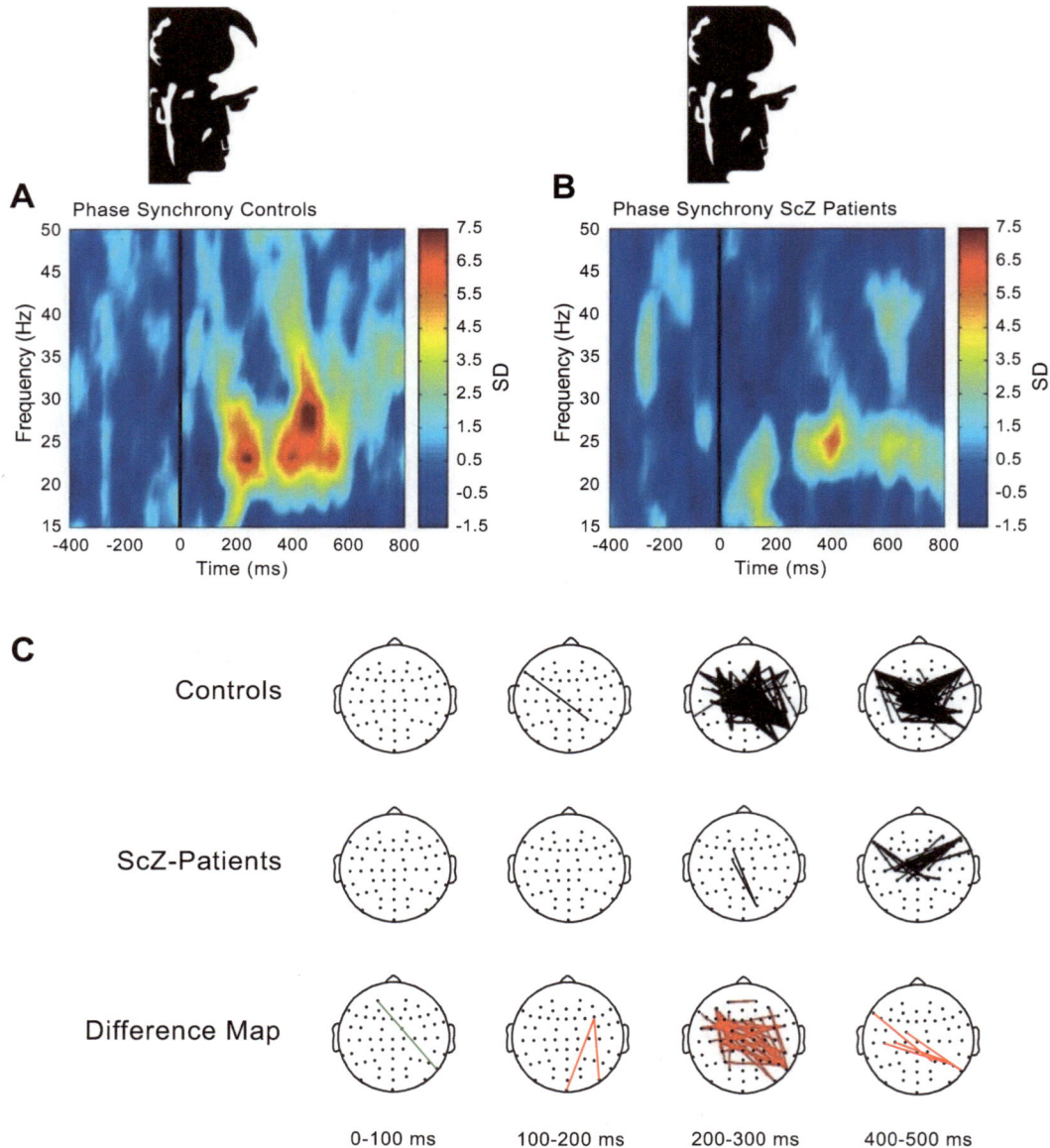

Fig. (7.1). Abnormalities in neural oscillations and synchrony in schizophrenia.

Panel (**B**) shows sensory evoked oscillations during a visual oddball task in patients with schizophrenia. The panel shows the phase locking factor (PLF), over the 20-100 Hz frequency range over occipital cortex (electrode O1) for healthy controls and patients with schizophrenia to the presentation of a target letter (x-axis: time; y-axis: PLF). PLF was tested by examining the variance of phases across trials over a single electrode (O1) that can range from 0 (random distribution) to 1 (perfect phase locking). Control participants show an increase in phase-locking for γ oscillations $\sim$ 100 ms after stimulus presentation. However, this is significantly reduced in patients with schizophrenia, indicating a dysfunction in early sensory processes. (This panel is adapted from referece [39]).

Panel (**C**) shows dysfunctional phase-synchrony during Gestalt perception in schizophrenia. Mooney faces were presented in an upright and inverted orientation and participants indicated whether a face was perceived. The middle panel shows the average phase synchrony over time for all electrodes during 'correct' trials. In patients with schizophrenia, phase synchrony between 200-300 ms was significantly reduced relatively to controls. In addition, patients with schizophrenia showed a pronounced desynchronization in the γ-band (30–55 Hz) in the 200–280 ms interval that was not present in the control. The right panel shows differences in the patterns of phase synchrony in the 20 and 30Hz frequency range between groups. Red lines indicate a decrease in synchrony between two electrodes in schizophrenia patients compared with controls. Green lines indicate increase in synchrony for patients with schizophrenia. (This panel is adapted from reference [47]).

Impairments in the ability of distributed networks to establish precise synchronization of neuronal assemblies oscillating at high frequencies can have many reasons. These comprise both a host of local factors that determine the time constants of synaptic and non-synaptic interactions within the oscillating microcircuits and the properties of long-distance connections that mediate interareal synchronization. Abnormalities have been identified for some of these candidate mechanisms in schizophrenia patients. *In vivo* anatomical examination with diffusion tensor imaging (DTI) has revealed white matter anomalies that might be related to deficiencies in long-range synchronization (for a review see reference [52]). Cortico-cortical connections were reduced in the frontal, temporal, and parietal lobes, and between the two hemispheres. However, there is also evidence for locally increased connectivity that is related to productive symptoms, such as auditory hallucinations [53]. One interpretation of these seemingly paradoxical findings is that hyperconnectivity between higher- and lower-order cortical areas favors backpropagation to the respective primary sensory cortices of oscillatory activity generated in higher sensory areas during visual and auditory imagery, thus generating activation patterns that resemble those induced by sensory stimulation. This interpretation receives some support by the finding that hallucinations are associated with the following: (1) increased γ-oscillations in the corresponding sensory areas of the cerebral cortex [54]; (2) long-range synchronization [49]; and (3) increased hemodynamic responses (blood oxygen level dependent (BOLD) signal) in the respective primary sensory areas [55]. For several reasons, this increased BOLD signal is likely to reflect the entrainment of neurons in the primary areas into synchronized, high-frequency oscillations. First, it is improbable that neurons in primary sensory areas exhibit major increases in discharge rates in the absence of sensory stimulation. Second, top-down effects, such as those associated with focused attention, cause an entrainment of selected neuronal populations into well-synchronized γ-oscillations without enhancing the discharge rates [56]. Third, increases of the BOLD signal correlate much better with the entrainment of neurons into synchronized high-frequency γ-oscillations than with increases in discharge rates [57].

Further candidate mechanisms for deficient synchronization in the high-frequency range are abnormalities in the rhythm-generating networks of inhibitory interneurons and abnormalities in the glutamatergic neurons mediating long-distance synchronization. Abnormalities in GABAergic inhibitory neurons [58] and NMDA-receptor dysregulation [59] have both been found in patients with schizophrenia. The possible role of NMDA-receptors in the pathophysiology of schizophrenia is supported by the acute effects of NMDA antagonists, such as ketamine or phencyclidine (PCP), on healthy volunteers. For example, sub-anesthetic doses of ketamine produce an acute psychosis that includes many of the symptoms and characteristic cognitive dysfunctions of schizophrenia [60]. Hypofunctioning of the NMDA-receptor in schizophrenia is also compatible with the dopamine hypothesis of schizophrenia, as NMDA antagonists can induce dopamine dysregulation [61]. Because the typical and atypical neuroleptics interfere with dopaminergic and serotonergic neurotransmission, respectively, abnormalities in these transmitter systems are thought to play a central role in the pathophysiology of schizophrenia. Whether these systems play a role in modulating neural synchrony has not been investigated yet.

In summary, there is consistent evidence that neural synchrony is impaired in patients with schizophrenia. This impairment is particularly pronounced for oscillatory activity in the β- and γ-frequency ranges and for the synchronization of these high-frequency oscillations over longer distances. Because synchronization of oscillatory activity in this frequency range is associated with cognitive functions that are disturbed in schizophrenia patients, it is conceivable that the relation between impaired synchrony and the symptomatology of schizophrenia is not merely correlative. Data on anatomical connectivity and neurotransmitter systems in schizophrenia suggest several potential causes for impaired neural synchrony, but more focused studies are required to distinguish between cause and effect.

NEURAL SYNCHRONY IN EPILEPSY

Epilepsy designates a group of heterogeneous disorders of the nervous system that differ with respect to etiology and symptomatology. Traditionally, epilepsy has been assumed to result from abnormal, typically too high and too extended, neural synchronization. Penfield *et al.*, for example, suggested that the high voltages recorded from epileptic cortex reflect hypersynchronous neural activity[2].

Etiologically, a wide range of factors can induce abnormal synchronization. These range from structural damage (encephalitis, craniocerebral trauma and tumors) to abnormal metabolic states (fever, sleep deprivation, alkalosis, etc.). Genetic predisposition also plays a role in epileptogenesis. Depending on etiology and disposition, seizures can be confined to restricted regions of the cortex (focal epilepsy). This leads to specific cognitive or motor symptoms, such as hallucinations, in the case of complex partial seizures within sensory areas, or myoclonia, if the focus is in motor areas. In contrast, in convulsive seizure disorders (grand-mal epilepsy), abnormal synchronization tends to spread over the whole neocortex, involving also subcortical structures, and leads to comatose states. In absence seizures, characteristic, highly synchronized low-frequency oscillations generated by thalamo-cortico-thalamic loops cause a breakdown of all higher cognitive functions[3]. Together with the evidence that synchronization of neural responses plays an important role in signal transduction and information processing (see Introduction), these well-established correlations between abnormal synchronization and the breakdown of neuronal functions are strong support for the hypothesis that temporal patterning of neural activity and a precisely regulated trade-off between correlated and decorrelated activation patterns are crucial for normal brain functions.

One of the hallmarks of epileptiform activity is abnormally high synchrony in extensive brain regions as reflected by large-amplitude fluctuations in the EEG both during and between seizures. For example, during absence seizures, the sudden arrest of ongoing behavior and the impairment of consciousness are accompanied by the abrupt occurrence of synchronous, low-frequency, three-per-second spike-and-wave discharges (SWDs) in the EEG over a wide range of cortical areas. Meeren *et al.* [62] showed in a genetic animal model of absence epilepsy that SWDs originate in the cortex and initiate oscillations in the thalamo-cortical-thalamic loop. These results are consistent with findings that cortical-spike wave seizures can still be recorded after ipsilateral thalamectomy [63], thus making it unlikely that seizure generation depends only on thalamic mechanisms.

Epilepsy is typically associated with a number of characteristic cognitive and behavioral phenomena. Complex partial seizures are frequently accompanied by auras that involve hallucinations in different modalities, unusual sensations, déjà vu experiences, emotional feelings, and recall of old memories [64]. After partial complex, generalized tonic-clonic, and certain other types of seizures, loss of short-term memories and retrograde amnesia has been reported. Depending on the involved cortical regions, specific cognitive dysfunctions are observed. Temporal lobe epilepsy (TLE) is typically associated with memory impairment, while focal epilepsy over the language-dominant hemisphere can cause word finding and naming difficulties [65]. These correlations suggest that abnormal temporal patterning of neural activity disrupts cognitive processes.

High-frequency oscillatory activity, especially in the γ-band, has been frequently observed in the EEG before and during epileptic events (for a review see reference [66]). Allen *et al.* [67] reported activity in the γ-band before and at the onset of seizures. High-frequency oscillations (100–500 Hz) were also found in intracerebral recordings in patients with focal epilepsy near the time of the onset of the seizure [68]. The presence of high-frequency oscillatory activity prior to the onset of ictal activity has also been observed in rodent models of epilepsy [69].

Several studies examined phase synchrony during interictal, ictal, and preictal activity and have provided further insights into the role of neural synchrony in the generation of seizure activity. These studies challenged the notion that neural synchrony is generally increased in epilepsy. Evidence from hippocampal slices shows that bursts in CA1 pyramidal neurons are caused by neuronal activity that is synchronized with high precision (<10 ms) in the β-band; however, during seizures, neuronal activity is no longer synchronous [70]. Garcia Dominguez *et al.* [71] analyzed MEG data from epileptic patients with generalized seizures in order to determine the extent of phase synchronization within and across distant cortical areas. The results revealed increased local synchrony in the β- and lower γ-band, whereas synchrony was normal, or even reduced, between distant regions. This is in agreement with the study by van Putten [72], which showed that only enhanced local phase synchronization is a significant correlate of seizure activity.

Analyzing phase synchrony during preictal EEG activity has also challenged the notion that neural synchrony is generally increased. Le Van Quyen *et al.* [73] examined phase synchrony with intracranial recordings from eight patients

---

[2]Penfield W, Jaspers H, McNaughton F. *Epilepsy and the Functional Anatomy of the Human Brain.* Little Brown, Boston: 1954.
[3]Niedermeyer E. Epileptic Seizure Disorders. In: E. Niedermeyer and F. Lopes Da Silva, Editors, *Electroencephalography: Basic Principles, Clinical Applications, And Related Fields* (Fifth Edition), Lippincott Williams and Wilkins, Philadelphia, 505–621: 2005.

exhibiting neocortical focal epilepsy. In 77% of the seizures, there was a preictal decrease in synchrony in the β-band. This reduction of synchrony between different electrode sites sometimes occurred before the actual seizure and was characterized by recurrent spatial patterns that were close to the actual sites of the epileptogenic focus. This suggests that preictal desynchronization may facilitate seizure activity through isolating the pathologically discharging neurons of the epileptic focus from the controlling influence of the embedding network. It is thus conceivable that reduction of coherence and the associated reduction in coupling allows the focus to engage in supracritical synchronous activity, which then spreads into the surrounding networks.

Data from functional and anatomical imaging studies support this view. Waites *et al.* [74] showed that during resting state, patients with TLE exhibit reduced functional connectivity between the brain areas involved in language generation. Likewise, in a recent DTI study, Dumas de la Roque *et al.* [75] reported that patients with intractable partial epilepsy had reduced connectivity between cortical areas surrounding the electric focus, as well as reduced connectivity between more distant cortical areas.

Experimental and clinical data suggest that convulsive epilepsy is often associated with an imbalance between excitatory and inhibitory neurotransmitter systems, causing enhanced excitability. GABAergic interneurons play a critical role in maintaining this balance [76] and accordingly, convulsive seizures can be suppressed or reduced by enhancing GABAergic transmission [77]. However, *in vitro* data indicate that seizure activity can be precipitated by the administration of GABAergic drugs [78]. In animal models of absence seizures, GABA(B) receptor agonists increase spiking activity, whereas blocking of GABA(B) receptors reduces the number of spiking episodes [79]. These heterogeneous effects of GABAergic drugs have to do with the multiple functional roles of inhibitory interneurons. On the one hand, their activity reduces network excitability; on the other hand, they contribute essentially to the oscillatory patterning and synchronization of neural activity (as described above). As synchronization increases the impact of neural activity in target structures, enhanced GABAergic transmission may, in certain cases, facilitate seizures by inducing synchronous population discharges that then spread very effectively across neighboring networks. In the case of absence seizures, GABA-mediated hyperpolarization is essential for the development of the synchronized, low-frequency oscillations because these depend on low-threshold $Ca2+$ channels that are only activatible when the membrane potential drops substantially below the average resting level [80]. However, there is also evidence that abnormalities in GABAergic transmission alone may not be sufficient for epileptogenesis in mature cortex and that seizure activity is likely to depend, in addition, upon synergistic alterations of glutamatergic transmission involving NMDA-receptors [81].

Furthermore, gap junctions have been proposed to play an important role in the synchronization and propagation of epileptic activity [33]. *In vitro* data show that the generation of the high-frequency oscillations associated with preictal EEG activity is facilitated by direct electrotonic coupling of neurons via gap junctions [82]. Accordingly, gap junction blockers have been shown to be effective in suppressing seizures in rat models of focal cortical epilepsy [83], in modifying the expression of rhythmical discharges, and in controlling the duration and propagation of individual seizures *in vivo* [84].

In conclusion, seizures are not only a consequence of heightened neuronal excitability such as results from an imbalance between excitatory and inhibitory mechanisms. Alterations of the mechanisms that support the oscillatory patterning and the synchronization of neuronal activity appear to be equally important. As synchronization enhances the coupling among distributed neuronal populations [85], reduced synchrony could contribute to the functional isolation of foci, allowing them to develop supracritical excitatory states, while synchronization could facilitate maintenance of supracritical excitatory activity in re-entrant loops and the spread of seizure activity. Both the reduced synchronization preceding some forms of epileptic activity and the enhanced synchronization associated with seizures proper go along with the disturbance of cognitive functions, supporting the notion that normal brain functions require not only appropriate adjustment of neuronal excitability, but also a subtle balance of synchrony.

NEURAL SYNCHRONY IN AUTISM

Autism is a developmental brain disorder characterized by a triad of impairments that affect social interaction, verbal and nonverbal communication, and the repertoire of interests and activities. Similar to recent work in schizophrenia [35], theories that account for the pervasive cognitive dysfunctions associated with autism have highlighted a deficit in the integration of cognitive mechanisms [86]. A number of studies have demonstrated in fact superior performance in tasks requiring recognition of details and directing attention to small elements as, for example, in visual search and in the identification of hidden figures. This reduced ability to integrate components into coherent representations is not confined to visual perception, but has also been found in the processing of auditory information, linguistic context, and social cues (for a review, see reference [86]).

Current theories and experimental data [87] converge on the notion that dysfunctional integrative mechanisms in autism may be the result of reduced neural synchronization. Recent fMRI and EEG studies have supported this view. Just *et al.* [88] examined functional connectivity by measuring the covariances of BOLD signals during sentence comprehension in high-functioning individuals with autism. The study showed systematic differences between groups with respect to the distribution of brain activation and functional connectivity. Compared to controls, subjects with autism were characterized by a marked reduction in functional connectivity throughout the cortical language system that was most pronounced during comprehension of sentences. In addition, individuals with autism showed reduced activation in the left inferior frontal gyrus (LIFG; also known as Broca's Areas), but enhanced activation in the left posterior superior temporal gyrus (LSTG) compared with the control group. This suggests that autistic subjects engaged more in extensive processing of the meaning of the individual words, as reflected in the activity in the LSTG, but reduced processing of syntactic and conceptual information.

A number of additional fMRI studies have supported the concept of reduced functional connectivity in autism. In a second study [89], Just *et al.* reported reduced functional connectivity between frontal and parietal areas during an executive task. Furthermore, there is evidence for reduced volume of the corpus callosum. fMRI studies of social cognition [90], working memory [91], and visuo-motor coordination [92] have further supported the notion that reduced functional connectivity may underlie a wide range of cognitive deficits in autism.

In analogy to the findings in schizophrenia patients, these data predict that autism should be associated with reduced neural synchrony. However, so far only a few studies have examined this possibility. Grice *et al.* [93] analyzed induced γ-band activity in individuals with autism and in a matched control group during the perception of face stimuli. In controls, an increase in induced γ-power differentiated responses to face from no-face stimuli, while subjects with autism showed no difference between the two experimental conditions. Analysis of auditory steady-state responses indicates that, similar to patients with schizophrenia, there is a reduction in the power of the stimulus-locked responses in the γ-band range in autism [94].

Several authors have recently proposed that cortical networks in autism may be characterized by an imbalance between excitation and inhibition, which leads to hyperexcitability and unstable cortical networks [95]. This hypothesis is consistent with abnormalities in GABAergic and glutamatergic transmitter systems. Indications for reduced GABAergic inhibition have been derived from the evidence that autism is associated with mutations of genes encoding subunits of the GABA(A) receptor, reduced expression of the GABA synthetic enzymes GAD65 and GAD67, and synthesis of abnormal isoforms of these enzymes [96]. Abnormal glutamatergic neurotransmission is supported by polymorphisms in genes that encode both metabotropic and ionotropic glutamate receptors [97], and a post mortem study has reported reduced AMPA-receptors in the cerebellum [97]. In addition, the serotonergic system may be dysregulated in autism [97]. To date, it is unclear how these abnormalities relate to the cognitive deficits in autism, whether they play a role in the hypothesized disruption of integrative processes, and whether there are electrographic correlates of reduced large-scale synchronization in this disorder.

Anatomically, there is evidence for both hyper- as well as hypo-connectivity in autism. During early development (between 7–11 years), white matter increases significantly more in autistic than in normal children. In the same age group, gray matter is reduced in a number of regions, including the hippocampus and amygdala [98]. Evidence for a transient hypertrophy of white matter has also been found in previous studies [99], and this finding has later been complemented by results suggesting exaggerated pruning to subnormal levels, consistent with evidence for anatomical hypoconnectivity [89]. These anatomical results also predict reduced or otherwise abnormal synchrony, but more EEG and MEG studies with advanced techniques for the identification of synchrony are required to clarify this issue.

NEURAL SYNCHRONY IN ALZHEIMER'S DISEASE

AD is the most common form of dementia, affecting approximately 11% of the world population older than 65 years of age[4]. AD is associated with a wide range of cognitive dysfunctions that typically start with characteristic memory impairment, followed by deficits in visuo-spatial and executive processes. These differential impairments in

---

[4]Hof PR, Morrison JH. The cellular basis of cortical disconnection in Alzheimer disease and related dementing conditions. In: R. Terry, R. Katzman, K.L. Bick and S. Sisodia, Editors, *Alzheimer Disease*. Lippincott Williams and Wilkins, New York: 197–229, 1999.

cognitive domains reflect the spread of cortical pathology from medial-temporal to parietal association areas [100]. Patients with AD show pronounced deficits while performing tasks that require interhemispheric transfer of information, executive processing, and episodic memory (for a review, see reference [101]). In contrast, in early stages of the disease, automatic processing is intact. Delbeuck *et al.* [101] have suggested that the profile of neuropsychological deficits is consistent with a disconnection syndrome.

A hallmark of the resting-state EEG in patients with AD is a relative increase in the θ- and Δ-band activity that co-occurs with a reduction in activity in the α- and β-band. The reduction in α-band activity correlates well with the severity of the disease and the cognitive deficits [102]. These power changes in distinct frequency bands are associated with impaired synchrony. Patients with AD show reduced coherence of oscillations in the α- and β-frequency band both for distant and nearby recording sites. More direct evidence comes from studies that have utilized more sensitive measures of synchrony. Stam and colleagues [103-105] have analyzed EEG resting data using a measure of synchronization likelihood (SL) [106] that is sensitive to linear and nonlinear interdependencies between EEG channels. The results indicate that patients with AD show a reduction in β- as well as α-band synchronization. Topographically, the reduction of synchrony is particularly pronounced for long-range synchronization [105]. In addition to lowered synchronization in the α- and β-band, patients with AD are also characterized by a reduction in γ-band synchronization in the resting state [107].

Thus, there is substantial evidence for reduced neural synchrony during the resting state, but relatively little research has been performed so far to link reductions in neural synchrony directly to impaired cognition by analyzing task- and performance-related changes of synchronization. The only task-related study is the investigation by Pijnenburg *et al.* [108]. The authors examined neural synchrony in patients with AD during a working memory task. Patients with AD showed a reduction of α- and β-band synchronization during maintenance of information in working memory compared with control subjects.

fMRI studies support this evidence of reduced coordination of neural activity in AD. By applying a working memory task, Grady *et al.* [109] found reduced functional connectivity between prefrontal cortex and hippocampus and suggested that this reflects impaired coupling and may underlie the typical memory breakdown associated with the disease. Bokde *et al.* [110] examined functional connectivity during a face-matching task in subjects with Mild Cognitive Impairment (MCI). Individuals with MCI have a higher risk of conversion to AD than cognitively normal subjects. Similar to the results by Grady and colleagues, MCI patients were characterized by a reduction in functional connectivity involving the fusiform gyrus (FG), the parietal lobes, and the dorsolateral prefrontal cortex (DLPFC). Interestingly, the groups did not differ in performance or activation. Also, the amplitudes of the BOLD signal were in the normal range, indicating that reduced functional connectivity might represent one of the earliest functional markers of AD.

The hypothesis that impaired neural synchrony underlies some of the cognitive deficits in AD is compatible with data suggesting that the degenerative processes caused by AD lead to a neocortical disconnection syndrome [101]. Neurofibrillary tangles (NFT) and neuritic plaques (NP) are particularly prominent in brain areas that give rise to long cortico-cortical tracts [111]. Accordingly, DTI studies [112] disclosed disintegration of white matter fiber tracts. Furthermore, neural synchrony in the high-frequency range is expected to be reduced because AD leads to a pronounced degeneration of the cholinergic projections to the cerebral cortex that originate in the basal forebrain and have been shown to be a necessary prerequisite for the generation of β- and γ-band oscillations and response synchronization in this frequency range [32]. The evidence that muscarinic antagonists, such as scopolamine, induce a pattern of memory and cognitive deficits characteristic of elderly subjects and shift EEG power toward lower frequencies [113] is compatible with this hypothesis.

Finally, there is evidence for alterations in glutamatergic neurotransmission, which may also affect neuronal synchronization in AD. Snyder *et al.* [114] demonstrated that NPs produce a persistent depression of NMDA-evoked currents in cortical neurons. Moreover, neurons from a genetically modified mouse model of AD expressed reduced amounts of NMDA-receptors. These findings suggest that AD-related alterations of cellular functions can cause depression of NMDA-receptor-mediated synaptic transmission. A more direct link between AD and impaired neural synchrony has been reported by Stern *et al.* [115]. Increased expression of amyloid precursor protein in transgenic mice produced an increased jitter in the timing of evoked action potentials in intracellular recordings from neocortical pyramidal neurons. These finding suggest the possibility that accumulation of AD-related proteins has specific effects on neural excitability and synaptic transmission that impair neural synchrony and, hence, also the propagation and temporal coordination of activity.

Taken together, these data suggest that the cognitive disturbances associated with AD may not solely be due to the loss of neurons, but also due to impairments in the temporal coordination of distributed neuronal activity. So far, studies have concentrated on neural synchrony in the lower frequency bands, especially in the α-band, and more investigations are required to examine the expected deficits of long-range synchrony in the higher frequency bands.

NEURAL SYNCHRONY IN PARKINSON'S DISEASE

Neural synchronization is not only relevant for cognitive functions; it also plays a major role in the temporal patterning of motor-related activity. For example, there is evidence for enhanced synchronized β-band activity prior to movement preparation and during visuo-motor coordination [116]. However, during the execution of movements this β-band synchronization disappears and gives way to synchronized γ-band oscillations [117]. These movement-related synchronization phenomena have been found in a widely distributed network comprising premotor and parietal areas of the neocortex, the cerebellum, the striatum, and subthalamic nucleus. Because we have focused this review on relations between synchrony and cognitive functions in selected brain disorders, we do not attempt to give a comprehensive overview of the numerous studies that have examined relations between oscillatory activity patterns, such as the μ or Piper rhythm, and motor processes. Instead, we review recent evidence on correlations between abnormal synchronization and movement disorders in PD.

This neurodegenerative disorder is due to the loss of dopaminergic neurons in the substantia nigra and causes changes in the patterning of neural activity in the basal ganglia (BG). Among the cardinal symptoms of PD are impaired motor activity, such as akinesia (inability to initiate movement and slowness of movement), rigidity (stiffness of muscles), and resting tremor. Evidence indicates that the pathophysiological mechanisms responsible for the akinesia and the tremor differ. Traditionally, BG dysfunctions were explained in terms of alterations in neural firing rates that underlie the spectrum of movement disorders [118]. However, recent research has emphasized a specific relation between large-scale synchronization of oscillations in the β-frequency band and akinesia (for a review see references [118-120]).

Increases in β-band activity in PD have been reported in the STN, globus pallidus externus (Gpe), and internus (Gpi) in single-unit activity and LFPs[5]. Moreover, noninvasive EEG and MEG recordings have yielded complementary data on increased long-range synchronization in the β-range between these structures and activity over cortical motor areas. This led to the hypothesis that enhanced synchronization in the β-band is responsible for the associated akinesia. This hypothesis is supported by the evidence that, in normal subjects, initiation of movements is associated with inhibition of β-rhythms in the STN and a burst of γ-oscillations. The duration of this β-suppression increases with the complexity of the intended movement, and the latency of β-suppression predicts the onset of movement; the earlier the suppression, the shorter the movement latency. In agreement with this hypothesis, therapeutic interventions reducing the akinetic symptoms have all been shown to reduce the enhanced synchronization in the β-band and to facilitate γ-oscillations. This holds for pharmacological treatments that enhance endogenous dopamine levels, for the stereotactic lesioning of the STN, and for the very effective electrical stimulation of the STN at high frequencies (>100 Hz) [121-122].

As expected, a direct relation exists between oscillatory neuronal activity and the tremor in PD. Levy *et al.* [123] examined the discharge patterns of STN neurons in PD patients with limb tremor who underwent functional stereotactic mapping. In patients who exhibited limb tremor during the recording session, neurons showed oscillatory activity that was coherent with the frequency of the tremor. Related results have been obtained with MEG recordings that have disclosed an extended tremor-related network exhibiting oscillatory activity that was harmonically related to the tremor frequency [124].

---

[5]Boroud T, Brown P, Goldberg JA, Graybiel AM, Magill PJ. Oscillations in the Basa Ganglia: The good, the bad, and the unexpected. In: J.P. Bolam, C.A. Ingham and P.J. Magill, Editors, *The Basal Ganglia VIII*. Springer, New York: 3–24, 2005.

DISCUSSION

Neural Synchrony and Pathological Brain States

The evidence reviewed suggests that schizophrenia, autism, epilepsy, AD, and PD are characterized by changes in neural synchrony that are likely to play an important role in the pathophysiology of the disorders (see Table **7.2** for a summary). There is consistent evidence across studies that disorders in schizophrenia, autism, and AD are associated with a reduction of neural synchrony that involves both local as well as long-range synchronization. In addition, the cognitive functions that are impaired have all been shown to be associated with neural synchronization, suggesting that abnormal synchrony could be one of the causes of the cognitive dysfunctions. The conditions in epilepsy and PD are more complex, as in these cases enhanced synchrony is responsible for some of the symptomatology.

The impairments of neural synchrony observed in schizophrenia, autism, and AD are consistent with current theories that emphasize a disconnection syndrome as the underlying pathophysiological mechanism. According to these theories, cognitive dysfunctions as well as the overt symptoms of these disorders arise from a dysfunction in the coordination of distributed neural activity between and within functionally specialized regions of the cerebral cortex. Reduced neural synchronization can be a consequence of disconnection, but it can also be the cause of impaired coupling between brain areas because synchronization of neural responses is essential for their propagation across sparsely connected networks[6]. At present, it is difficult to differentiate between these possibilities.

In contrast, epilepsy and PD are characterized by a large variety of abnormalities in the temporal patterning of neural activity, involving changes in the frequency of oscillatory activity and increases as well as decreases in synchronization. Each of these abnormalities is associated with specific impairments of cognitive or motor functions, supporting the notion that normal brain functions depend to a crucial extent on the appropriate adjustment and coordination of temporally structured activity. This fine-tuning appears to involve selection of oscillation frequencies as well as a delicate balance between synchronization and desynchronization of interacting cell assemblies.

Table 7.2   Summarizes Neural Synchrony in Pathological Brain States

Disorder	Neural Synchrony	Cognitive Dysfunctions	Anatomical Connectivity	Neurotransmitters
Schizophrenia	Consistent evidence for a reduction of local- and long-range synchronization	Preception, Executive for reduced anatomical connectivity	Glutamate, GABA, Dopamine	
Epilepsy	Increrase in local synchrony, evidnce for a reduction in long-range synchronization	Specific cognitive deficits in relationship to seizure fous	Reduced connectivity between seizure focus and surrounding cortical areas	GABA, Glutamate
Autism	Reduced functional connectivity, Perception, Executive Functions, Social Cognition, Attention, Memory	Increased connectivity during early development but possibly hypoconneectivity in mature cortex	GABA, Glutamate, Serotonin	
Alzheimer's Disease	Reduced neural synchrony during resting state, evidence for reduced funcational connectivity	Working Memory, Perception, Attention, Executive Process	Reduction in anatomical connectivity	Acetycholine, Glutamate

Neural Synchrony and Pathological Brain States: Implications for Normal Brain Functioning

A wide range of cognitive functions requires the coordination of distributed neural activity, and current theories highlight neural synchrony as a putative mechanism for this coordination. The findings summarized in this review provide further support for this hypothesis by demonstrating a correlation between abnormal synchronization and specific cognitive deficits in a variety of neuropsychiatric disorders.

---

[6]Abeles A. Corticonics: Neural Circuits of the Cerebral Cortex, Cambridge University Press, Cambridge (1991).

These data also suggest that deficits of mainly large-scale integration correlate with cognitive impairments. In schizophrenia [49], AD [105, 110], and autism [88], large-scale integration was found to be more impaired than local synchronization, as reflected by the amplitude of local oscillatory activity and BOLD activation. Furthermore, cognitive dysfunctions were particularly pronounced for tasks requiring interactions between widely distributed brain areas, such as integration of polymodal stimulus attributes, dynamic perceptual grouping, working memory, and executive processes [35, 101]. This agrees with the proposals of several authors that complex cognitive processes, such as attention, memory, dynamic grouping, and awareness require large-scale integration of activity [48, 85, 119].

Future Perspectives of Research on Neural Synchrony in Pathological Brain States

The data reviewed here suggest that measures of neural synchronization may be of importance for the diagnosis of neuropsychiatric disorders. As measurements of neuronal synchrony are noninvasive and quantifiable in an objective way that is largely immune to observer bias, advanced methods of time series analysis may provide valuable diagnostic tools for the assessment of disease progression and efficiency of therapeutic interventions. For example, analysis of phase synchronization has been applied to the EEG data of patients with epilepsy, and the results suggest that seizures can be predicted based on changes in synchronization [73]. Aberrant large-scale integration of neural activity may also turn out to be a predictor of incipient AD. The study by Bokde et al. [110] showed that the covariance of BOLD responses during a face-matching task was a more sensitive measure for impaired brain functioning in patients with MCI than behavioral performance or the amplitude of regional brain activation, suggesting that reduced functional connectivity might represent one of the earliest markers of changes in brain functioning in AD. Prospective longitudinal studies of phase synchronization with EEG, and preferably MEG, methodology are required to examine whether changes of synchrony in the high-frequency bands can be used as an early predictor of AD.

Impaired neural synchrony may also guide further research into the pathophysiological mechanisms underlying neuropsychiatric disorders. For example, there is increasing interest in the role of GABAergic neurotransmission in schizophrenia and autism. These efforts have already led to the investigation of therapeutic effects of GABAergic modulators in these disorders. We believe that further research into neurotransmitter systems and other mechanisms involved in the generation of oscillatory activity and its synchronization could ultimately help develop more precise pharmacological interventions for these disorders.

Besides pathological brain states such as AD, schizophrenia, epilepsy, autism, and PD, neural synchrony is also of relevance for several other disorders that have not been reviewed here. One case is multiple sclerosis (MS) because it is to be expected that axonal damage and demyelination interfere with the temporal coordination of neuronal activity. In particular, long-distance synchronization is likely to be impaired by prolongation of conduction times as has been recently demonstrated by Cover *et al.* [125].

Future studies could also consider the use of measures of neural synchrony rather than just the power of EEG or MEG signals as biofeedback signals. Evidence indicates that biofeedback can be used to modify brain states in neuropsychiatric disorders [126]. So far, the therapeutic effects of this approach have been variable, but it is conceivable that more advanced measures of the temporal coordination of distributed activity will be more effective in helping the patients bring aberrant activity under voluntary control.

CONCLUSIONS

Theoretical considerations and experimental results suggest that synchronization of neuronal activity within and across different brain regions is a fundamental property of cortical and subcortical networks and serves a variety of functions in cognitive processes (for reviews see references [3, 5, 48, 85]). The data reviewed here suggest, in addition, that neuronal synchrony is altered in a number of pathological brain states, such as schizophrenia, epilepsy, autism, AD, and PD, and that these alterations in neural synchrony may account for some of the cognitive and motor dysfunctions associated with these diseases. Some of the disease-related alterations of anatomical conditions and neurotransmitter systems interfere directly with mechanisms that support synchronization of neuronal responses. These correlations between changes in neuronal substrate, synchrony, and cognitive performance support the hypothesis that temporal coordination of distributed neuronal activity through precise synchronization plays an important role in normal brain functions. Furthermore, these correlations suggest that a focused search for abnormalities in the temporal patterning and coordination of neuronal responses may be of potential clinical relevance both for the diagnosis and eventually for the treatment of those disorders as well.

REFERENCES

[1] Gray CM, Konig P, Engel AK, Singer W. Oscillatory responses in cat visual cortex exhibit inter-columnar synchronization which reflects global stimulus properties. Nature 1989; 338(6213): 334-7.

[2] Fries P, Nikolic D, Singer W. The gamma cycle. Trends Neurosci 2007; 30(7): 309-16.

[3] Singer W. Neuronal synchrony: a versatile code for the definition of relations? Neuron 1999; 24(1): 49-65, 111-25.

[4] von Stein A, Chiang C, Konig P. Top-down processing mediated by interareal synchronization. Proc Natl Acad Sci USA. 2000; 97(26): 14748-53.

[5] Uhlhaas PJ, Pipa G, Lima B, et al. Neural synchrony in cortical networks: history, concept and current status. Front Integr Neurosci 2009; 3: 17.

[6] Volgushev M, Chistiakova M, Singer W. Modification of discharge patterns of neocortical neurons by induced oscillations of the membrane potential. Neuroscience 1998; 83(1): 15-25.

[7] Fries P, Neuenschwander S, Engel AK, Goebel R, Singer W. Rapid feature selective neuronal synchronization through correlated latency shifting. Nat Neurosci 2001; 4(2): 194-200.

[8] Kreiter AK, Singer W. Stimulus-dependent synchronization of neuronal responses in the visual cortex of the awake macaque monkey. J Neurosci 1996; 16(7): 2381-96.

[9] Neuenschwander S, Engel AK, Konig P, Singer W, Varela FJ. Synchronization of neuronal responses in the optic tectum of awake pigeons. Vis Neurosci 1996; 13(3): 575-84.

[10] Engel AK, Konig P, Gray CM, Singer W. Stimulus-Dependent Neuronal Oscillations in Cat Visual Cortex: Inter-Columnar Interaction as Determined by Cross-Correlation Analysis. Eur J Neurosci 1990; 2(7): 588-606.

[11] Neuenschwander S, Singer W. Long-range synchronization of oscillatory light responses in the cat retina and lateral geniculate nucleus. Nature 1996; 379(6567): 728-32.

[12] Brecht M, Singer W, Engel AK. Correlation analysis of corticotectal interactions in the cat visual system. J Neurophysiol 1998; 79(5): 2394-407.

[13] Roelfsema PR, Engel AK, Konig P, Singer W. Visuomotor integration is associated with zero time-lag synchronization among cortical areas. Nature 1997; 385(6612): 157-61.

[14] Fries P, Roelfsema PR, Engel AK, Konig P, Singer W. Synchronization of oscillatory responses in visual cortex correlates with perception in interocular rivalry. Proc Natl Acad Sci USA. 1997; 94(23): 12699-704.

[15] Munk MH, Roelfsema PR, Konig P, Engel AK, Singer W. Role of reticular activation in the modulation of intracortical synchronization. Science 1996; 272(5259): 271-4.

[16] Herculano-Houzel S, Munk MH, Neuenschwander S, Singer W. Precisely synchronized oscillatory firing patterns require electroencephalographic activation. J Neurosci 1999; 19(10): 3992-4010.

[17] Biederlack J, Castelo-Branco M, Neuenschwander S, Wheeler DW, Singer W, Nikolic D. Brightness induction: rate enhancement and neuronal synchronization as complementary codes. Neuron 2006; 52(6): 1073-83.

[18] Mitzdorf U, Singer W. Excitatory synaptic ensemble properties in the visual cortex of the macaque monkey: a current source density analysis of electrically evoked potentials. J Comp Neurol 1979; 187(1): 71-83.

[19] Bertrand O, Bohorquez J, Pernier J. Time-frequency digital filtering based on an invertible wavelet transform: an application to evoked potentials. IEEE Trans Biomed Eng 1994; 41(1): 77-88.

[20] Mitra PP, Pesaran B. Analysis of dynamic brain imaging data. Biophys J. 1999; 76(2): 691-708.

[21] Tallon-Baudry C, Bertrand O. Oscillatory gamma activity in humans and its role in object representation. Trends Cogn Sci 1999; 3(4): 151-62.

[22] Herrmann CS, Munk MH, Engel AK. Cognitive functions of gamma-band activity: memory match and utilization. Trends Cogn Sci 2004; 8(8): 347-55.

[23] Lachaux JP, Rodriguez E, Martinerie J, Varela FJ. Measuring phase synchrony in brain signals. Hum Brain Mapp 1999; 8(4): 194-208.

[24] Andrew C, Pfurtscheller G. Event-related coherence as a tool for studying dynamic interaction of brain regions. Electroencephalogr Clin Neurophysiol 1996; 98(2): 144-8.

[25] Schoffelen JM, Gross J. Source connectivity analysis with MEG and EEG. Hum Brain Mapp 2009; 30(6): 1857-65.

[26] Friston KJ, Frith CD, Liddle PF, Frackowiak RS. Functional connectivity: the principal-component analysis of large (PET) data sets. J Cereb Blood Flow Metab 1993; 13(1): 5-14.

[27] Engel A, Konig P, Kreiter A, Singer W. Interhemispheric synchronization of oscillatory neuronal responses in cat visual cortex. Science 1991; 252(5009): 1177-9.

[28] Lowel S, Singer W. Selection of intrinsic horizontal connections in the visual cortex by correlated neuronal activity. Science 1992; 255(5041): 209-12.

[29] Schmidt KE, Goebel R, Lowel S, Singer W. The perceptual grouping criterion of colinearity is reflected by anisotropies of connections in the primary visual cortex. Eur J Neurosci 1997; 9(5): 1083-9.

[30] Schmidt KE, Kim DS, Singer W, Bonhoeffer T, Lowel S. Functional specificity of long-range intrinsic and interhemispheric connections in the visual cortex of strabismic cats. J Neurosci 1997; 17(14): 5480-92.

[31] Bartos M, Vida I, Jonas P. Synaptic mechanisms of synchronized gamma oscillations in inhibitory interneuron networks. Nat Rev Neurosci 2007; 8(1): 45-56.

[32] Rodriguez R, Kallenbach U, Singer W, Munk MH. Short- and long-term effects of cholinergic modulation on gamma oscillations and response synchronization in the visual cortex. J Neurosci 2004; 24(46): 10369-78.

[33] Traub RD, Whittington MA, Buhl EH, et al. A possible role for gap junctions in generation of very fast EEG oscillations preceding the onset of, and perhaps initiating, seizures. Epilepsia 2001; 42(2): 153-70.

[34] Green MF. What are the functional consequences of neurocognitive deficits in schizophrenia? Am J Psychiatry 1996; 153(3): 321-30.

[35] Phillips WA, Silverstein SM. Convergence of biological and psychological perspectives on cognitive coordination in schizophrenia. Behav Brain Sci 2003; 26(1): 65-82; discussion -137.

[36] Kwon JS, O'Donnell BF, Wallenstein GV, Greene RW, Hirayasu Y, Nestor PGet al. Gamma frequency-range abnormalities to auditory stimulation in schizophrenia. Arch Gen Psychiatry 1999; 56(11): 1001-5.

[37] Brenner CA, Sporns O, Lysaker PH, O'Donnell BF. EEG synchronization to modulated auditory tones in schizophrenia, schizoaffective disorder, and schizotypal personality disorder. Am J Psychiatry 2003; 160(12): 2238-40.

[38] Krishnan GP, Vohs JL, Hetrick WP, et al. Steady state visual evoked potential abnormalities in schizophrenia. Clin Neurophysiol 2005; 116(3): 614-24.

[39] Spencer KM, Nestor PG, Niznikiewicz MA, Salisbury DF, Shenton ME, McCarley RW. Abnormal neural synchrony in schizophrenia. J Neurosci 2003; 23(19): 7407-11.

[40] Spencer KM, Niznikiewicz MA, Shenton ME, McCarley RW. Sensory-evoked gamma oscillations in chronic schizophrenia. Biol Psychiatry 2008; 63(8): 744-7.

[41] Johannesen JK, Bodkins M, O'Donnell BF, Shekhar A, Hetrick WP. Perceptual anomalies in schizophrenia co-occur with selective impairments in the gamma frequency component of midlatency auditory ERPs. J Abnorm Psychol 2008; 117(1): 106-18.

[42] Roach BJ, Mathalon DH. Event-related EEG time-frequency analysis: an overview of measures and an analysis of early gamma band phase locking in schizophrenia. Schizophr Bull 2008; 34(5): 907-26.

[43] Hirano S, Hirano Y, Maekawa T, et al. Abnormal neural oscillatory activity to speech sounds in schizophrenia: a magnetoencephalography study. J Neurosci 2008; 28(19): 4897-903.

[44] Ferrarelli F, Massimini M, Peterson MJ, et al. Reduced evoked gamma oscillations in the frontal cortex in schizophrenia patients: a TMS/EEG study. Am J Psychiatry 2008; 165(8): 996-1005.

[45] Schmiedt C, Brand A, Hildebrandt H, Basar-Eroglu C. Event-related theta oscillations during working memory tasks in patients with schizophrenia and healthy controls. Brain Res Cogn Brain Res 2005; 25(3): 936-47.

[46] Haenschel C, Bittner RA, Waltz J, et al. Cortical oscillatory activity is critical for working memory as revealed by deficits in early-onset schizophrenia. J Neurosci 2009; 29(30): 9481-9.

[47] Winterer G, Coppola R, Goldberg TE, et al. Prefrontal broadband noise, working memory, and genetic risk for schizophrenia. Am J Psychiatry 2004; 161(3): 490-500.

[48] Varela F, Lachaux JP, Rodriguez E, Martinerie J. The brainweb: phase synchronization and large-scale integration. Nat Rev Neurosci 2001; 2(4): 229-39.

[49] Uhlhaas PJ, Linden DE, Singer W, et al. Dysfunctional long-range coordination of neural activity during Gestalt perception in schizophrenia. J Neurosci 2006; 26(31): 8168-75.

[50] Linkenkaer-Hansen K, Smit DJ, Barkil A, et al. Genetic contributions to long-range temporal correlations in ongoing oscillations. J Neurosci 2007; 27(50): 13882-9.

[51] Hong LE, Summerfelt A, Mitchell BD, McMahon RP, Wonodi I, Buchanan RWet al. Sensory gating endophenotype based on its neural oscillatory pattern and heritability estimate. Arch Gen Psychiatry 2008; 65(9): 1008-16.

[52] Kubicki M, McCarley R, Westin CF, et al. A review of diffusion tensor imaging studies in schizophrenia. J Psychiatr Res 2007; 41(1-2): 15-30.

[53] Hubl D, Koenig T, Strik W, et al. Pathways that make voices: white matter changes in auditory hallucinations. Arch Gen Psychiatry 2004; 61(7): 658-68.

[54] Lee SH, Wynn JK, Green MF, et al. Quantitative EEG and low resolution electromagnetic tomography (LORETA) imaging of patients with persistent auditory hallucinations. Schizophr Res 2006; 83(2-3): 111-9.

[55] Dierks T, Linden DE, Jandl M, et al. Activation of Heschl's gyrus during auditory hallucinations. Neuron 1999; 22(3): 615-21.

[56] Fries P, Reynolds JH, Rorie AE, Desimone R. Modulation of oscillatory neuronal synchronization by selective visual attention. Science 2001; 291(5508): 1560-3.

[57]   Niessing J, Ebisch B, Schmidt KE, Niessing M, Singer W, Galuske RA. Hemodynamic signals correlate tightly with synchronized gamma oscillations. Science 2005; 309(5736): 948-51.

[58]   Lewis DA, Hashimoto T, Volk DW. Cortical inhibitory neurons and schizophrenia. Nat Rev Neurosci 2005; 6(4): 312-24.

[59]   Moghaddam B. Bringing order to the glutamate chaos in schizophrenia. Neuron 2003; 40(5): 881-4.

[60]   Krystal JH, Karper LP, Seibyl JP, et al. Subanesthetic effects of the noncompetitive NMDA antagonist, ketamine, in humans. Psychotomimetic, perceptual, cognitive, and neuroendocrine responses. Arch Gen Psychiatry 1994; 51(3): 199-214.

[61]   Jentsch JD, Roth RH. The neuropsychopharmacology of phencyclidine: from NMDA receptor hypofunction to the dopamine hypothesis of schizophrenia. Neuropsychopharmacology 1999; 20(3): 201-25.

[62]   Meeren HK, Pijn JP, Van Luijtelaar EL, Coenen AM, Lopes da Silva FH. Cortical focus drives widespread corticothalamic networks during spontaneous absence seizures in rats. J Neurosci 2002; 22(4): 1480-95.

[63]   Steriade M, Contreras D. Spike-wave complexes and fast components of cortically generated seizures. I. Role of neocortex and thalamus. J Neurophysiol 1998; 80(3): 1439-55.

[64]   Medvedev AV. Epileptiform spikes desynchronize and diminish fast (gamma) activity of the brain. An "anti-binding" mechanism? Brain Res Bull 2002; 58(1): 115-28.

[65]   Motamedi G, Meador K. Epilepsy and cognition. Epilepsy Behav 2003; 4(Suppl 2): S25-38.

[66]   Rampp S, Stefan H. Fast activity as a surrogate marker of epileptic network function? Clin Neurophysiol 2006; 117(10): 2111-7.

[67]   Allen PJ, Fish DR, Smith SJ. Very high-frequency rhythmic activity during SEEG suppression in frontal lobe epilepsy. Electroencephalogr Clin Neurophysiol 1992; 82(2): 155-9.

[68]   Jirsch JD, Urrestarazu E, LeVan P, Olivier A, Dubeau F, Gotman J. High-frequency oscillations during human focal seizures. Brain 2006; 129(Pt 6): 1593-608.

[69]   Bragin A, Engel J, Jr., Wilson CL, Fried I, Mathern GW. Hippocampal and entorhinal cortex high-frequency oscillations (100--500 Hz) in human epileptic brain and in kainic acid--treated rats with chronic seizures. Epilepsia 1999; 40(2): 127-37.

[70]   Netoff TI, Schiff SJ. Decreased neuronal synchronization during experimental seizures. J Neurosci. 2002; 22(16): 7297-307.

[71]   Garcia Dominguez L, Wennberg RA, Gaetz W, Cheyne D, Snead OC, 3rd, Perez Velazquez JL. Enhanced synchrony in epileptiform activity? Local versus distant phase synchronization in generalized seizures. J Neurosci 2005; 25(35): 8077-84.

[72]   van Putten MJ. Nearest neighbor phase synchronization as a measure to detect seizure activity from scalp EEG recordings. J Clin Neurophysiol 2003; 20(5): 320-5.

[73]   Le Van Quyen M, Navarro V, Martinerie J, Baulac M, Varela FJ. Toward a neurodynamical understanding of ictogenesis. Epilepsia 2003; 44 Suppl 12: 30-43.

[74]   Waites AB, Briellmann RS, Saling MM, Abbott DF, Jackson GD. Functional connectivity networks are disrupted in left temporal lobe epilepsy. Ann Neurol 2006; 59(2): 335-43.

[75]   Dumas de la Roque A, Oppenheim C, Chassoux F, et al. Diffusion tensor imaging of partial intractable epilepsy. Eur Radiol 2005; 15(2): 279-85.

[76]   Levitt P. Disruption of interneuron development. Epilepsia 2005; 46(Suppl 7): 22-8.

[77]   Snead OC, 3rd. Evidence for GABAB-mediated mechanisms in experimental generalized absence seizures. Eur J Pharmacol 1992; 213(3): 343-9.

[78]   von Krosigk M, Bal T, McCormick DA. Cellular mechanisms of a synchronized oscillation in the thalamus. Science 1993; 261(5119): 361-4.

[79]   Marrosu F, Santoni F, Fa M, et al. Beta and gamma range EEG power-spectrum correlation with spiking discharges in DBA/2J mice absence model: role of GABA receptors. Epilepsia 2006; 47(3): 489-94.

[80]   McCormick DA, Williamson A. Convergence and divergence of neurotransmitter action in human cerebral cortex. Proc Natl Acad Sci USA 1989; 86(20): 8098-102.

[81]   Khalilov I, Le Van Quyen M, Gozlan H, Ben-Ari Y. Epileptogenic actions of GABA and fast oscillations in the developing hippocampus. Neuron 2005; 48(5): 787-96.

[82]   Draguhn A, Traub RD, Schmitz D, Jefferys JG. Electrical coupling underlies high-frequency oscillations in the hippocampus in vitro. Nature 19989; 394(6689): 189-92.

[83]   Nilsen KE, Kelso AR, Cock HR. Antiepileptic effect of gap-junction blockers in a rat model of refractory focal cortical epilepsy. Epilepsia 2006; 47(7): 1169-75.

[84]   Gajda Z, Gyengesi E, Hermesz E, Ali KS, Szente M. Involvement of gap junctions in the manifestation and control of the duration of seizures in rats in vivo. Epilepsia 2003; 44(12): 1596-600.

[85]   Fries P. A mechanism for cognitive dynamics: neuronal communication through neuronal coherence. Trends Cogn Sci 2005; 9(10): 474-80.

[86]   Happe F, Frith U. The weak coherence account: detail-focused cognitive style in autism spectrum disorders. J Autism Dev Disord 2006; 36(1): 5-25.

[87]   Uhlhaas PJ, Singer W. What do disturbances in neural synchrony tell us about autism? Biol Psychiatry 2007; 62(3): 190-1.

[88]   Just MA, Cherkassky VL, Keller TA, Minshew NJ. Cortical activation and synchronization during sentence comprehension in high-functioning autism: evidence of underconnectivity. Brain 2004; 127(Pt 8): 1811-21.

[89]   Just MA, Cherkassky VL, Keller TA, Kana RK, Minshew NJ. Functional and anatomical cortical underconnectivity in autism: evidence from an FMRI study of an executive function task and corpus callosum morphometry. Cereb Cortex 2007; 17(4): 951-61.

[90]   Castelli F, Frith C, Happe F, Frith U. Autism, Asperger syndrome and brain mechanisms for the attribution of mental states to animated shapes. Brain 2002; 125(Pt 8): 1839-49.

[91]   Koshino H, Carpenter PA, Minshew NJ, Cherkassky VL, Keller TA, Just MA. Functional connectivity in an fMRI working memory task in high-functioning autism. Neuroimage 2005; 24(3): 810-21.

[92]   Villalobos ME, Mizuno A, Dahl BC, Kemmotsu N, Muller RA. Reduced functional connectivity between V1 and inferior frontal cortex associated with visuomotor performance in autism. Neuroimage 2005; 25(3): 916-25.

[93]   Grice SJ, Spratling MW, Karmiloff-Smith A, et al. Disordered visual processing and oscillatory brain activity in autism and Williams syndrome. Neuroreport 2001; 12(12): 2697-700.

[94]   Wilson TW, Rojas DC, Reite ML, Teale PD, Rogers SJ. Children and adolescents with autism exhibit reduced MEG steady-state gamma responses. Biol Psychiatry 2007; 62(3): 192-7.

[95]   Rubenstein JL, Merzenich MM. Model of autism: increased ratio of excitation/inhibition in key neural systems. Genes Brain Behav 2003; 2(5): 255-67.

[96]   Polleux F, Lauder JM. Toward a developmental neurobiology of autism. Ment Retard Dev Disabil Res Rev 2004; 10(4): 303-17.

[97]   Purcell AE, Jeon OH, Zimmerman AW, Blue ME, Pevsner J. Postmortem brain abnormalities of the glutamate neurotransmitter system in autism. Neurology 2001; 57(9): 1618-28.

[98]   Herbert MR, Ziegler DA, Deutsch CK, et al. Dissociations of cerebral cortex, subcortical and cerebral white matter volumes in autistic boys. Brain 2003; 126(Pt 5): 1182-92.

[99]   Courchesne E, Karns CM, Davis HR, et al. Unusual brain growth patterns in early life in patients with autistic disorder: an MRI study. Neurology 2001; 57(2): 245-54.

[100]   Braak H, Braak E. Neuropathological stageing of Alzheimer-related changes. Acta Neuropathol 1991; 82(4): 239-59.

[101]   Delbeuck X, Van der Linden M, Collette F. Alzheimer's disease as a disconnection syndrome? Neuropsychol Rev 2003; 13(2): 79-92.

[102]   Jeong J. EEG dynamics in patients with Alzheimer's disease. Clin Neurophysiol 2004; 115(7): 1490-505.

[103]   Stam CJ, Montez T, Jones BF, et al. Disturbed fluctuations of resting state EEG synchronization in Alzheimer's disease. Clin Neurophysiol 2005; 116(3): 708-15.

[104]   Stam CJ, van der Made Y, Pijnenburg YA, Scheltens P. EEG synchronization in mild cognitive impairment and Alzheimer's disease. Acta Neurol Scand 2003; 108(2): 90-6.

[105]   Stam CJ, Jones BF, Nolte G, Breakspear M, Scheltens P. Small-world networks and functional connectivity in Alzheimer's disease. Cereb Cortex 2007; 17(1): 92-9.

[106]   Stam CJ, Dijk BWv. Synchronization likelihood: an unbiased measure of generalized synchronization in multivariate data sets. Phys D 2002; 163(3): 236-51.

[107]   Koenig T, Prichep L, Dierks T, et al. Decreased EEG synchronization in Alzheimer's disease and mild cognitive impairment. Neurobiol Aging 2005; 26(2): 165-71.

[108]   Pijnenburg YA, v d Made Y, van Cappellen van Walsum AM, Knol DL, Scheltens P, Stam CJ. EEG synchronization likelihood in mild cognitive impairment and Alzheimer's disease during a working memory task. Clin Neurophysiol 2004; 115(6): 1332-9.

[109]   Grady CL, Furey ML, Pietrini P, Horwitz B, Rapoport SI. Altered brain functional connectivity and impaired short-term memory in Alzheimer's disease. Brain 2001; 124(Pt 4): 739-56.

[110]   Bokde AL, Lopez-Bayo P, Meindl T, et al. Functional connectivity of the fusiform gyrus during a face-matching task in subjects with mild cognitive impairment. Brain 2006; 129(Pt 5): 1113-24.

[111]   Pearson RC, Esiri MM, Hiorns RW, Wilcock GK, Powell TP. Anatomical correlates of the distribution of the pathological changes in the neocortex in Alzheimer disease. Proc Natl Acad Sci USA 1985; 82(13): 4531-4.

[112]   Naggara O, Oppenheim C, Rieu D, et al. Diffusion tensor imaging in early Alzheimer's disease. Psychiatry Res 2006; 146(3): 243-9.

[113]   Ebert U, Kirch W. Scopolamine model of dementia: electroencephalogram findings and cognitive performance. Eur J Clin Invest 1998; 28(11): 944-9.

[114]   Snyder EM, Nong Y, Almeida CG, et al. Regulation of NMDA receptor trafficking by amyloid-beta. Nat Neurosci 2005; 8(8): 1051-8.

[115]   Stern EA, Bacskai BJ, Hickey GA, Attenello FJ, Lombardo JA, Hyman BT. Cortical synaptic integration in vivo is disrupted by amyloid-beta plaques. J Neurosci 2004; 24(19): 4535-40.

[116]   Murthy VN, Fetz EE. Oscillatory activity in sensorimotor cortex of awake monkeys: synchronization of local field potentials and relation to behavior. J Neurophysiol 1996; 76(6): 3949-67.

[117]   Schoffelen JM, Oostenveld R, Fries P. Neuronal coherence as a mechanism of effective corticospinal interaction. Science 2005; 308(5718): 111-3.

[118]   Brown P. Oscillatory nature of human basal ganglia activity: relationship to the pathophysiology of Parkinson's disease. Mov Disord 2003; 18(4): 357-63.

[119]   Schnitzler A, Gross J. Normal and pathological oscillatory communication in the brain. Nat Rev Neurosci 2005; 6(4): 285-96.

[120]   Hutchison WD, Dostrovsky JO, Walters JR, et al. Neuronal oscillations in the basal ganglia and movement disorders: evidence from whole animal and human recordings. J Neurosci 2004; 24(42): 9240-3.

[121]   Brown P, Oliviero A, Mazzone P, Insola A, Tonali P, Di Lazzaro V. Dopamine dependency of oscillations between subthalamic nucleus and pallidum in Parkinson's disease. J Neurosci 2001; 21(3): 1033-8.

[122]   Sharott A, Magill PJ, Harnack D, Kupsch A, Meissner W, Brown P. Dopamine depletion increases the power and coherence of beta-oscillations in the cerebral cortex and subthalamic nucleus of the awake rat. Eur J Neurosci 2005; 21(5): 1413-22.

[123]   Levy R, Hutchison WD, Lozano AM, Dostrovsky JO. High-frequency synchronization of neuronal activity in the subthalamic nucleus of parkinsonian patients with limb tremor. J Neurosci 2000; 20(20): 7766-75.

[124]   Timmermann L, Gross J, Dirks M, Volkmann J, Freund HJ, Schnitzler A. The cerebral oscillatory network of parkinsonian resting tremor. Brain 2003; 126(Pt 1): 199-212.

[125]   Cover KS, Vrenken H, Geurts JJ, et al. Multiple sclerosis patients show a highly significant decrease in alpha band interhemispheric synchronization measured using MEG. Neuroimage 2006; 29(3): 783-8.

[126]   Sterman MB, Egner T. Foundation and practice of neurofeedback for the treatment of epilepsy. Appl Psychophysiol Biofeedback 2006; 31(1): 21-35.

CHAPTER 8

Brain Stimulation Techniques and Network Studies of Brain Function

Mouhsin Shafi[1,*] and Alvaro Pascual-Leone[2]

[1]*Neurology Department, 55 Fruit Street, Wang 8, Massachusetts General Hospital, Boston, MA, 02114, USA and* [2]*Department of Neurology, Berenson-Allen Center for Noninvasive Brain Stimulation Beth Israel Deaconess Medical Center Harvard Medical School, 330 Brookline Ave, KS 454, Boston MA 02215, USA*

Abstract: Recently developed brain stimulation techniques such as transcranial magnetic stimulation (TMS) and transcranial direct current stimulation (tDCS) use electromagnetic principles to noninvasively alter brain activity, with the precise effects varying as a function of stimulus intensity, frequency and duration, as well as the target location. The ability to manipulate brain activity in a temporally and spatially specific manner has helped delineate the time-varying contributions of various brain regions to normal cortical function. When combined with other brain imaging technologies such as MRI, PET and EEG, these brain stimulation techniques can also provide additional insights into the network dynamics and functional connectivity of different brain regions. Such studies have played an important role in advancing our understanding of the processes that underlie normal brain functions such as sleep and language, and the alterations that occur in pathological conditions such as depression. Furthermore, these techniques have also been used to study the brain's response to injury, such as in motor recovery after ischemic stroke. Because brain stimulation techniques can also be used to noninvasively produce potentially long-lasting, predictable changes in cortical activity, their utility in the treatment of various neuropsychiatric disorders is also being actively explored, with some encouraging results. Consequently, brain stimulation techniques are promising and important new tools in the understanding of cortical function and treatment of brain pathology.

Keywords: Transcranial magnetic stimulation, transcranial direct current stimulation, non-invasive, multi-modal, plasticity, mechanisms, depression, sleep, stroke.

INTRODUCTION

In the past several decades, a variety of techniques to explore brain function have been developed and applied. Most of these techniques either passively measure brain activity in different ways, or else require invasive procedures. Recently, however, a number of noninvasive techniques for manipulating brain activity have been developed. These noninvasive techniques provide a valuable tool for human interventional neurophysiology studies, permitting targeted interventions on human brain function and behavior. Combination of brain stimulation techniques with other methods such as EEG, fMRI and PET enable even more sophisticated studies of the mechanisms and dynamics of brain activity, and the relationship with specific cognitive processes. Furthermore, by producing potentially long-lasting changes in cortical function, brain stimulation techniques provide a new therapeutic modality whose utility is being explored in a variety of neuropsychiatric diseases. The two most common noninvasive brain stimulation techniques, transcranial magnetic stimulation (TMS) and transcranial direct current stimulation (tDCS), both rely on electromagnetic principles to influence brain activity.

In TMS, a large but spatially restricted magnetic flux is used to induce an electrical field in a target cortical area. The induced currents can be sufficient to depolarize neurons and produce spiking; as such, TMS can be either neurostimulatory or neuromodulatory. The effects of TMS vary based on a variety of different parameters, including the number, frequency and intensity of the TMS pulse, as well as the location of the target. When a train of TMS stimuli are applied (a procedure called repetitive TMS, or rTMS), changes in cortical activity can persist long after the end of stimulation [1-3]. Consequently, TMS has been increasingly applied in a variety of experimental settings [4] aimed at elucidating the network architecture of various cognitive processes, as well as in network dysfunctions and adaptations in various disease states. Furthermore, because of the ability to produce long-lasting changes in cortical function, rTMS is also being explored as a therapeutic intervention in a number of neuropsychiatric diseases [5-6].

Address correspondence to Mouhsin Shafi: Neurology Department, 55 Fruit Street, Wang 8, Massachusetts General Hospital, Boston, MA, 02114, USA; Email: mshafi@partners.org

In contrast, in tDCS, low-amplitude direct currents are applied *via* scalp electrodes and penetrate the skull to enter the brain. While these currents are usually not sufficient to induce action potentials, they do modulate the membrane potential, thus altering the excitability of neurons in response to additional inputs. When tDCS is applied for a sufficient duration, the modulation of cortical excitability persists beyond the duration of stimulation [7]. For these reasons, tDCS has also been used as a research and therapeutic device.

TRANSCRANIAL MAGNETIC STIMULATION: BASIC BIOPHYSICS

Magnetic stimulation is based on the principle of electromagnetic induction (Fig. **8.1**). A changing electric current in the stimulation coil produces a magnetic flux, which in turn induces electric currents in conducting materials such as human brain tissue. Consequently, the basic TMS stimulator design involves a capacitive high-voltage, high-current charge-discharge system connected *via* a switch (usually a thyristor or a silicon-controlled rectifier to prevent ringing in the circuit) to the inductor of the stimulation coil. Current TMS machines are capable of producing a pulsed magnetic field of up to several Tesla, with a pulse duration as brief as a quarter of a millisecond. Single pulse devices are capable of delivering a stimulus every several seconds, while the rapid stimulators used in repetitive TMS (rTMS) are capable of delivering stimuli at up to 100 Hz.

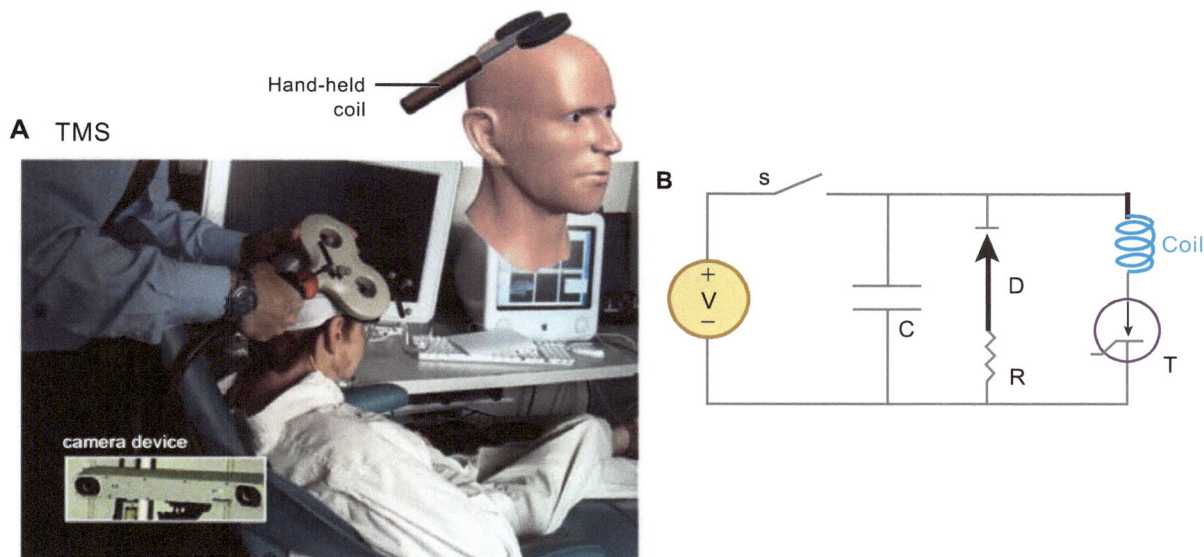

Fig. (8.1). The experimental setup for TMS stimulation. The patient is wearing a device that permits targeted administration of the TMS pulse. A simplified circuit diagram of a single-pulse magnetic stimulator is illustrated below. In this diagram, *V* is the voltage source, *S* is a switch, *C* is a capacitor, *R* is the resistor, *D* is the diode, and T is the thyristor (with permission from Wagner *et al*, 2007).

The effect of a TMS pulse on cortical activity is dependent on a number of different factors, including the strength of the magnetic flux, the shape of the stimulation coil, the shape and duration of the pulse, the distance and angle between the coil and the cortical surface, the direction of the induced electrical currents, the precise stimulation sequence, and the underlying cortical architecture and activity. The TMS pulse configuration can be either monophasic or biphasic, with differential effects on the cortex. The shape of the stimulation coil determines the induced current distribution, and thus influences the site of stimulation. The first stimulation coil to be used was a simple circle several centimeters in diameter, containing up to twenty turns of copper wire. The induced current in the underlying tissue is maximal near the outer edge of the coil; as such, a relatively large region of cortex is stimulated. To address this issue, another commonly used coil design is the "figure-8" or "butterfly", in which two round coils are placed side by side such that the currents flow in the same direction at the junction point. As a result, the induced electric fields add up to a maximum in the region below the junction of the two coils, thereby limiting the area in which the induced currents are sufficient to significantly alter neuronal activity (Fig. **8.2**). The area of the cortical surface that is intensely stimulated has been debated, but models and some experimental data on evoked responses suggest that it is on the order of approximately 1 cm^2 [8-9]. Other coil designs have also been developed in order to achieve greater focality or to stimulate deeper regions; however, it has been shown analytically that the induced current will always be greatest at the cortical surface [10].

TMS

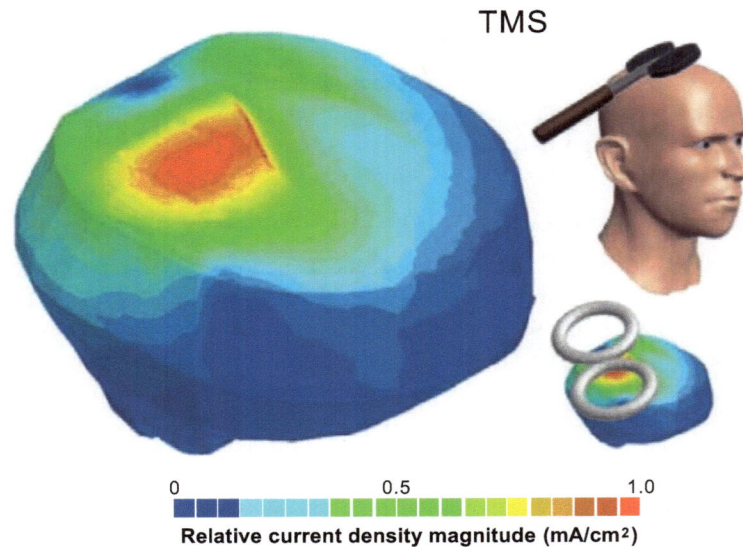

0   0.5   1.0

Relative current density magnitude (mA/cm²)

Fig. (8.2). Current density magnitude on the cortical surface. Relative current density is shown in pseudo-color according to the scale. The coil position is shown over the head, as well as a schematic of the current induced beneath it (Modified with permission from Wagner *et al*, 2007).

Unfortunately, little is known about the precise mechanisms of TMS activation of neural tissue *in vivo*. One model used to study the effects of TMS is the Roth peripheral nerve model, an active-cable-type model incorporating Hodgkin-Huxley conductances. Using this model, some studies have predicted that the site of neural stimulation (the initiation of action potentials) occurs at the point where the spatial derivative of the induced electric field is maximal [11-13]. However, this model applies only to peripheral nerve stimulation. Another model that attempted to more accurately incorporate cortical microanatomy suggested that excitation occurs at either the axon terminal or at the cell body where the neural axons begin [14-16].

TMS PARADIGMS: PHYSIOLOGICAL EFFECTS AND MECHANISMS OF ACTION

Relatively few studies have investigated the physiological effects of TMS on single-unit and neuronal population activity. One study utilizing extracellular recordings in the visual cortex of anesthetized cats assessed the effects of single-pulse TMS on neuronal activity [17]. They demonstrated that a single TMS pulse was associated with a strong facilitation of spontaneous and visual-evoked spiking activity during the first 500ms after the TMS pulse. This was followed by a subsequent long-lasting (several second) suppression of activity, the duration of which increased with increasing stimulus strength. In addition, stronger TMS pulses increasingly evoked an early suppression of activity for 100–200ms, which was followed by the previously described facilitation and then inhibition. In another study utilizing different TMS pulse trains (1 to 4 seconds, 1 to 8 Hz), TMS increased the spontaneous activity for up to sixty seconds; in contrast, visual evoked responses were significantly decreased for approximately five minutes [18]. As such, these experiments suggest that the effects of TMS on cortical circuits are complex, depending on an interaction between the specific stimulation parameters (which may be specific to the experimental preparation) and the underlying cortical state.

Despite the uncertainty regarding the precise cellular mechanisms by which TMS exerts its effects, TMS continues to be used to probe and to alter cortical excitability in a variety of different experimental paradigms. TMS of motor cortex produces muscle responses, termed motor-evoked potentials (MEPs), which provide a particularly useful metric for measuring cortical responses to TMS. The MEP size varies with the intensity of stimulus, with stronger TMS stimuli producing larger MEPs [19]. TMS-evoked MEPs are also facilitated if the subject voluntarily contracts the target muscle slightly [20-22]. Another commonly studied metric is the motor threshold, usually defined as the minimum stimulus intensity necessary to produce MEPs of a particular size (usually 50 μV) in 50% of trials [23]; the change in motor threshold in various disease states is usually interpreted as evidence of altered cortical excitability. Paired-pulse TMS studies can be helpful in further localizing and characterizing excitation/inhibition balance intracortically [24]. After the initial MEP, TMS during voluntary muscle contraction also produces a subsequent period of suppressed activity lasting up to 100-300 ms, termed the cortical silent period [25-26], which is believed to be mediated *via* interneuron activity at GABA-B receptors [27]; the duration of the silent period can be modulated by the TMS intensity, number and timing of pulses, and various pathological states, including for example, epilepsy [28].

As mentioned above, paired-pulse stimulation protocols can provide further insights into excitation/inhibition balance. A conditioning stimulus is applied to the brain prior to the test stimulus delivered, for example over motor cortex. Studies have shown that a subthreshold conditioning stimulus to motor cortex decreases the MEP produced by the test stimulus when the interstimulus interval (fISI) is from 1-5 ms [29-31]. This inhibition, termed short-interval intracortical inhibition, is believed to be mediated at the level of local interneurons, likely *via* GABA-A receptors [29, 32-33]. Paired-pulse TMS with two suprathreshold stimuli also results in inhibition of the test MEP at ISIs of 50-200 ms [34-35]; however, this long-interval intracortical inhibition is believed to be mediated *via* GABA-B receptors [36]. As such, different GABAergic inhibitory mechanisms can be studied in the brain using different paired-pulse TMS protocols. Particularly important is the discovery that a conditioning stimulus applied to one motor cortex inhibits the response to a subsequent test stimulus delivered to the contralateral motor cortex [37-38]; similarly, TMS of motor cortex suppresses voluntary contraction of the ipsilateral hand for a short period of time [37-39]. In patients with agenesis of the corpus callosum, no such inhibition was seen [39]. The inter-hemispheric inhibition noted in these studies provided the motivation for subsequent experiments evaluating the therapeutic potential of rTMS to modulate the excitability of the unaffected hemisphere in stroke patients (see below). In addition to the inhibition described above, intracortical facilitation in response to paired-pulse TMS at specific intervals has also been noted.

Another common stimulation method is repetitive TMS (rTMS), which involves the delivery of trains of TMS pulses, often at high frequencies. These protocols produce changes in cortical excitability that persist beyond the duration of the stimulus. The specific effect depends on stimulus frequency, intensity and duration, the total number of stimuli, the structure of the pulse train, and the pre-existing cortical state. The mechanisms through which these protocols alter excitability are unknown, but are believed to involve processes similar to synaptic long-term potentiation and long-term depression [40]. In one of the earliest studies of the effects of rTMS, Pascual-Leone *et al.* demonstrated that high-frequency (>5 Hz) rTMS trains generally increased cortical excitability, as measured *via* MEP size [2]. Significantly, these effects persisted for 3-4 minutes after the end of stimulation. In contrast, rTMS at frequencies of 1 Hz or below generally decreases cortical excitability. One of the first studies of low-frequency rTMS demonstrated that low-frequency rTMS at 0.9 Hz at 115% of resting motor threshold for 15 minutes led to a decrease of MEP amplitude of approximately 20%; this effect persisted for over 15 minutes [3]. Subsequent studies have confirmed and extended these findings. A recent review of studies of the effects of rTMS on cortical excitability (as measured with simultaneous EEG) notes that both low-frequency and high-frequency rTMS produce an approximately 30% change in TMS-evoked response (depression with low-frequency rTMS, and facilitation with high-frequency rTMS), with the excitability changes persisting for a mean of about 30 minutes [41]. Significantly however, one study demonstrated that if an identical rTMS protocol was repeated on consecutive days, the evoked change in cortical excitability was larger on day 2, implying some type of carryover effect [42]. Indeed, the presence of some long-term effects with repeated rTMS underlies its use as a therapeutic modality in various neuropsychiatric disorders.

More recently, Huang *et al.* developed a patterned repetitive stimulation protocol to rapidly induce changes in cortical plasticity [1]. The stimulation protocols they devised are based on rodent microelectrode experiments in which a "theta-burst" stimulation pattern was used to induce synaptic long-term potentiation and long-term depression. The "theta-burst" pattern they developed consisted of 3 pulses at 50 Hz and intensity of 80% active motor threshold, repeated every 200 ms (ie. at 5 Hz). In the continuous protocol, a 40-second train of uninterrupted theta-burst stimulation was applied, for a total of 600 pulses; the result was a maximum decrease in MEP amplitude of over 40%, with suppression persisting for as long as 60 minutes. In the intermittent theta burst protocol, a two-second train of theta burst stimulation was repeated every 10 seconds, also for a total of 600 pulses; the maximum increase in MEP amplitude was 75%, with the facilitation lasting for about 15 to 20 minutes. In the studies of rTMS with EEG, theta-burst effects on evoked responses persisted for up to 90 minutes, longer than for conventional (fixed-rate) rTMS protocols.

Previous studies in animals combined electrical stimulation of motor cortex with recordings from the dorsolateral surface of the spinal cord [43-44]. These studies demonstrated that a single suprathreshold electrical stimulus to motor cortex resulted in a series of high-frequency waves in the downstream electrodes. The first wave was thought to result from direct activation of the axons of fast pyramidal tract neurons, and was therefore called the D-wave. Later waves were thought to originate from indirect trans-synaptic activation of pyramidal neurons, and were therefore termed I-waves. Based on these findings, a number of recent studies have evaluated the effect of TMS on motor cortex during epidural recordings from human patients with electrodes implanted in the spinal cord for treatment of chronic pain (see Di Lazzaro for review [33]). These studies have demonstrated that single pulse TMS produces primarily I-waves, "indirect" waves elicited *via* trans-synaptic mechanisms, with the number and magnitude of the waves a function of stimulus intensity, induced current direction, pre-existing voluntary muscle contraction. The interpeak interval between successive I-waves is approximately 1.4 ms, consistent with a discharge frequency of 700 Hz. Furthermore, these studies have indicated that the various inhibitory and facilitating processes identified in paired-pulse experiments tend to affect the later I-waves, suggesting that they are operating at the level of intracortical circuits. Similar recordings in subjects undergoing rTMS have demonstrated that suprathreshold 5 Hz stimulation leads to an increase in the size and number of descending corticospinal volleys evoked by each TMS pulse, and this increase persists after the end of stimulation. Meanwhile, continuous theta-burst stimulation leads to a significant decrease in the very first I-wave, with later waves much less affected. Thus, the various TMS protocols all produce effects that are believed to be mediated primarily *via* trans-synaptic intracortical pathways, rather than by direct axonal activation.

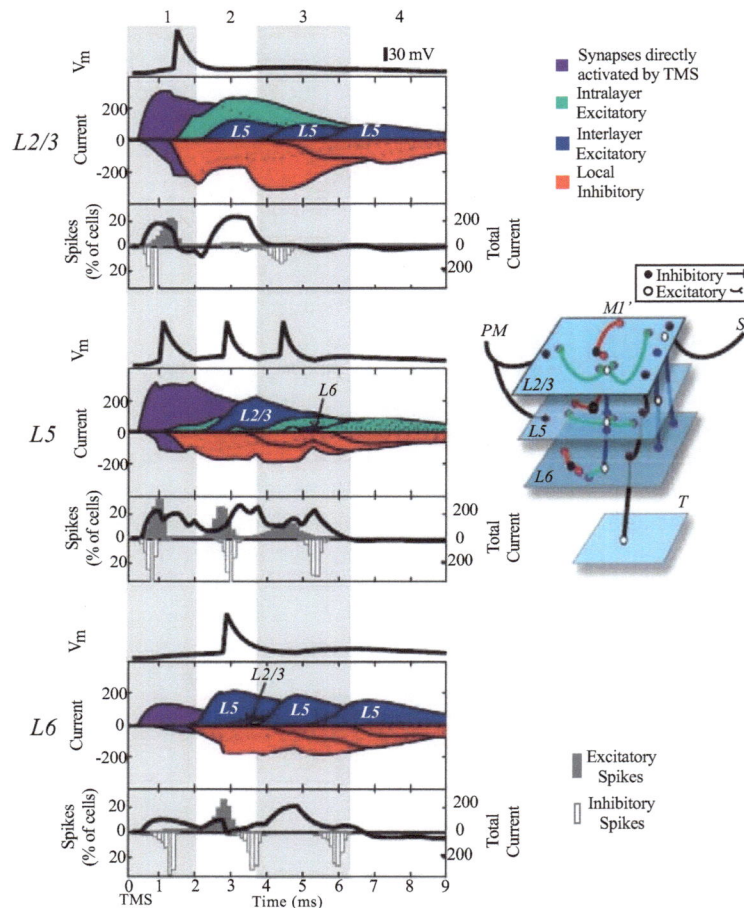

Fig. (8.3). The cortical response to a single TMS pulse, sorted by layer (with permission from Esser *et al*, 2005). The top solid line trace in each layer depicts the typical membrane potential change in an excitatory cell within that layer. The colored graphs represent the various synaptic currents within this cell sorted by their source; the interlayer excitatory currents are labeled according to the source layer. Once activated, the currents take many milliseconds to decay, as illustrated by the dotted lines that continue from each wave of activity. The solid black line below the current sections depicts the total summated (excitatory minus inhibitory) current to that cell. The gray and white bars demonstrate the total number of excitatory and inhibitory spikes within that layer. In the figure shown below, a single TMS pulse strong enough to activate 20% of the fibers in primary motor cortex (area MP in the circuit diagram on the right) results in three waves of excitatory output from the pyramidal cells in layer 5. These distinct waves are a result of a complex interplay of excitatory and inhibitory interactions within and between layers, with distinct segments of current activity indicated by the numbers on top. A schematic of the circuit is included on the right; the interactions between the three layers in primary motor cortex (MP) are shown in the center, with inputs from the thalamus (T), somatosensory cortex (SI) and premotor cortex (PM) also illustrated.

To help understand the mechanisms by which TMS exerts its effects, Esser *et al.* constructed a detailed computational model of motor cortex, and then simulated the effects of a TMS pulse [45] (Fig. **8.3**). Their model consisted of a 33,000 neuron, 3-layer cortex with spiking integrate-and-fire units with individual glutamate (AMPA and NMDA) and GABA conductances, and with over 5 million synaptic connections structured according to current literature. Their model replicated many previous experimental findings, such as a sequence of I-waves similar to those produced by real TMS pulses, and the cortical response to TMS in the presence of GABA antagonists. They demonstrated that the I-waves produced by a TMS pulse result from a complex interplay of intra-laminar and inter-laminar excitatory and inhibitory connections, with individual I-waves resulting from spiking activity in different cortical layers, but primarily from layer 5.

tDCS: BIOPHYSICS AND MECHANISMS OF ACTION

In transcranial direct current stimulation (tDCS), static weak polarizing electrical currents are applied to the scalp and penetrate to cortical regions of the brain (Fig. **8.4**). These currents preferentially modulate the activity of neurons with axons that are oriented longitudinally in the plane of the applied electric field, producing changes in the activity of individual cortical neurons [46-48]. The induced changes in excitability occur primarily *via* modulation of voltage-sensitive cation channels [49]. Unlike in TMS, tDCS modulates the firing rate of neurons, but does not directly induce firing. Anodal stimulation of the cortex generally increases the excitability of underlying neurons by depolarizing cell membranes, while cathodal stimulation decreases cortical excitability *via* hyperpolarization (although this is not always the case [47]. More recent studies have combined tDCS with single-pulse TMS to assess the excitability changes produced by tDCS [7, 50-52]. These studies demonstrated that anodal tDCS significantly increases the size of the TMS evoked MEP, while cathodal tDCS decreases MEP size. Furthermore, these excitability changes persisted after the end of the tDCS stimulation, with the duration and magnitude of the effects varying as a function of the current intensity and duration of tDCS [50]. A subsequent study demonstrated that if tDCS is applied at 1 milli-ampere (mA) for at least 9 minutes, the induced excitability changes after cessation of stimulation were long-lasting (90 minutes when anodal tDCS was applied for 13 minutes) [7]. These long-lasting changes are believed to occur at an intracortical level, perhaps mediated through NMDA receptor activity [51-55].

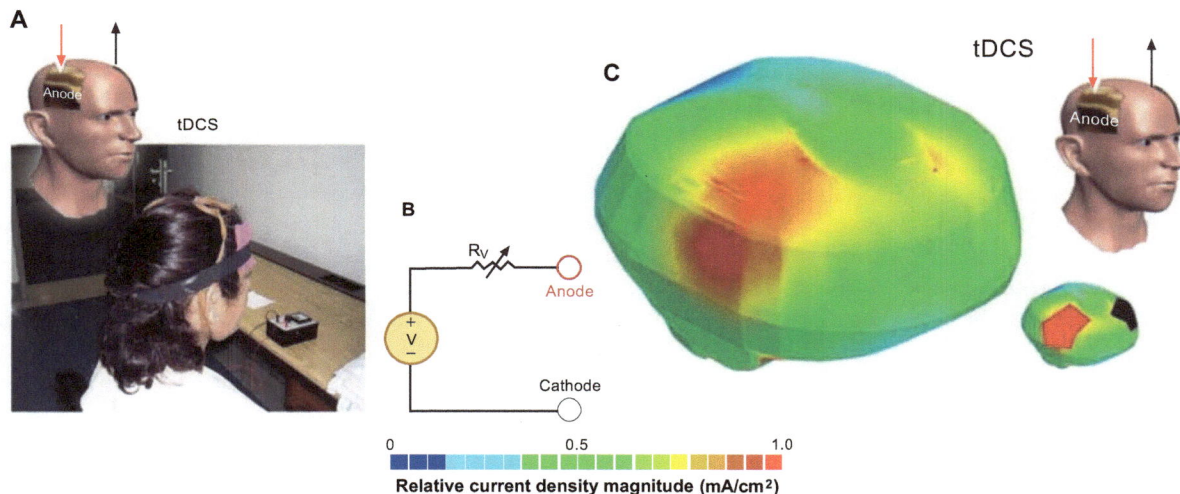

Fig. (8.4). The experimental setup for tDCS. A constant low-amplitude DC current is applied to the cortex *via* large scalp electrodes (**A**), along with the corresponding circuit (**B**). V represents the voltage source, and Rv is the variable resistor. Panel **C** shows the current density magnitude on the cortical surface. Relative current density is shown in pseudo-color according to the scale. (Modified with permission from Wagner *et al*, 2007).

CLINICAL UTILITY OF BRAIN STIMULATION TECHNIQUES

Brain stimulation techniques such as TMS and tDCS possess a number of advantages that make them excellent tools for human research. Both are noninvasive techniques that can be applied in a relatively brief period of time; a typical rTMS or tDCS session takes on the order of 20 minutes. The machinery required for both techniques is relatively affordable; single-pulse TMS machines cost less than $10,000, while more sophisticated rTMS systems, capable of applying patterned TMS protocols, incorporating MRI data and recording online EEG and EMG, cost less than $200,000. tDCS systems are even less expensive. Both are quite portable, and thus have the advantage that they can be moved around a hospital or clinic setting, and brought to patients with limited mobility. Furthermore, a significant benefit of brain stimulation techniques is that they are relatively benign, in that the "virtual lesion" effects usually don't persist. Consequently, brain stimulation techniques can be used to create "virtual lesions", thereby safely permitting the exploration of the role of different cortical regions in a variety of human cognitive functions. Furthermore, the adverse effect profile of both techniques is quite favorable. While TMS can provoke seizures at high frequencies/intensities, especially in susceptible individuals, the risk of seizures is quite small if appropriate safety guidelines are followed [56]. There are little to no long-term persistent effects from single sessions (or from sessions separated by long periods of time), and thus the long-term risks are felt to be negligible. TMS in particular is relatively focal, capable of altering cortical excitability directly over a relatively small region (although the activity changes provoked in the stimulated region will then be propagated to other regions; see below). As such, it offers a powerful tool for achieving spatially targeted changes in cortical activity, or for targeting focal pathologies. Finally, brain stimulation techniques can be combined with other tools such as EEG, fMRI and PET. By inducing targeted changes in brain activity, and then studying how those changes are propagated throughout the brain, it becomes possible to causally test network theories of brain function in humans, and to study the dynamics of cortical activity. For all of these reasons, noninvasive brain stimulation techniques hold significant promise in the study of human cognition, and the treatment of neuropsychiatric disease. In the following sections such applications are described in greater detail.

TRANSCRANIAL BRAIN STIMULATION AND NETWORK ANALYSIS

Traditionally, insights into brain function have been largely derived from studying the deficits caused by specific brain lesions. The view emerging from this approach posits a relatively simple structure-function relationship, in which anatomically distinct brain regions perform specialized, relatively independent computations (*e.g.* visual cortex is responsible for vision). More recently, this approach has been significantly extended by studies using brain imaging (*e.g.* functional MRI) to obtain evidence correlating brain activity in certain brain regions with specific behaviors. However, it has become increasingly apparent that complex brain functions, such as coordinated movement, memory and language, depend critically on dynamic interactions between brain areas, leading to the concept of functional connectivity networks - distributed brain regions transiently interacting to perform a particular neural function [57-59]. Abnormalities in the interactions of network components play a critical role in common and devastating neurological and psychiatric disorders ranging from depression to epilepsy [60-62], and damage to specific functional connectivity networks can lead to distinct neurological syndromes [63]. Furthermore, both the deficits and functional recovery after damage from strokes or traumatic brain injury may depend on the architecture and adaptability of these networks [64-67]. Despite the increasing implication of network dysfunction in the clinical setting, functional network analysis currently has only a minimal role currently in clinical neuropsychiatry. The reasons for this are two-fold: 1) the techniques currently used in functional connectivity studies are primarily correlational, and the interactions they identify have not been validated in experiments that directly manipulate neural activity, and 2) therapeutic interventions that modulate neural networks in a specific and targeted fashion have not been developed. Noninvasive brain stimulation techniques offer a unique set of tools to potentially address both of these issues. TMS changes neural activity directly in a spatially and temporally focused manner. By studying how the changes induced by TMS are then propagated throughout the rest of the brain, the connectivity of the stimulated brain region can be causally assessed, and the results compared with the findings of traditional functional connectivity analysis [68-73]. Furthermore, since different rTMS and tDCS protocols produce somewhat long-lasting changes in neural activity in a relatively predictable manner, noninvasive brain stimulation techniques permit the directed manipulation of neural activity. The potential implications for our understanding and treatment of network dysfunction in neuropsychiatric diseases are significant.

TMS enables the assessment of dynamical changes in the manner in which different cortical regions interact. One of the earliest uses of TMS involved producing a "virtual lesion" to assess the temporal relationship of involvement of different cortical regions in specific cognitive functions [4]. For example, Amassian *et al.* demonstrated that TMS to the occipital pole was effective in abolishing visual perception of a letter if the pulse was administered between 80 and 100ms after stimulus onset; pulses administered significantly before or after this interval had no such effect [74]. Such studies can reveal surprising results; for example, Chambers *et al.* demonstrated that the right angular gyrus is involved in the reorienting of spatial attention at two distinctly different time points (between 90 and 120 ms after stimulus onset, and again between 210 and 240 ms after stimulus onset), suggesting that the same cortical region can be involved at different time points during a single task [75]. Furthermore, experiments with TMS can delineate the time-course of interactions between different cortical regions. As an example, Silvanto *et al.* studied the effects of single-pulse stimulation to the frontal eye fields (FEF) on the excitability of area V5/MT (as measured by phosphene threshold, the minimum TMS intensity required to produce a phosphene) [76]. They demonstrated that FEF stimulation 20 to 40 milliseconds before stimulation of area V5/MT lowered the phosphene threshold significantly. Stimulation of the frontal eye fields at other time points had no such effects.

The combination of TMS with other technologies such as PET, EEG and fMRI permits more detailed analyses of the interactions between a number of different cortical regions, thereby permitting a causal assessment of functional connectivity networks. One seminal early study performed PET scanning while rTMS pulse trains of varying lengths were applied to the frontal eye fields [77]. They demonstrated a significant positive relationship between blood flow and TMS in the region being stimulated (the left frontal eye fields), as well as in a number of distant cortical regions, including the left medial parieto-occipital cortex, the bilateral superior parietal cortex, and the right supplementary eye field. Thus, TMS produced changes in cerebral blood flow not only at the site of stimulation, but in a distributed network of functionally connected regions. A subsequent study showed that the pattern of blood flow changes varies as a function of the stimulated region [78]. rTMS to premotor cortex modulated a widespread network, including several regions in the prefrontal and parietal cortices; in contrast, rTMS to motor cortex modulated activity in a smaller number of brain regions, primarily confined to the cortical and subcortical motor systems. More recent studies combining TMS with fMRI have confirmed and extended the above findings (Fig. **8.5**), demonstrating that even subthreshold TMS can activate a widespread cortical and subcortical network [79-81].

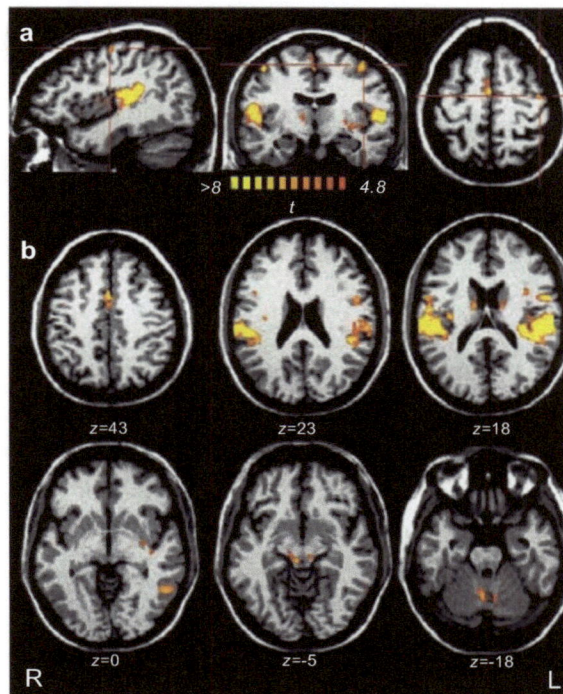

Fig. (8.5). BOLD MRI responses to rTMS of left premotor cortex (with permission from Bestmann *et al.* 2005), based on a t-score pseudocolor scaling. Panel **A** demonstrates the sagittal, coronal and axial view of activity in the targeted left dorsal premotor cortex (cross-hairs). Panel **B** shows six transverse sections showing activity changes in the cingulated gyrus, ventral premotor cortex, auditory cortex, caudate nucleus, left posterior temporal lobe, medial geniculate and cerebellum.

Similarly, early studies combining TMS with EEG demonstrated that single-pulse TMS to the motor cortex produced a complex sequence of successive activations, with EEG activity changes under the TMS coil occurring immediately, then spreading over a few milliseconds to ipsilateral motor, premotor and parietal regions, and then spreading several milliseconds later to the contralateral motor cortex [82-83] (Fig. **8.6**). Furthermore, subsequent studies utilizing EEG functional connectivity measures such as coherence have provided quantitative evidence that rTMS can actually alter the strength of the connection between different cortical regions [84-85]; the behavioral significance of these changes is as yet unknown.

a)

b)

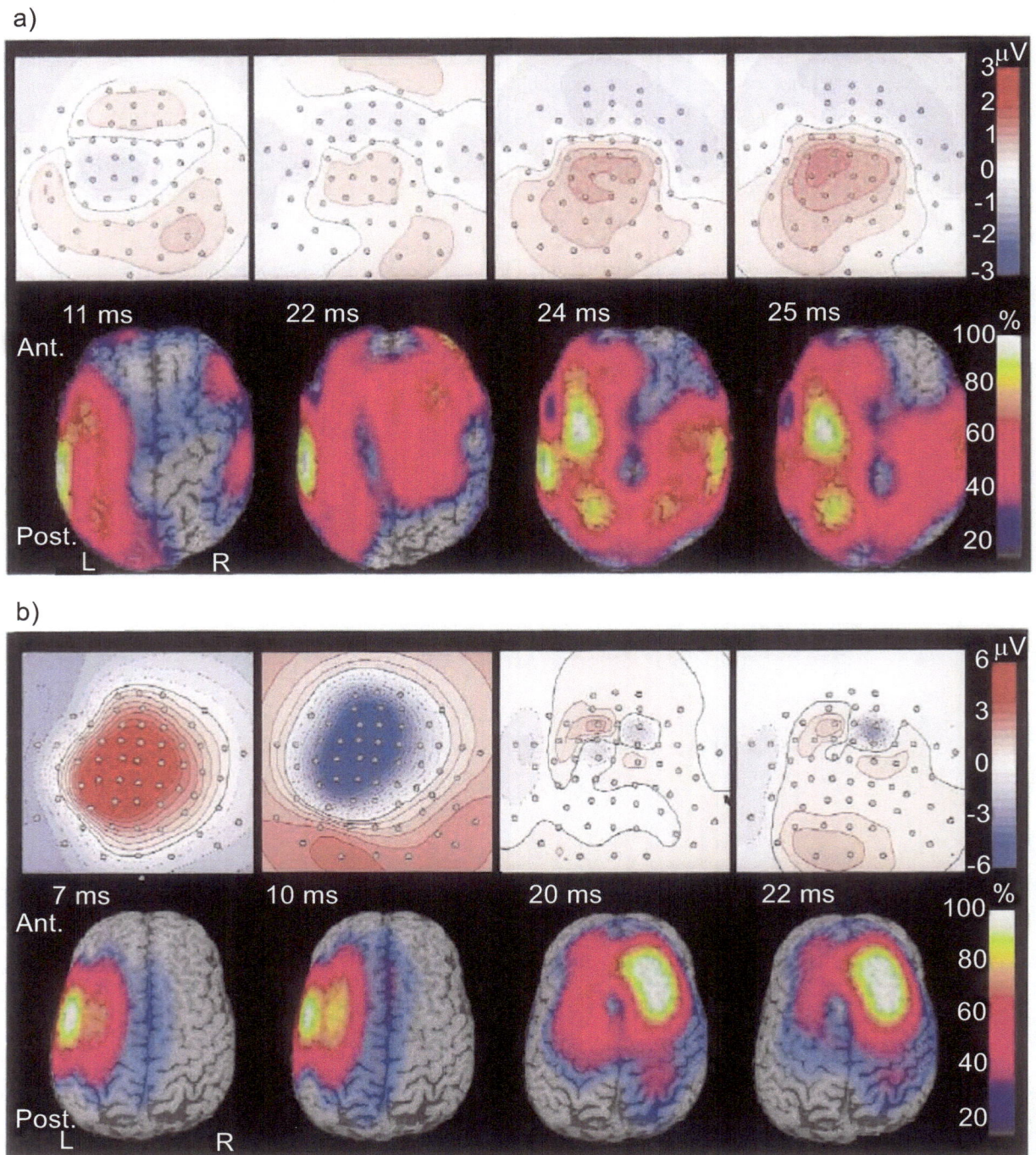

Fig. (8.6). The spread of activation after stimulation of right motor cortex, illustrated as scalp potential maps and current density distributions, in two subjects (with permission from Komssi *et al.* 2002). On the scalp potential maps (top panels in **A** and **B**), the head is shown as a two dimensional projections. The contour lines depict constant potentials; positive potentials are red, negative potentials are blue. In the current-density distributions (bottom panels in **A** and **B**), the calculated current-density at each time point is depicted as a percentage of the maximum current-density at that time point. For the subject depicted in panel **A**, at 11 ms, the activation had spread from below the coil center to involve the surrounding frontal and parietal cortices. Contralateral activation emerged at 22 ms, and peaked at 24 ms. For the subject depicted in panel **B**, the spread of activation is similar, although the regions of activation are more confined.

The combination of TMS with other technologies also permits more sophisticated analysis of the dynamics of interactions between different cortical regions. For example, in one novel study, the TMS-evoked response was studied using functional connectivity analysis of EEG data in the awake and sleeping state [86]. It was shown that while the local TMS-evoked response is similar in the two states, the activity in remote cortical regions differed markedly, (see below, *"Brain stimulation and sleep"* for more details). Furthermore, such combined-modality studies permit analysis of precisely how different regions interact. For example, in a recent study, TMS was applied to the left motor hand region while brain activity was imaged with PET [87]. Structural equation modeling was then applied to the PET data to evaluate the connectivity, focusing on regions that were known to be activated during TMS to motor cortex (Fig. 8.7). Since TMS was being applied to a single (known) location at a specific time point, the sequence and direction of interactions with other cortical regions could be precisely delineated, permitting the construction of a detailed activity-path model. In this study, after TMS of left motor cortex, activity initially propagated to five regions: the supplementary motor area, the cingulate gyrus, the left ventral nucleus of the thalamus, the right secondary somatosensory cortex, and the right cerebellum. From these initial points, activity then propagated through a number of additional regions.

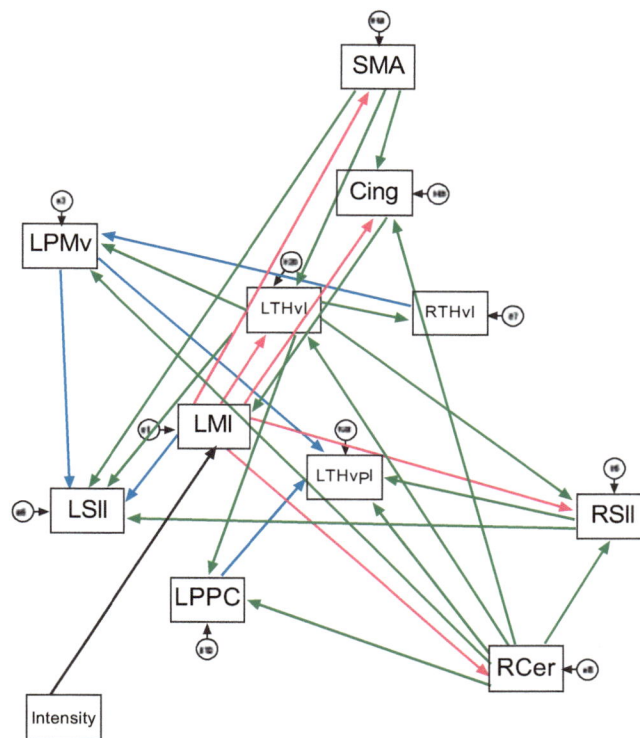

Fig. (8.7). Connectivity of left M1 hand region, based on structural equation modeling of PET data after TMS (with permission, from Laird *et al*. 2008). This map was created by applying TMS stimulation to the left primary motor cortex, and PET was used to measure changes in blood flow. Connectivity of regions in this case is based on the temporal relationship of changes in activity (using a technique called structural equation modeling). First order paths are shown in pink, meaning that the TMS "signal" propagates immediately after motor cortex stimulation. The second-order paths are green, indicating propagation of activity changes from the first-order targets (and similarly, the third order paths are shown in blue). Regions are as follows: LMI - Left primary sensorimotor cortex; LPPC = Left posterior parietal cortex; LTHvpl - Left ventral posterolateral nucleus of the thalamus; LTHvl - Left ventral lateral nucleus of the thalamus; LPMv - Left ventral premotor area; Cing - Cingulate gyrus; SMA - Supplementary motor area; RSII - Right secondary somatosensory Cortex; LSII - Left secondary somatosensory cortex; RTHvl - Right ventrolateral thalamus; Rcer - Right cerebellum.

In addition, combined-modality studies involving TMS can be used to assess how the neural functional connectivity changes during different cognitive tasks. In one particularly interesting recent study combining TMS and EEG, single-pulse TMS was applied to the human FEF while subjects performed either a face discrimination or motion discrimination task [88]. Notably, there was a significant difference between the two tasks in the TMS event-related potentials in the right parieto-occipital region. Furthermore, the TMS pulse during the motion task preferentially activated a current source in the region corresponding to area MT (known from fMRI studies to be involved in face perception), while the fusiform face area was the preferential source of the currents evoked by the TMS pulse during the face task. Taken together, these results suggest that the activity provoked by FEF TMS propagated along different pathways depending on which visual task was being performed, and that the functional connectivity of the FEF varied dynamically as a function of the task parameters.

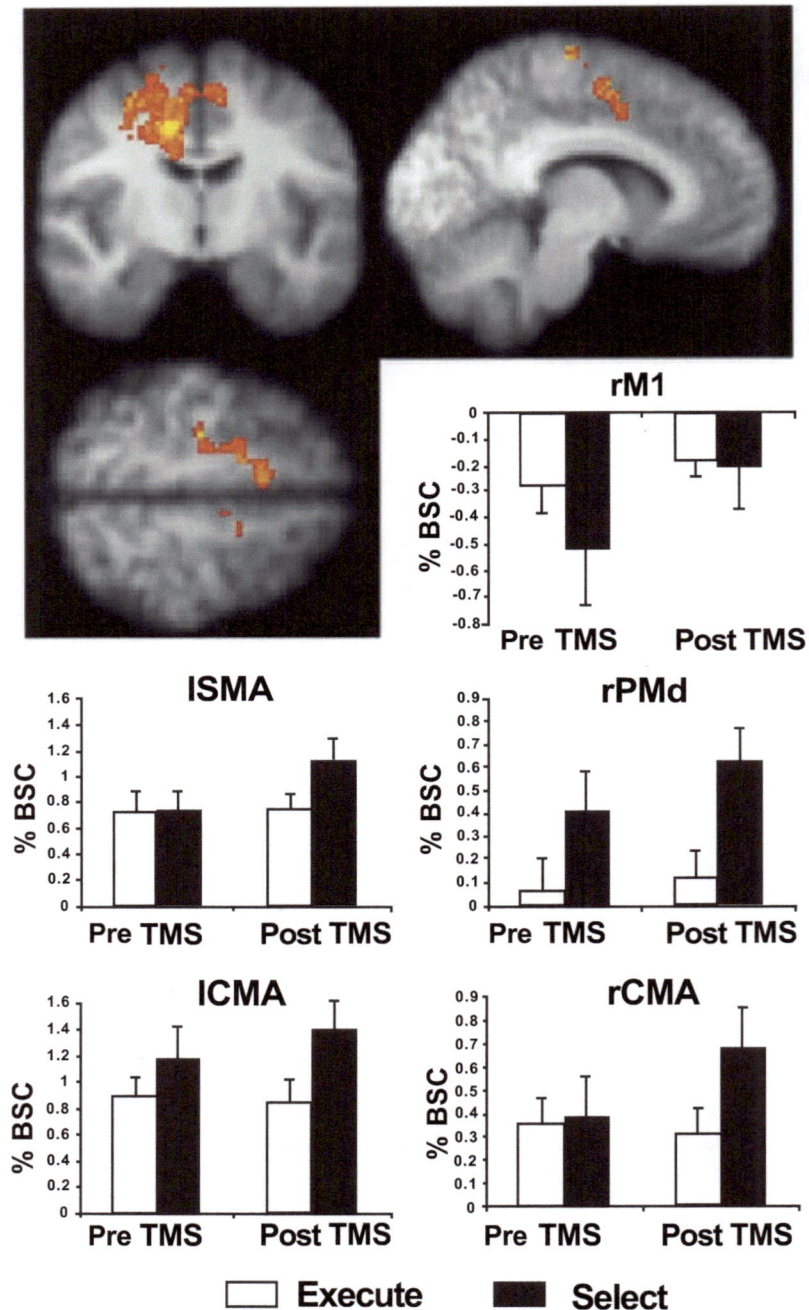

Fig. (8.8). Compensatory activation increases in the action selection network after left dorsal premotor cortex rTMS (with permission, from O'Shea *et al.* 2007). 1Hz rTMS of left dorsal premotor cortex (lPMd), and inhibitory frequency, caused increased activation most prominent in right dorsal premotor cortex (rPMd) and right cingulate motor area (rCMA); lesser changes occurred in right primary motor cortex (rM1), left supplementary motor area (lSMA), and left cingulate motor area (lCMA). BOLD signal changes accompanied action selection (black bars) compared to the control action execution (white bars).

TMS can also be used to study the dynamic mechanisms that the brain utilizes to compensate for focal disruptions in activity. In one elegant study, O'Shea *et al.* used repetitive TMS to induce mild, transient disruptions to a focal cortical region, and then used fMRI to study compensatory changes in the brain [89] (Fig. **8.8**). They focused on the left dorsal premotor region, an area which shows increased activation after motor stroke, and is involved in action selection. Inhibitory rTMS applied to the left dorsal premotor cortex initially resulted in a disruption in performance on an action selection task; within a few minutes, however, performance returned to baseline. fMRI demonstrated that during task performance prior to rTMS, blood flow increased to a left-hemisphere dominant premotor-parietal network. fMRI several minutes after rTMS of the left premotor cortex, after behavioral performance had recovered to baseline, demonstrated increased activation in the right premotor cortex, left supplementary motor area, and bilateral cingulated motor areas

Thus, recovery of task performance was associated with increased activity in multiple other cortical regions. Importantly, these compensatory increases in activity were not seen when subjects performed a control motor task that does not involve the left premotor cortex, and these changes were also not seen when rTMS was applied to primary motor cortex, suggesting that the observed compensatory changes are occurring in a task- and region-specific manner. To show that this compensatory activity in right premotor cortex is behaviorally relevant, TMS was then also applied to the right premotor cortex. TMS to the right premotor cortex alone had no effect on task performance, suggesting that right premotor cortex is usually not critical for task performance; however, if right premotor cortex was stimulated after rTMS of left premotor cortex, task performance was impaired. Thus, the results suggest that the compensatory increase in right premotor activity seen after inhibitory rTMS of left premotor cortex is casually involved in behavioral recovery, a finding with significant clinical implications for motor recovery after stroke (see below, *Brain stimulation and stroke*).

ASSESSING THE ROLE OF OSCILLATIONS

When combined with EEG, brain stimulation techniques also have a potentially significant role in elucidating the origin and function of cortical oscillatory activity. This is partly because single TMS pulses induce transient changes in power and coherence in specific frequency bands, with the precise frequency and magnitude of effects varying as a function of stimulus intensity and location [90-93]. One early study demonstrated that suprathreshold stimulation of motor cortex led to an increase in beta-frequency EEG oscillations in motor and premotor cortices [94]. A follow-up study demonstrated that there was an increase in phase-synchronization in the beta frequency range after the TMS pulse, with no significant amplitude modulation, suggesting that the beta oscillatory response seen after single-pulse TMS is due to phase resetting and synchronization of existing oscillatory activity, rather than the induction of new oscillations [91-92]. Furthermore, the amplitude of the induced beta oscillation was significantly higher in primary motor than in premotor cortex, suggesting that the oscillatory response is related to the intrinsic rhythmicity of the underlying cortex. Intriguingly, the authors also demonstrated that inhibitory rTMS to the motor cortex did not affect subsequent single-pulse induced beta oscillations, suggesting that the generation of beta oscillations was not significantly dependent on the local intracortical connections modulated by inhibitory rTMS. The importance of thalamocortical connections in generation of the beta rhythm was demonstrated by another study that utilized TMS in combination with EEG in Parkinsonian patients that had undergone a unilateral thalamotomy [91-92]. The study demonstrated that the oscillatory activity induced by single-pulse TMS was significantly greater in the intact than in the operated hemisphere; specifically, both the amplitude and duration of the TMS-evoked beta activity was greater in the intact hemisphere. Furthermore, the TMS-evoked beta oscillatory activity in the intact hemisphere was also significantly greater than the activity in normal controls (whereas the beta activity was similar in the lesioned hemisphere of parkinsonian patients and normal controls). Taken together, these studies demonstrated the utility of TMS in elucidating the mechanism of oscillatory activity in the cortex, as well as its alteration in neurologic disease.

Another recent study utilized TMS to demonstrate that different cortical regions are tuned to oscillate at different characteristic frequencies [93]. In this study, the authors applied single pulse TMS to three different cortical regions (occipital, parietal and frontal cortex; Brodmann areas 19, 7 and 6). Intriguingly, TMS of occipital cortex produced primarily alpha activity (mean frequency of dominant oscillation 11 Hz), while that of parietal cortex produced oscillatory activity in the beta-1 range (18 Hz) and prefrontal stimulation produced low gamma activity (29 Hz). Furthermore, each region produced approximately the same oscillatory response, regardless of which specific area was stimulated: TMS applied to area 6 resulted in 10.6 Hz activity in area 19, 19 Hz activity in area 7, and 29 Hz activity in area 6. These differential preferred frequencies were consistent across all normal subjects. Intriguingly, however, TMS applied to frontal cortex of schizophrenic patients produced reduced high-frequency oscillatory activity [95], suggesting that the intrinsic rhythmicity of different cortical regions might be altered in various pathological states.

Brain stimulation techniques can also be utilized to study how the presence of oscillatory activity affects the cortical reactivity to external stimuli. For example, in visual cortex, a variety of different studies in both animals and humans have suggested that the baseline activity is related to the size or latency of cortical responses to a subsequent visual stimulus, and also to the probability of whether a threshold stimulus is detected [96-101]. Indeed, several studies have suggested that alpha-band EEG activity is related to perception [98, 100-101]. To explore this issue further, Romei *et al.* applied single-pulse TMS at phosphene threshold to human visual cortex, while simultaneously recording EEG [102]. They found that instantaneous alpha activity (in the 250ms prior to TMS administration) was significantly lower on trials in which phosphenes were elicited versus trials in which no phosphenes were produced. The alpha activity in a given region (and thus the likelihood of a perceptual response to TMS) fluctuated on a relatively rapid (sub-second) time scale. A separate study, found that individual phosphene threshold was directly correlated with individual alpha power in parieto-occipital cortex; subjects with higher alpha power required higher stimulation intensities to generate phosphenes, and the authors were unable to elicit phosphenes in the subjects with the highest alpha power, even at maximum stimulator intensity [103]. These experiments thus directly demonstrated that alpha activity in visual cortex is associated with decreased cortical excitability (as defined by the MEP). A subsequent study demonstrated similar findings (increased local alpha power associated with decreased cortical excitability to stimulation) in motor cortex; no association was found between activity in any other frequency band and the motor response [104]. These studies demonstrate how brain stimulation techniques can be utilized to study the functional consequences of oscillatory activity.

The effects of rTMS may also be mediated through changes in cortical oscillatory activity. Several studies have demonstrated that rTMS at different frequencies modulates EEG power and coherence in different frequency bands [105-108]. Hamidi *et al.* investigated how rTMS affected alpha power in individual subjects, and whether the TMS-induced changes in power was correlated with behavioral performance in a working memory task [109]. Performance on a spatial working memory task (and a control object working memory task) was assessed with and without delivery of 10Hz rTMS to superior parietal lobule (and a control location in primary somatosensory cortex) during the delay period. When rTMS was delivered to the superior parietal lobule during the spatial working memory task, the authors found a clear negative correlation between rTMS-induced change in alpha-band power and subsequent behavioral performance. Subjects in whom rTMS decreased alpha power had improved performance, while subjects in whom rTMS increased alpha power performed more poorly; in contrast, there was a *positive* correlation between alpha activity and task performance in the three control conditions. Thus, the authors demonstrated that the behavioral effects of rTMS in this task are associated with modulation of oscillatory activity. This experiment thus demonstrates how rTMS may be a useful technique in exploring how oscillatory activity contributes to behavior and cognition.

BRAIN STIMULATION AND SLEEP

Noninvasive brain stimulation techniques have also been used to investigate the mechanisms and purpose of sleep. One recent study explored the question of why consciousness fades during sleep [86]. The authors hypothesized that consciousness is based on the brain's ability to integrate information from disparate sources, which in turn is contingent on effective connectivity between different specialized regions of the thalamocortical system. As a consequence of this hypothesis, they predicted that effective connectivity decreases during sleep. To test this issue, they applied single-pulse TMS to the frontal cortex of subjects in either wakefulness or different sleep stages, and studied the resulting TMS-evoked potential using EEG (Fig. **8.9**). The authors found that during wakefulness, TMS induced a sustained response of recurrent waves of activity, with the underlying cortical currents shifting over time to different regions across the cortex. In contrast, during NREM sleep, TMS induced a much larger immediate local response that then terminated rapidly; furthermore, the TMS-evoked potential was confined to the region of stimulation, and did not propagate to any other cortical region. These results thus supported the hypothesis that the loss of consciousness during sleep is associated with a breakdown in effective connectivity between different cortical regions. A recent follow-up study utilizing TMS demonstrated a similar breakdown in effective connectivity during the loss of consciousness induced by midazolam anesthesia [110].

Brain stimulation techniques have also been used to explore the relationship between sleep (especially slow wave sleep), synaptic plasticity and learning. Specifically, brain stimulation techniques have been used to study the hypothesis of synaptic homeostasis [111] that slow-wave activity increases after local synaptic potentiation, and decreases after local synaptic depression. In one study, 5Hz rTMS or sham stimulation was applied to motor cortex, with a resulting potentiation of both the motor-evoked potentials and the EEG TMS-evoked response in the subjects receiving 5Hz rTMS; the maximum increase in the TMS-evoked currents was in premotor cortex [112]. Subjects were then allowed to fall asleep, and the first NREM sleep episode recorded (likely mixed sub-stages present). Subjects who had received 5Hz stimulation had an increase in total slow-wave activity as compared to subjects who received sham stimulation, with the maximum increase in slow-wave activity occurring at the same electrode (premotor cortex) with the largest increase in the TMS-evoked currents. Furthermore, the change in the TMS-evoked response was significantly correlated with the increase in slow wave activity in frontal electrodes. In a follow-up study, another TMS protocol called paired associative stimulation was used to either potentiate or depress the excitability of motor cortex (as measured by motor-evoked potentials and TMS-evoked EEG response) [113]. In subjects in whom cortical excitability was increased, local slow-wave activity increased during subsequent NREM sleep; in contrast, in subjects with decreased cortical excitability, low slow-wave activity also decreased during NREM sleep. The magnitude of the change in cortical excitability was significantly correlated with subsequent changes in slow wave-activity. Taken together, these studies provided support for the notion that changes in local cortical excitability lead to changes in local slow-wave activity during subsequent sleep period, suggesting that slow-wave sleep is involved in synaptic plasticity and learning.

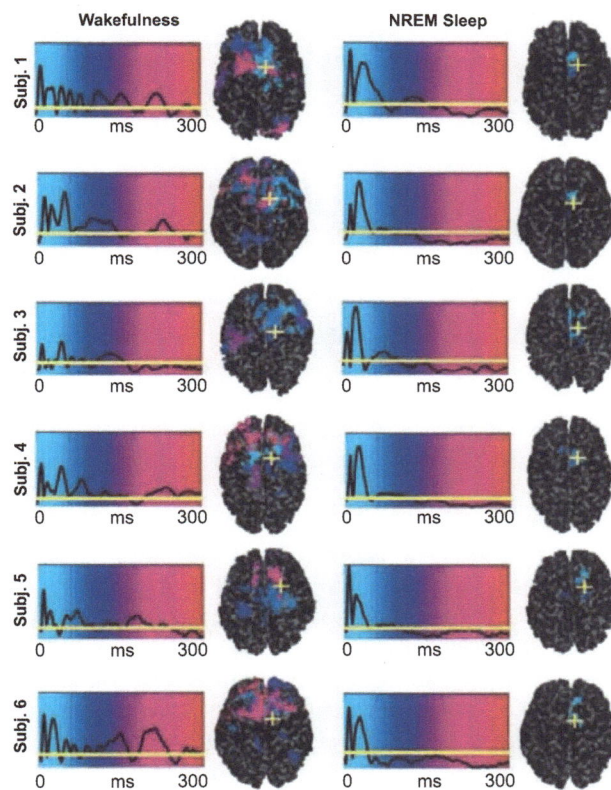

Fig. (8.9). Spatiotemporal TMS-evoked current maps during wakefulness and NREM sleep in six subjects. The black traces represent the global mean field power at each time point; when the black line is above the horizontal yellow line, the global power of the evoked field was significantly higher (>6 SD) than the mean prestimulus level. For each significant time sample, maximum current sources were plotted and color-coded according to their latency of activation (light blue, 0 ms; red, 300 ms). The yellow cross marks the TMS target on the cortical surface.

This hypothesis is further strengthened by a study that applied transcranial oscillating electrical potentials at a frequency of 0.75 Hz to human subjects during periods of NREM sleep [114]. In this study, the subjects were trained on a declarative memory (paired-association word learning) task, and then allowed to fall asleep. Transcranial oscillating potentials at 0.75 Hz were then applied (with the anodal electrodes applied frontolaterally, and the cathodes at the mastoids) during stage N2 sleep. Application of the transcranial oscillating potentials led to an increase in slow oscillations and slow spindle activity over the frontal electrodes. Importantly, subjects undergoing transcranial stimulation had a significantly greater improvement in performance of the declarative memory task the following morning than subjects undergoing sham stimulation; no such difference was noted in subjects performing a procedural memory task. Thus, the authors demonstrated that boosting slow-wave activity during NREM sleep directly improved performance on a declarative memory task, thereby providing strong evidence for the association between slow-wave sleep and learning.

BRAIN STIMULATION AND DEPRESSION

To date, the strongest support for brain stimulation techniques in clinical neuropsychiatry (and the only FDA-approved indication) is in the treatment of depression. The use of brain stimulation techniques in depression has been predicated on the hypothesis that depression is driven by widespread network dysfunction. Neuroimaging studies have suggested that one of the changes seen in depressed subjects is a relative hypoactivity of the left dorsal prefrontal cortex [115-117], with a normalization of activity with response to treatment [118-119].

The potential utility of brain stimulation techniques was illustrated in several early studies that demonstrated that rTMS to prefrontal cortex had effects on mood [120-121]. Based on these findings, Pascual-Leone *et al.* conducted a trial of daily high-frequency or sham rTMS to left or right dorsolateral prefrontal cortex, with each site stimulated for five consecutive days [122]; they showed that only high-frequency rTMS to the left dorsolateral prefrontal cortex significantly improved depression scores, with the effects lasting for approximately two weeks. A large number of subsequent trials have been carried out, with the majority finding high-frequency rTMS to the left dorsolateral prefrontal cortex to be effective in relieving symptoms of depression. More recently, several studies have also looked at the effects of low-frequency (inhibitory) rTMS to the right prefrontal cortex, with most finding that inhibitory rTMS to the right prefrontal cortex is also efficacious in the treatment of depression [40, 123-124]. A recent meta-analysis found a total of 34 randomized, placebo-controlled, parallel-group studies of rTMS to prefrontal cortex in depression, involving a total of 1383 patients [125]; 28/34 studies demonstrated a benefit with rTMS, with a mean weighted effect size (mean difference / standard deviation) for all studies of 0.55 (p < 0.001). The single largest randomized placebo-controlled trial conducted to date involved the application of high-frequency (10 Hz) rTMS to the left prefrontal cortex, in daily sessions occurring five times a week for a maximum of 30 sessions over six weeks [126]. A total of 301 patients were enrolled; all patients were medication-free at the time of enrollment, and had previously failed 1-4 adequate medication trials. The authors found that active rTMS was consistently and significantly superior to sham treatment on a variety of different outcome measures. They also found that a longer duration of treatment was associated with a better response. Based on the findings of this trial, rTMS was approved by the FDA for the treatment of medication-resistant depression in October 2008.

The neural mechanisms by which rTMS modulates depression are unknown, but two (non-exclusive) hypothesis are that 1) rTMS directly modulates activity (*e.g. via* synaptic plasticity mechanisms) in the frontocingulate network that is associated with depression, or 2) rTMS may facilitate monoaminergic transmission (with likely diverse impact on neurochemical milieu [127]. To explore how rTMS of frontal cortex affects cortical activity in other regions, Paus *et al.* [94] conducted a study combining rTMS of dorsolateral prefrontal cortex with PET. Intriguingly, the authors demonstrated that an initial test stimulus (double-pulse TMS) caused decreased blood flow in both the area being stimulated, and a number of other regions (including the anterior cingulate). After excitatory rTMS, the same double-pulse TMS now caused an increase in blood flow in the same regions, thereby demonstrating the rTMS effects modulate activity in a widespread cortical network. Another study studied changes in regional blood flow in depressed patients after 10 daily treatments of either 20-Hz or 1-Hz rTMS to the left dorsolateral prefrontal cortex [128] (Fig. **8.10**)l. As predicted, 20-Hz rTMS increased blood flow in a widespread network including the L>R prefrontal cortex, the L>R cingulate gyrus, limbic cortex, thalamus and cerebellum. In contrast, low-frequency rTMS caused significant decreases in blood flow in right prefrontal cortex, left mesial temporal lobe, left basal ganglia and left amygdala. Importantly, patients whose mood improved after 20-Hz rTMS had worsening of their mood after 1-Hz rTMS – and for uncertain reasons, the reverse pattern was also observed in some patients. In a follow-up study, it was demonstrated that depressed patients with global baseline hypoperfusion had improvement after 20-Hz rTMS and worsening after 1-Hz rTMS; conversely, patients with hyperperfusion in specific cortical regions showed improvement after 1-Hz rTMS (no relationship was found for 20-Hz rTMS in this subpopulation) [129]. Another study looking at blood flow changes after rTMS also demonstrated relatively increased blood flow in prefrontal cortex after high-frequency stimulation, and relatively decreased blood flow after low-frequency stimulation [130]; however, the pattern of changes in other cortical regions after high or low frequency rTMS was complex, with increases in some regions and decreases in others.

Regardless, these studies all demonstrated that prefrontal rTMS modulates the activity of a widespread network, thereby raising the possibility that rTMS may exert its effects *via* a normalization of network activity.

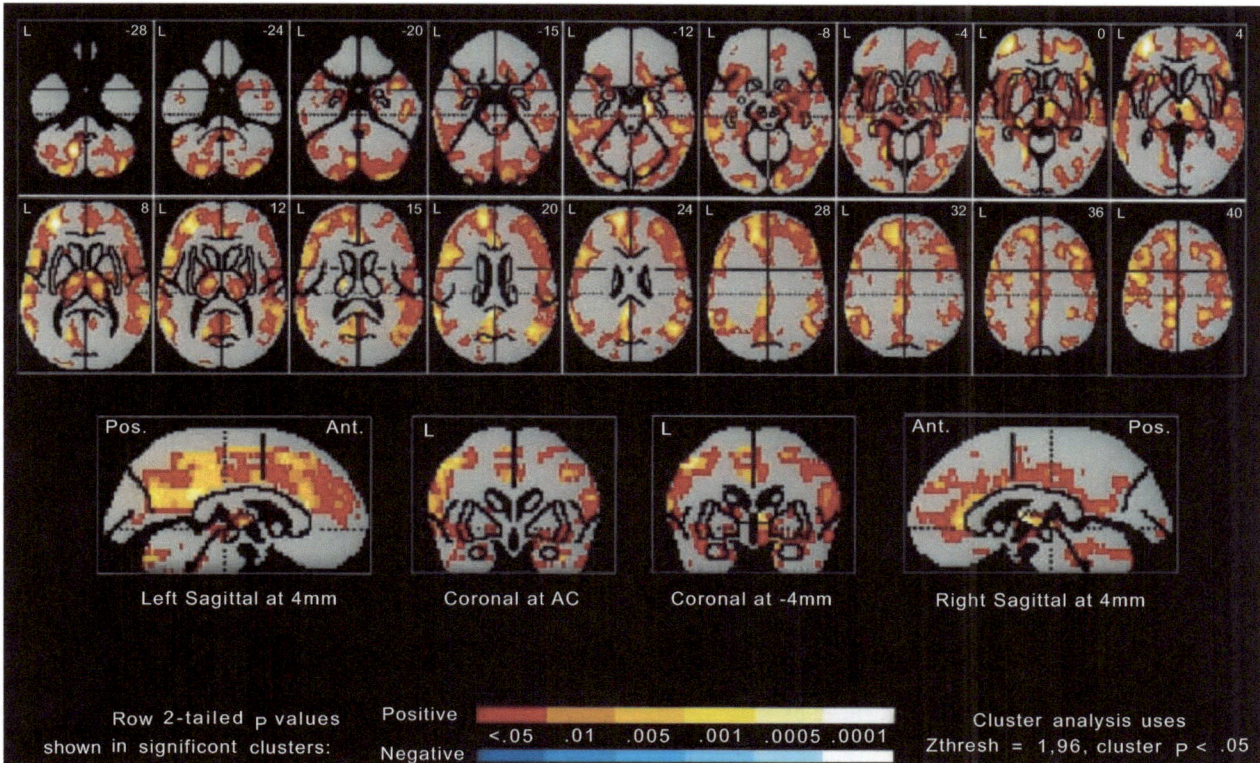

Fig. (8.10). The spatial distribution of significantly increased regional cerebral blood flow (rCBF) from a group of 10 depressed subjects who underwent 2 weeks of 20-Hz rTMS over the left prefrontal cortex (with permission, from Speer et al., 2000). The measurements were taken 72 hrs after this block of stimulation, which was conducted at 100% of motor threshold. Changes are shown relative to the pre-treatment baseline. The pseudocolor mapping corresponds to the *p* value of each voxel (with increased CBF shown in yellow/red scale). The position of each axial slice, relative to the level of the anterior commissure – posterior commissure plane, is given by a number (in millimeters) in the upper right of each panel. 20 Hz rTMS caused widespread increases in rCBF: prefrontal cortex, cingulate gyrus, bilateral insula, basal ganglia, uncus, hippocampus, parahippocampus, thalamus, cerebellum, and left amygdala.

Similarly, several recent studies have also begun to investigate the role of tDCS in the treatment of depression. In the first randomized, double-blinded sham-controlled study, 10 patients were randomized to either anodal left prefrontal tDCS or sham for 5 sessions of 20 minutes each [131-132]. After real but not sham stimulation, patients had a significant improvement in their depression scores. A subsequent study replicated and extended these findings, demonstrating that 10 days of left prefrontal anodal tDCS, but not occipital or sham stimulation, produced a significant improvement in mood, with the benefits sustained for at least one month after the last stimulation [133].

MOTOR RECOVERY AFTER STROKE

Noninvasive brain stimulation techniques have been applied to both explore and promote motor recovery after stroke. A number of early studies utilized single and paired-pulse TMS metrics, such as MEP size and motor threshold, to assess the excitability of ipsilesional and contralesional motor cortex after stroke [134-143]. Such studies have demonstrated that the MEPs produced by ipsilesional TMS are smaller (if present at all) than the MEPs produced contralesionally. Furthermore, in patients with plegia or severe paresis after strokes, these studies have also demonstrated that the absence of ipsilesional TMS-evoked MEPs has utility in the prediction of poor motor and functional recovery [138-140, 143-144]. Some studies have suggested that MEPs are larger in patients with milder deficits [137, 140, 145]. In patients with MEPs, motor threshold in the lesioned hemisphere is generally higher than in the intact hemisphere or in normal subjects, suggesting decreased cortical excitability [135, 142, 146]. Other studies using TMS have shown that the optimum location for producing TMS-evoked MEPs for hand muscles can shift up to a few centimeters during the reorganization period (well beyond the normal variability of 2-3 mm), suggesting a remapping of motor cortical somatotopy [147-151].

In addition, experiments utilizing TMS have also provided insights into the network mechanisms of stroke recovery, as well as factors that may inhibit this process. Intriguingly, studies using paired-pulse TMS have demonstrated that in cortical strokes, short-interval intracortical inhibition is decreased in the acute stage, whereas intracortical facilitation is unchanged; this suggests that the balance of excitability in these cortical circuits is shifted towards excitation [141-142, 148-149, 152]. However, other studies have demonstrated that the cortical silent period is initially prolonged, suggesting increased inhibition [142, 149, 153-155]; this prolongation normalizes with clinical recovery [150, 155-157]. Stroke patients undergoing rehabilitation also demonstrate an increase in the number of cortical sites from where an MEP of the paretic hand can be obtained [148, 155, 158-159]. Another study demonstrated that TMS pulses to ipsilesional dorsal premotor cortex can produce much greater delays in reaction time in stroke patients with infarcts in motor cortex but preserved premotor cortices than in healthy controls [160]. Furthermore, TMS to the premotor cortex in the intact cortex produces MEPs in the ipsilateral (paretic) hand [161], suggesting that the contralesional premotor cortex also plays a role in motor activation after stroke. The importance of the contralesional hemisphere was also demonstrated in a study by Lotze et al., who evaluated the impact of inhibitory rTMS to various locations in the contralesional hemisphere in patients who had recovered fully from subcortical strokes [162]. They demonstrated that stimulation of the contralesional M1, dorsal premotor cortex, and superior parietal lobule all produced significant decreases in performance of motor tasks by the ipsilateral hand (that was affected by the stroke). Taken together, these studies suggest that the excitability of the lesioned hemisphere is altered after a stroke, and non-primary motor cortices can be recruited to compensate for the decrease in motor cortex activity.

One clinically significant study assessed the impact of interhemispheric inhibition from the unaffected hemisphere to the affected hemisphere. In normal subjects, the amount of transcallosal inhibition from the "resting" hemisphere to the "active" hemisphere decreases and actually becomes facilitation just before movement onset (stimulation of one hemisphere leads to a larger response in contralateral stimulation); however, in stroke patients, interhemispheric inhibition remained significant [163]. Furthermore, the degree of interhemispheric inhibition to the lesioned cortex was also correlated with slower performance on a finger-tapping task. Based on these results, the authors postulated that interhemispheric inhibition from the unaffected hemisphere might actually inhibit motor activity from the lesioned hemisphere after stroke.

Such studies motivated research investigating the therapeutic potential of noninvasive brain stimulation techniques in stroke recovery. Based on the results described above, one approach aims to increase the excitability of the ipsilesional motor cortex. In one early study, anodal tDCS (which increases cortical excitability) was applied to ipsilesional motor cortex of six patients with chronic subcortical strokes [164]. Real but not sham tDCS led to an improvement in performance of tests of hand motor function, with a greater benefit on distal hand performance; importantly, improvement was seen in all six patients tested, and persisted for at least 25 minutes after the end of stimulation. In another study, Khedr et al. applied high-frequency (3 Hz) rTMS to the motor cortex of the lesioned hemisphere for 10 consecutive days, beginning soon (5 to 10 days) after the stroke [165]. They found that patients assigned to real rTMS had significantly better outcomes (more patients with functional independence and only mild disability) 10 days after the end of treatment than patients assigned to sham rTMS. Thus, these studies provided evidence for the use of brain stimulation techniques to increase the excitability of ipsilesional motor cortex.

Another approach has been to decrease the excitability of contralesional motor cortex, and thereby decrease the reported interhemispheric inhibition [163]. A study utilizing cathodal (inhibitory) tDCS to the unaffected hemisphere of chronic stroke patients demonstrated a significant improvement in motor performance of the paretic hand [166]. Similarly, in one double-blind study in chronic stroke patients, 1 Hz rTMS to contralesional M1 reduced the transcallosal inhibition to the lesioned cortex, and produced some improvement on functional measures in the paretic hand [167]. In a follow-up study applying 1-Hz rTMS to the contralesional motor cortex on five consecutive days, the improvement in various measures of hand function persisted for at least two weeks after the end of the treatment protocol [131]. Subsequent studies have replicated these findings [168], including in a pediatric stroke population [169]. Another recent study demonstrated that the benefit persists for at least 10 weeks after the end of treatment [170]. Thus, in sum, these studies suggest that excitatory brain stimulation to the lesioned hemisphere, or inhibitory brain stimulation to the unaffected hemisphere, may have beneficial effects in promoting recovery after stroke.

In a particularly intriguing recent study, Grefkes *et al.* utilized fMRI and functional connectivity analysis techniques to explore the network changes produced by rTMS of the contralesional hemisphere in stroke patients [171]. This study was motivated by previous work that demonstrated significant disturbances in the effective connectivity between different cortical regions in stroke patients: reduced coupling between ipsilesional SMA and M1, reduced coupling between the bilateral SMAs, and increased interhemispheric inhibition from contralesional M1 to ipsilesional M1 during movements with the paretic hand [172]. Interestingly, the weaker the coupling between ipsilesional SMA and M1, and the greater the interhemispheric inhibition from contralesional M1 to ipsilesional M1, the worse the performance is in the paretic hand. After 1Hz rTMS to the contralesional cortex, motor performance of the paretic hand improved. rTMS was also associated with an increase in the endogenous coupling of ipsilesional SMA and M1, and a significant decrease of the pathologic inhibition from contralesional M1 to ipsilesional M1 with movement of the paretic hand. The magnitude of the reduction in this pathologic inhibition was correlated with the improvement in motor performance of the paretic hand [171]. Thus, this study demonstrated that rTMS might promote more efficient network interactions in both ipsilesional and contralesional cortex. The techniques utilized in this study hold significant potential in understanding how brain stimulation techniques affect cortical networks, and thus enable the development of more effective therapeutic protocols.

CONCLUSIONS

In recent decades, a range of noninvasive techniques for manipulating brain activity have been developed. The most prominent of these include Transcranial magnetic stimulation and Transcranial direct current stimulation. Both of these techniques rely on electromagnetic principles to modulate brain activity. Furthermore, both techniques can produce long-lasting changes in cortical excitability, with the direction of change often predictable as a function of the stimulation parameters. In addition, numerous studies have demonstrated that TMS and tDCS affect not only the focal region to which stimulation is being applied, but also widespread cortical networks that are connected to the target region. Furthermore, these techniques can be combined with other neurophysiologic assessment modalities such as EEG, fMRI and PET to study how brain activity is affected by focal cortical stimulation. As such, these techniques provide powerful tools for probing the connectivity of different cortical regions, and for causally investigating the role of network activity in various cognitive functions. Furthermore, because brain stimulation techniques can produce sustained alterations in cortical excitability, they are also under investigation as therapeutic modalities in a number of neuropsychiatric disease states including depression and stroke recovery. Thus, noninvasive brain stimulation techniques offer considerable promise in our understanding and treatment of human brain function and pathology.

REFERENCES

[1]   Huang Y-Z, Edwards MJ, Rounis E, Bhatia KP, Rothwell JC. Theta burst stimulation of the human motor cortex. Neuron 2005; 45(2): 201-6.

[2]   Pascual-Leone A, Valls-Solé J, Wassermann EM, Hallett M. Responses to rapid-rate transcranial magnetic stimulation of the human motor cortex. Brain 1994; 117(Pt 4): 847-58.

[3]   Chen R, Classen J, Gerloff C, *et al.* Depression of motor cortex excitability by low-frequency transcranial magnetic stimulation. Neurology 1997; 48(5): 1398-403.

[4]   Walsh V, Pascual-Leone A. Transcranial Magnetic Stimulation: A Neurochronometrics of Mind. New edition ed: The MIT Press; 2005.

[5]   Fregni F, Pascual-Leone A. Technology insight: noninvasive brain stimulation in neurology-perspectives on the therapeutic potential of rTMS and tDCS. Nat Clin Pract Neurol 2007; 3(7): 383-93.

[6]   Ridding MC, Rothwell JC. Is there a future for therapeutic use of transcranial magnetic stimulation? Nat Rev Neurosci 2007; 8(7): 559-67.

[7]   Nitsche MA, Paulus W. Sustained excitability elevations induced by transcranial DC motor cortex stimulation in humans. Neurology 2001; 57(10): 1899-901.

[8]   Cowey A, Walsh V. Magnetically induced phosphenes in sighted, blind and blindsighted observers. Neuroreport 2000; 11(14): 3269-73.

[9]   Wagner TA, Zahn M, Grodzinsky AJ, Pascual-Leone A. Three-dimensional head model simulation of transcranial magnetic stimulation. IEEE Trans Biomed Eng 2004; 51(9): 1586-98.

[10]   Heller L, van Hulsteyn DB. Brain stimulation using electromagnetic sources: theoretical aspects. Biophys J 1992; 63(1): 129-38.

[11]   Roth BJ, Basser PJ. A model of the stimulation of a nerve fiber by electromagnetic induction. IEEE Trans Biomed Eng 1990; 37(6): 588-97.

[12]   Roth BJ, Cohen LG, Hallett M. The electric field induced during magnetic stimulation. Electroencephalogr Clin Neurophys Suppl 1991; 43: 268-78.

[13]   Roth BJ, Saypol JM, Hallett M, Cohen LG. A theoretical calculation of the electric field induced in the cortex during magnetic stimulation. Electroencephalogr Clin Neurophys 1991; 81(1): 47-56.

[14]   Nagarajan SS, Durand DM, Warman EN. Effects of induced electric fields on finite neuronal structures: a simulation study. IEEE Trans Biomed Eng 1993; 40(11): 1175-88.

[15]   Nagarajan SS, Durand DM. Analysis of magnetic stimulation of a concentric axon in a nerve bundle. IEEE Trans Biomed Eng 1995; 42(9): 926-33.

[16]   Nagarajan SS, Durand DM. A generalized cable equation for magnetic stimulation of axons. IEEE Trans Biomed Eng 1996; 43(3): 304-12.

[17]   Moliadze V, Zhao Y, Eysel U, Funke K. Effect of transcranial magnetic stimulation on single-unit activity in the cat primary visual cortex. J Physiol 2003; 553(Pt 2): 665-79.

[18]   Allen EA, Pasley BN, Duong T, Freeman RD. Transcranial magnetic stimulation elicits coupled neural and hemodynamic consequences. Science 2007; 317(5846): 1918-21.

[19]   van der Kamp W, Zwinderman AH, Ferrari MD, van Dijk JG. Cortical excitability and response variability of transcranial magnetic stimulation. J Clin Neurophys 1996; 13(2): 164-71.

[20]   Hess CW, Mills KR, Murray NMF. Magnetic stimulation of the human brain: Facilitation of motor responses by voluntary contraction of ipsilateral and contralateral muscles with additional observations on an amputee. Neurosci Lett 1986; 71(2): 235-40.

[21]   Hess CW, Mills KR, Murray NM. Responses in small hand muscles from magnetic stimulation of the human brain. J Physiol 1987; 388(1): 397-419.

[22]   Andersen B, Rösler KM, Lauritzen M. Nonspecific facilitation of responses to transcranial magnetic stimulation. Muscle & Nerve 1999; 22(7): 857-63.

[23]   Rossini PM, Berardelli A, Deuschl G, *et al.* Applications of magnetic cortical stimulation. Electroencephalogr Clin Neurophysiol Suppl 1999; 52: 171-85.

[24]   Kobayashi M, Pascual-Leone A. Transcranial magnetic stimulation in neurology. Lancet Neurol 2003; 2(3): 145-56.

[25]   Calancie B, Nordin M, Wallin U, Hagbarth KE. Motor-unit responses in human wrist flexor and extensor muscles to transcranial cortical stimuli. J Neurophys 1987; 58(5): 1168-85.

[26]   Roick H, von Giesen HJ, Benecke R. On the origin of the postexcitatory inhibition seen after transcranial magnetic brain stimulation in awake human subjects. Exp Brain Res 1993; 94(3): 489-98.

[27]   Siebner HR, Dressnandt J, Auer C, Conrad B. Continuous intrathecal baclofen infusions induced a marked increase of the transcranially evoked silent period in a patient with generalized dystonia. Muscle Nerve 1998; 21(9): 1209-12.

[28]   Tataroglu C, Ozkiziltan S, Baklan B. Motor cortical thresholds and cortical silent periods in epilepsy. Seizure 2004; 13(7): 481-5.

[29]   Kujirai T, Caramia MD, Rothwell JC, *et al.* Corticocortical inhibition in human motor cortex. J Physiol 1993; 471: 501-19.

[30]   Ziemann U, Lönnecker S, Steinhoff BJ, Paulus W. The effect of lorazepam on the motor cortical excitability in man. Exp Brain Res 1996; 109(1): 127-35.

[31]   Orth M, Snijders AH, Rothwell JC. The variability of intracortical inhibition and facilitation. Clin Neurophysiol 2003; 114(12): 2362-9.

[32]   Ziemann U, Rothwell JC, Ridding MC. Interaction between intracortical inhibition and facilitation in human motor cortex. J Physiol 1996; 496 (Pt 3): 873-81.

[33]   Di Lazzaro V, Oliviero A, Saturno E, *et al.* Effects of lorazepam on short latency afferent inhibition and short latency intracortical inhibition in humans. J Physiol 2005; 564(Pt 2): 661-8.

[34]   Claus D, Weis M, Jahnke U, Plewe A, Brunhölzl C. Corticospinal conduction studied with magnetic double stimulation in the intact human. J Neurol Sci 1992; 111(2): 180-8.

[35]   Valls-Solé J, Pascual-Leone A, Wassermann EM, Hallett M. Human motor evoked responses to paired transcranial magnetic stimuli. Electroencephalogr Clin Neurophysiol 1992; 85(6): 355-64.

[36]   McDonnell M, Orekhov Y, Ziemann U. The role of GABAB receptors in intracortical inhibition in the human motor cortex. Exp Brain Res 2006; 173(1): 86-93.

[37]   Ferbert A, Priori A, Rothwell JC, Day BL, Colebatch JG, Marsden CD. Interhemispheric inhibition of the human motor cortex. J Physiol 1992; 453: 525-46.

[38]   Chen R, Yung D, Li J-Y. Organization of ipsilateral excitatory and inhibitory pathways in the human motor cortex. J Neurophysiol. 2003; 89(3): 1256-64.

[39]   Meyer BU, Röricht S, Gräfin von Einsiedel H, Kruggel F, Weindl A. Inhibitory and excitatory interhemispheric transfers between motor cortical areas in normal humans and patients with abnormalities of the corpus callosum. Brain 1995; 118 (Pt 2): 429-40.

[40]   Fitzgerald PB, Brown TL, Marston NAU, Daskalakis ZJ, De Castella A, Kulkarni J. Transcranial magnetic stimulation in the treatment of depression: a double-blind, placebo-controlled trial. Arch Gen Psychiatry 2003; 60(10): 1002-8.

[41]   Thut G, Pascual-Leone A. A review of combined TMS-EEG studies to characterize lasting effects of repetitive TMS and assess their usefulness in cognitive and clinical neuroscience. Brain Topogr 2010; 22(4): 219-32.

[42] Maeda F, Keenan JP, Tormos JM, Topka H, Pascual-Leone A. Modulation of corticospinal excitability by repetitive transcranial magnetic stimulation. Clin Neurophysiol 2000; 111(5): 800-5.

[43] Adrian ED, Moruzzi G. Impulses in the pyramidal tract. J Physiol 1939; 97(2): 153-99.

[44] Patton HD, Amassian VE. Single and multiple-unit analysis of cortical stage of pyramidal tract activation. J Neurophysiol 1954; 17(4): 345-63.

[45] Esser SK, Hill SL, Tononi G. Modeling the effects of transcranial magnetic stimulation on cortical circuits. J Neurophysiol 2005; 94(1): 622-39.

[46] Bindman LJ, Lippold OC, Redfearn JW. Long-lasting changes in the level of the electrical activity of the cerebral cortex produced bypolarizing currents. Nature 1962; 196: 584-5.

[47] Creutzfeldt OD, Fromm GH, Kapp H. Influence of transcortical d-c currents on cortical neuronal activity. Exp Neurol 1962; 5: 436-52.

[48] Purpura DP, McMurtry JG. Intracellular activities and evoked potential changes during polarization of motor cortex. J Neurophysiol 1965; 28: 166-85.

[49] Lopez L, Chan CY, Okada YC, Nicholson C. Multimodal characterization of population responses evoked by applied electric field *in vitro*: extracellular potential, magnetic evoked field, transmembrane potential, and current-source density analysis. J Neurosci 1991; 11(7): 1998-2010.

[50] Nitsche MA, Paulus W. Excitability changes induced in the human motor cortex by weak transcranial direct current stimulation. J Physiol 2000; 527 Pt 3: 633-9.

[51] Nitsche MA, Nitsche MS, Klein CC, Tergau F, Rothwell JC, Paulus W. Level of action of cathodal DC polarisation induced inhibition of the human motor cortex. Clin Neurophysiol 2003; 114(4): 600-4.

[52] Nitsche MA, Seeber A, Frommann K, *et al.* Modulating parameters of excitability during and after transcranial direct current stimulation of the human motor cortex. J Physiol 2005; 568(Pt 1): 291-303.

[53] Liebetanz D, Nitsche MA, Tergau F, Paulus W. Pharmacological approach to the mechanisms of transcranial DC-stimulation-induced after-effects of human motor cortex excitability. Brain 2002; 125(Pt 10): 2238-47.

[54] Nitsche MA, Jaussi W, Liebetanz D, Lang N, Tergau F, Paulus W. Consolidation of human motor cortical neuroplasticity by D-cycloserine. Neuropsychopharm 2004; 29(8): 1573-8.

[55] Nitsche MA, Grundey J, Liebetanz D, Lang N, Tergau F, Paulus W. Catecholaminergic consolidation of motor cortical neuroplasticity in humans. Cereb Cortex 2004; 14(11): 1240-5.

[56] Rossi S, Hallett M, Rossini PM, Pascual-Leone A. Safety, ethical considerations, and application guidelines for the use of transcranial magnetic stimulation in clinical practice and research. Clin Neurophysiol 2009; 120(12): 2008-39.

[57] Pessoa L. On the relationship between emotion and cognition. Nat Rev Neurosci 2008; 9(2): 148-58.

[58] Sporns O, Tononi G, Edelman GM. Connectivity and complexity: the relationship between neuroanatomy and brain dynamics. Neural Networks 2000; 13(8-9): 909-22.

[59] Schlösser RGM, Wagner G, Sauer H. Assessing the working memory network: studies with functional magnetic resonance imaging and structural equation modeling. Neuroscience 2006; 139(1): 91-103.

[60] Mayberg HS, Lozano AM, Voon V, et al. Deep brain stimulation for treatment-resistant depression. Neuron 2005; 45(5): 651-60.

[61] Greicius M. Resting-state functional connectivity in neuropsychiatric disorders. Curr Opin Neurol 2008; 21(4): 424-30.

[62] Lytton WW. Computer modelling of epilepsy. Nature Reviews Neuroscience 2008; 9(8): 626-37.

[63] Seeley WW, Crawford RK, Zhou J, Miller BL, Greicius MD. Neurodegenerative diseases target large-scale human brain networks. Neuron 2009; 62(1): 42-52.

[64] Kumar S, Rao SL, Chandramouli BA, Pillai SV. Reduction of functional brain connectivity in mild traumatic brain injury during working memory. J Neurotrauma 2009; 26(5): 665-75.

[65] He BJ, Snyder AZ, Vincent JL, Epstein A, Shulman GL, Corbetta M. Breakdown of functional connectivity in frontoparietal networks underlies behavioral deficits in spatial neglect. Neuron 2007; 53(6): 905-18.

[66] Ween JE. Functional imaging of stroke recovery: an ecological review from a neural network perspective with an emphasis on motor systems. J Neuroimaging 2008; 18(3): 227-36.

[67] Wang L, Yu C, Chen H, *et al.* Dynamic functional reorganization of the motor execution network after stroke. Brain 2010; 133(Pt 4): 1224-38.

[68] O'Shea J, Taylor PCJ, Rushworth MFS. Imaging causal interactions during sensorimotor processing. Cortex 2008; 44(5): 598-608.

[69] Pascual-Leone A, Walsh V, Rothwell J. Transcranial magnetic stimulation in cognitive neuroscience--virtual lesion, chronometry, and functional connectivity. Curr Opin Neurobiol 2000; 10(2): 232-7.

[70] Paus T. Inferring causality in brain images: a perturbation approach. Philos Trans R Soc Lond B Biol Sci 2005; 360(1457): 1109-14.

[71] Lee L, Siebner H, Bestmann S. Rapid modulation of distributed brain activity by Transcranial Magnetic Stimulation of human motor cortex. Behav Neurol 2006; 17(3-4): 135-48.

[72] Bestmann S, Ruff CC, Blankenburg F, Weiskopf N, Driver J, Rothwell JC. Mapping causal interregional influences with concurrent TMS-fMRI. Exp Brain Res 2008; 191(4): 383-402.

[73] Miniussi C, Thut G. Combining TMS and EEG offers new prospects in cognitive neuroscience. Brain Topogr 2010; 22(4): 249-56.

[74]   Amassian VE, Cracco RQ, Maccabee PJ, Cracco JB, Rudell A, Eberle L. Suppression of visual perception by magnetic coil stimulation of human occipital cortex. Electroencephalogr Clin Neurophysiol 1989; 74(6): 458-62.

[75]   Chambers CD, Payne JM, Stokes MG, Mattingley JB. Fast and slow parietal pathways mediate spatial attention. Nat Neurosci 2004; 7(3): 217-8.

[76]   Silvanto J, Lavie N, Walsh V. Stimulation of the human frontal eye fields modulates sensitivity of extrastriate visual cortex. J Neurophysiol 2006; 96(2): 941-5.

[77]   Paus T, Jech R, Thompson CJ, Comeau R, Peters T, Evans AC. Transcranial magnetic stimulation during positron emission tomography: a new method for studying connectivity of the human cerebral cortex. J Neurosci 1997; 17(9): 3178-84.

[78]   Chouinard PA, Van Der Werf YD, Leonard G, Paus T. Modulating neural networks with transcranial magnetic stimulation applied over the dorsal premotor and primary motor cortices. J Neurophysiol 2003; 90(2): 1071-83.

[79]   Bestmann S, Baudewig J, Siebner HR, Rothwell JC, Frahm J. Subthreshold high-frequency TMS of human primary motor cortex modulates interconnected frontal motor areas as detected by interleaved fMRI-TMS. Neuroimage 2003; 20(3): 1685-96.

[80]   Bestmann S, Baudewig J, Siebner HR, Rothwell JC, Frahm J. Functional MRI of the immediate impact of transcranial magnetic stimulation on cortical and subcortical motor circuits. Eur J Neurosci 2004; 19(7): 1950-62.

[81]   Bestmann S, Baudewig J, Siebner HR, Rothwell JC, Frahm J. BOLD MRI responses to repetitive TMS over human dorsal premotor cortex. Neuroimage 2005; 28(1): 22-9.

[82]   Komssi S, Aronen HJ, Huttunen J, *et al.* Ipsi- and contralateral EEG reactions to transcranial magnetic stimulation. Clin Neurophysiol 2002; 113(2): 175-84.

[83]   Ilmoniemi RJ, Virtanen J, Ruohonen J, *et al.* Neuronal responses to magnetic stimulation reveal cortical reactivity and connectivity. Neuroreport 1997; 8(16): 3537-40.

[84]   Jing H, Takigawa M. Observation of EEG coherence after repetitive transcranial magnetic stimulation. Clin Neurophysiol 2000; 111(9): 1620-31.

[85]   Plewnia C, Rilk AJ, Soekadar SR, *et al.* Enhancement of long-range EEG coherence by synchronous bifocal transcranial magnetic stimulation. Eur J Neurosci 2008; 27(6): 1577-83.

[86]   Massimini M, Ferrarelli F, Huber R, Esser SK, Singh H, Tononi G. Breakdown of cortical effective connectivity during sleep. Science 2005; 309(5744): 2228-32.

[87]   Laird AR, Robbins JM, Li K, *et al.* Modeling motor connectivity using TMS/PET and structural equation modeling. Neuroimage 2008; 41(2): 424-36.

[88]   Morishima Y, Akaishi R, Yamada Y, Okuda J, Toma K, Sakai K. Task-specific signal transmission from prefrontal cortex in visual selective attention. Nat Neurosci 2009; 12(1): 85-91.

[89]   O'Shea J, Johansen-Berg H, Trief D, Göbel S, Rushworth MFS. Functionally specific reorganization in human premotor cortex. Neuron 2007; 54(3): 479-90.

[90]   Fuggetta G, Fiaschi A, Manganotti P. Modulation of cortical oscillatory activities induced by varying single-pulse transcranial magnetic stimulation intensity over the left primary motor area: a combined EEG and TMS study. Neuroimage 2005; 27(4): 896-908.

[91]   Van Der Werf YD, Sadikot AF, Strafella AP, Paus T. The neural response to transcranial magnetic stimulation of the human motor cortex. II. Thalamocortical contributions. Exp Brain Res 2006; 175(2): 246-55.

[92]   Van Der Werf YD, Paus T. The neural response to transcranial magnetic stimulation of the human motor cortex. I. Intracortical and cortico-cortical contributions. Exp Brain Res 2006; 175(2): 231-45.

[93]   Rosanova M, Casali A, Bellina V, Resta F, Mariotti M, Massimini M. Natural frequencies of human corticothalamic circuits. J Neurosci 2009; 29(24): 7679-85.

[94]   Paus T, Sipila PK, Strafella AP. Synchronization of neuronal activity in the human primary motor cortex by transcranial magnetic stimulation: an EEG study. J Neurophysiol 2001; 86(4): 1983-90.

[95]   Ferrarelli F, Massimini M, Peterson MJ, *et al.* Reduced evoked gamma oscillations in the frontal cortex in schizophrenia patients: a TMS/EEG study. Am J Psychiatry 2008; 165(8): 996-1005.

[96]   Arieli A, Sterkin A, Grinvald A, Aertsen A. Dynamics of ongoing activity: explanation of the large variability in evoked cortical responses. Science 1996; 273(5283): 1868-71.

[97]   Azouz R, Gray CM. Cellular mechanisms contributing to response variability of cortical neurons in vivo. J Neurosci. 1999; 19(6): 2209-23.

[98]   Ergenoglu T, Demiralp T, Bayraktaroglu Z, Ergen M, Beydagi H, Uresin Y. Alpha rhythm of the EEG modulates visual detection performance in humans. Brain Res Cogn Brain Res 2004; 20(3): 376-83.

[99]   van der Togt C, Spekreijse H, Supèr H. Neural responses in cat visual cortex reflect state changes in correlated activity. Eur J Neurosci 2005; 22(2): 465-75.

[100]   Hanslmayr S, Klimesch W, Sauseng P, *et al.* Visual discrimination performance is related to decreased alpha amplitude but increased phase locking. Neurosci Lett 2005; 375(1): 64-8.

[101]   Hanslmayr S, Aslan A, Staudigl T, Klimesch W, Herrmann CS, Bäuml K-H. Prestimulus oscillations predict visual perception performance between and within subjects. Neuroimage 2007; 37(4): 1465-73.

[102]   Romei V, Rihs T, Brodbeck V, Thut G. Resting electroencephalogram alpha-power over posterior sites indexes baseline visual cortex excitability. Neuroreport 2008; 19(2): 203-8.

[103]   Romei V, Brodbeck V, Michel C, Amedi A, Pascual-Leone A, Thut G. Spontaneous fluctuations in posterior alpha-band EEG activity reflect variability in excitability of human visual areas. Cerebr Cortex 2008; 18(9): 2010-8.

[104]   Sauseng P, Klimesch W, Gerloff C, Hummel FC. Spontaneous locally restricted EEG alpha activity determines cortical excitability in the motor cortex. Neuropsychologia 2009; 47(1): 284-8.

[105]   Griskova I, Ruksenas O, Dapsys K, Herpertz S, Höppner J. The effects of 10 Hz repetitive transcranial magnetic stimulation on resting EEG power spectrum in healthy subjects. Neurosci Lett 2007; 419(2): 162-7.

[106]   Brignani D, Manganotti P, Rossini PM, Miniussi C. Modulation of cortical oscillatory activity during transcranial magnetic stimulation. Hum Brain Mapp 2008; 29(5): 603-12.

[107]   Fuggetta G, Pavone EF, Fiaschi A, Manganotti P. Acute modulation of cortical oscillatory activities during short trains of high-frequency repetitive transcranial magnetic stimulation of the human motor cortex: a combined EEG and TMS study. Hum Brain Mapp 2008; 29(1): 1-13.

[108]   Oliviero A, Strens LHA, Di Lazzaro V, Tonali PA, Brown P. Persistent effects of high frequency repetitive TMS on the coupling between motor areas in the human. Exp Brain Res 2003; 149(1): 107-13.

[109]   Hamidi M, Slagter HA, Tononi G, Postle BR. Repetitive Transcranial Magnetic Stimulation Affects behavior by Biasing Endogenous Cortical Oscillations. Front Integr Neurosci 2009; 3: 14.

[110]   Ferrarelli F, Massimini M, Sarasso S, et al. Breakdown in cortical effective connectivity during midazolam-induced loss of consciousness. Pro Natl Acad Sci USA 2010; 107(6): 2681-6.

[111]   Tononi G, Cirelli C. Sleep function and synaptic homeostasis. Sleep Med Rev 2006; 10(1): 49-62.

[112]   Huber R, Esser SK, Ferrarelli F, Massimini M, Peterson MJ, Tononi G. TMS-induced cortical potentiation during wakefulness locally increases slow wave activity during sleep. PLoS One 2007; 2(3): e276.

[113]   Huber R, Määttä S, Esser SK, et al. Measures of cortical plasticity after transcranial paired associative stimulation predict changes in electroencephalogram slow-wave activity during subsequent sleep. J Neurosci 2008; 28(31): 7911-8.

[114]   Marshall L, Helgadóttir H, Mölle M, Born J. Boosting slow oscillations during sleep potentiates memory. Nature 2006; 444(7119): 610-3.

[115]   Baxter LR, Schwartz JM, Phelps ME, et al. Reduction of prefrontal cortex glucose metabolism common to three types of depression. Arch Gen Psychiatry 1989; 46(3): 243-50.

[116]   Martinot JL, Hardy P, Feline A, et al. Left prefrontal glucose hypometabolism in the depressed state: a confirmation. Am J Psychiatry 1990; 147(10): 1313-7.

[117]   Drevets WC. Functional anatomical abnormalities in limbic and prefrontal cortical structures in major depression. Prog Brain Res 2000; 126: 413-31.

[118]   Bench CJ, Frackowiak RS, Dolan RJ. Changes in regional cerebral blood flow on recovery from depression. Psychol Med 1995; 25(2): 247-61.

[119]   Mayberg HS, Brannan SK, Tekell JL, et al. Regional metabolic effects of fluoxetine in major depression: serial changes and relationship to clinical response. Biol Psychiatry 2000; 48(8): 830-43.

[120]   George MS, Wassermann EM, Williams WA, et al. Changes in mood and hormone levels after rapid-rate transcranial magnetic stimulation (rTMS) of the prefrontal cortex. J Neuropsychiatry Clin Neurosci 1996; 8(2): 172-80.

[121]   Pascual-Leone A, Rubio B, Pallardó F, Catalá MD. Rapid-rate transcranial magnetic stimulation of left dorsolateral prefrontal cortex in drug-resistant depression. Lancet 1996; 348(9022): 233-7.

[122]   Pascual-Leone A, Catalá MD, Pascual-Leone Pascual A. Lateralized effect of rapid-rate transcranial magnetic stimulation of the prefrontal cortex on mood. Neurology 1996; 46(2): 499-502.

[123]   Klein E, Kreinin I, Chistyakov A, et al. Therapeutic efficacy of right prefrontal slow repetitive transcranial magnetic stimulation in major depression: a double-blind controlled study. Arch Gen Psychiatry 1999; 56(4): 315-20.

[124]   Januel D, Dumortier G, Verdon C-M, et al. A double-blind sham controlled study of right prefrontal repetitive transcranial magnetic stimulation (rTMS): therapeutic and cognitive effect in medication free unipolar depression during 4 weeks. Prog Neuropsychopharmacol Biol Psychiatry 2006; 30(1): 126-30.

[125]   Slotema CW, Blom JD, Hoek HW, Sommer IEC. Should we expand the toolbox of psychiatric treatment methods to include Repetitive Transcranial Magnetic Stimulation (rTMS)? a meta-analysis of the efficacy of rTMS in psychiatric disorders. J Clin Psychiatry 2010.

[126]   O'Reardon JP, Solvason HB, Janicak PG, et al. Efficacy and safety of transcranial magnetic stimulation in the acute treatment of major depression: a multisite randomized controlled trial. Biol Psychiatry 2007; 62(11): 1208-16.

[127]   Paus T, Barrett J. Transcranial magnetic stimulation (TMS) of the human frontal cortex: implications for repetitive TMS treatment of depression. J Psychiatry Neurosci 2004; 29(4): 268-79.

[128]   Speer AM, Kimbrell TA, Wassermann EM, et al. Opposite effects of high and low frequency rTMS on regional brain activity in depressed patients. Biol Psychiatry 2000; 48(12): 1133-41.

[129]   Speer AM, Benson BE, Kimbrell TK, et al. Opposite effects of high and low frequency rTMS on mood in depressed patients: relationship to baseline cerebral activity on PET. J Affect Disord 2009; 115(3): 386-94.

[130]   Loo CK, Sachdev PS, Haindl W, et al. High (15 Hz) and low (1 Hz) frequency transcranial magnetic stimulation have different acute effects on regional cerebral blood flow in depressed patients. Psychol Med 2003; 33(6): 997-1006.

[131] Fregni F, Boggio PS, Valle AC, *et al.* A sham-controlled trial of a 5-day course of repetitive transcranial magnetic stimulation of the unaffected hemisphere in stroke patients. Stroke 2006; 37(8): 2115-22.

[132] Fregni F, Boggio PS, Nitsche MA, Marcolin MA, Rigonatti SP, Pascual-Leone A. Treatment of major depression with transcranial direct current stimulation. Bipolar Disord 2006; 8(2): 203-4.

[133] Boggio PS, Rigonatti SP, Ribeiro RB, *et al.* A randomized, double-blind clinical trial on the efficacy of cortical direct current stimulation for the treatment of major depression. Int J Neuropsychopharmacol 2008; 11(2): 249-54.

[134] Berardelli A, Inghilleri M, Manfredi M, Zamponi A, Cecconi V, Dolce G. Cortical and cervical stimulation after hemispheric infarction. J Neurol Neurosurg Psychiatry 1987; 50(7): 861-5.

[135] Abbruzzese G, Morena M, Dall'Agata D, Abbruzzese M, Favale E. Motor evoked potentials (MEPs) in lacunar syndromes. Electroencephalogr Clin Neurophysiol 1991; 81(3): 202-8.

[136] Heald A, Bates D, Cartlidge NE, French JM, Miller S. Longitudinal study of central motor conduction time following stroke. 2. Central motor conduction measured within 72 h after stroke as a predictor of functional outcome at 12 months. Brain 1993; 116 (Pt 6): 1371-85.

[137] Araç N, Sağduyu A, Binai S, Ertekin C. Prognostic value of transcranial magnetic stimulation in acute stroke. Stroke 1994; 25(11): 2183-6.

[138] Rapisarda G, Bastings E, de Noordhout AM, Pennisi G, Delwaide PJ. Can motor recovery in stroke patients be predicted by early transcranial magnetic stimulation? Stroke 1996; 27(12): 2191-6.

[139] Escudero JV, Sancho J, Bautista D, Escudero M, López-Trigo J. Prognostic value of motor evoked potential obtained by transcranial magnetic brain stimulation in motor function recovery in patients with acute ischemic stroke. Stroke 1998; 29(9): 1854-9.

[140] Cruz Martínez A, Tejada J, Díez Tejedor E. Motor hand recovery after stroke. Prognostic yield of early transcranial magnetic stimulation. Electromyogr Clin Neurophysiol 1999; 39(7): 405-10.

[141] Manganotti P, Patuzzo S, Cortese F, Palermo A, Smania N, Fiaschi A. Motor disinhibition in affected and unaffected hemisphere in the early period of recovery after stroke. Clin Neurophysiol 2002; 113(6): 936-43.

[142] Nardone R, Tezzon F. Inhibitory and excitatory circuits of cerebral cortex after ischaemic stroke: prognostic value of the transcranial magnetic stimulation. Electromyogr Clin Neurophysiol 2002; 42(3): 131-6.

[143] Hendricks HT, Pasman JW, van Limbeek J, Zwarts MJ. Motor evoked potentials in predicting recovery from upper extremity paralysis after acute stroke. Cerebrovasc Dis 2003; 16(3): 265-71.

[144] Hendricks HT, Zwarts MJ, Plat EF, van Limbeek J. Systematic review for the early prediction of motor and functional outcome after stroke by using motor-evoked potentials. Arch Phys Med Rehabil 2002; 83(9): 1303-8.

[145] Palliyath S. Role of central conduction time and motor evoked response amplitude in predicting stroke outcome. Electromyogr Clin Neurophysiol 2000; 40(5): 315-20.

[146] Catano A, Houa M, Caroyer JM, Ducarne H, Noël P. Magnetic transcranial stimulation in acute stroke: early excitation threshold and functional prognosis. Electroencephalogr Clin Neurophysiol 1996; 101(3): 233-9.

[147] Cicinelli P, Traversa R, Rossini PM. Post-stroke reorganization of brain motor output to the hand: a 2-4 month follow-up with focal magnetic transcranial stimulation. Electroencephalogr Clin Neurophysiol 1997; 105(6): 438-50.

[148] Liepert J, Storch P, Fritsch A, Weiller C. Motor cortex disinhibition in acute stroke. Clin Neurophysiol 2000; 111(4): 671-6.

[149] Liepert J, Bauder H, Wolfgang HR, Miltner WH, Taub E, Weiller C. Treatment-induced cortical reorganization after stroke in humans. Stroke 2000; 31(6): 1210-6.

[150] Byrnes ML, Thickbroom GW, Phillips BA, Mastaglia FL. Long-term changes in motor cortical organisation after recovery from subcortical stroke. Brain Res 2001; 889(1-2): 278-87.

[151] Bastings EP, Greenberg JP, Good DC. Hand motor recovery after stroke: a transcranial magnetic stimulation mapping study of motor output areas and their relation to functional status. Neurorehabil Neural Repair 2002; 16(3): 275-82.

[152] Cicinelli P, Pasqualetti P, Zaccagnini M, Traversa R, Oliveri M, Rossini PM. Interhemispheric asymmetries of motor cortex excitability in the postacute stroke stage: a paired-pulse transcranial magnetic stimulation study. Stroke 2003; 34(11): 2653-8.

[153] Braune HJ, Fritz C. Transcranial magnetic stimulation-evoked inhibition of voluntary muscle activity (silent period) is impaired in patients with ischemic hemispheric lesion. Stroke 1995; 26(4): 550-3.

[154] Ahonen JP, Jehkonen M, Dastidar P, Molnár G, Häkkinen V. Cortical silent period evoked by transcranial magnetic stimulation in ischemic stroke. Electroencephalogr Clin Neurophysiol 1998; 109(3): 224-9.

[155] Traversa R, Cicinelli P, Bassi A, Rossini PM, Bernardi G. Mapping of motor cortical reorganization after stroke. A brain stimulation study with focal magnetic pulses. Stroke 1997; 28(1): 110-7.

[156] Classen J, Schnitzler A, Binkofski F, *et al.* The motor syndrome associated with exaggerated inhibition within the primary motor cortex of patients with hemiparetic. Brain 1997; 120 (Pt 4): 605-19.

[157] Cicinelli P, Mattia D, Spanedda F, *et al.* Transcranial magnetic stimulation reveals an interhemispheric asymmetry of cortical inhibition in focal epilepsy. Neuroreport 2000; 11(4): 701-7.

[158] Liepert J, Miltner WH, Bauder H, *et al.* Motor cortex plasticity during constraint-induced movement therapy in stroke patients. Neurosci Lett 1998; 250(1): 5-8.

[159] Wittenberg GF, Chen R, Ishii K, *et al.* Constraint-induced therapy in stroke: magnetic-stimulation motor maps and cerebral activation. Neurorehabil Neural Repair 2003; 17(1): 48-57.

[160] Fridman EA, Hanakawa T, Chung M, Hummel F, Leiguarda RC, Cohen LG. Reorganization of the human ipsilesional premotor cortex after stroke. Brain 2004; 127(Pt 4): 747-58.

[161] Caramia MD, Palmieri MG, Giacomini P, Iani C, Dally L, Silvestrini M. Ipsilateral activation of the unaffected motor cortex in patients with hemiparetic stroke. Clin Neurophysiol 2000; 111(11): 1990-6.

[162] Lotze M, Markert J, Sauseng P, Hoppe J, Plewnia C, Gerloff C. The role of multiple contralesional motor areas for complex hand movements after internal capsular lesion. J Neurosci 2006; 26(22): 6096-102.

[163] Murase N, Duque J, Mazzocchio R, Cohen LG. Influence of interhemispheric interactions on motor function in chronic stroke. Ann Neurol 2004; 55(3): 400-9.

[164] Hummel F, Celnik P, Giraux P, *et al*. Effects of non-invasive cortical stimulation on skilled motor function in chronic stroke. Brain 2005; 128(Pt 3): 490-9.

[165] Khedr EM, Ahmed MA, Fathy N, Rothwell JC. Therapeutic trial of repetitive transcranial magnetic stimulation after acute ischemic stroke. Neurology 2005; 65(3): 466-8.

[166] Fregni F, Boggio PS, Mansur CG, *et al*. Transcranial direct current stimulation of the unaffected hemisphere in stroke patients. Neuroreport 2005; 16(14): 1551-5.

[167] Takeuchi N, Chuma T, Matsuo Y, Watanabe I, Ikoma K. Repetitive transcranial magnetic stimulation of contralesional primary motor cortex improves hand function after stroke. Stroke 2005; 36(12): 2681-6.

[168] Nowak DA, Grefkes C, Ameli M, Fink GR. Interhemispheric competition after stroke: brain stimulation to enhance recovery of function of the affected hand. Neurorehabil Neural Repair 2009; 23(7): 641-56.

[169] Kirton A, Chen R, Friefeld S, Gunraj C, Pontigon A-M, Deveber G. Contralesional repetitive transcranial magnetic stimulation for chronic hemiparesis in subcortical paediatric stroke: a randomised trial. Lancet Neurol 2008; 7(6): 507-13.

[170] Emara TH, Moustafa RR, Elnahas NM, *et al*. Repetitive transcranial magnetic stimulation at 1Hz and 5Hz produces sustained improvement in motor function and disability after ischaemic stroke. Eur J Neurol 2010; 17(9): 1203-9.

[171] Grefkes C, Nowak DA, Wang LE, Dafotakis M, Eickhoff SB, Fink GR. Modulating cortical connectivity in stroke patients by rTMS assessed with fMRI and dynamic causal modeling. Neuroimage 2010; 50(1): 233-42.

[172] Grefkes C, Nowak DA, Eickhoff SB, *et al*. Cortical connectivity after subcortical stroke assessed with functional magnetic resonance imaging. Ann Neurol 2008; 63(2): 236-46.

SUBJECT INDEX

acetylcholine, 10, 82, 85, 92, 94

actigraphy, 51, 58-60

alpha oscillation, 5, 24, 25, 55, 68-70, 84, 112, 113

Alzheimer's Disease, 7, 8, 40, 41, 59, 65, 81, 91, 94

anesthesia, 54, 55, 88, 102, 114

artifact, 66, 67, 71, 72, 84,

attention (cognitive), 27, 53, 54, 68, 81-83, 85, 87, 90, 94, 95, 108

attention deficit disorder, 7, 28

auditory, 9. 22. 28, 40. 41, 53, 54, 70, 71, 85-87, 90, 91, 108

autism, 3, 7, 9, 28, 81, 90, 91, 93-95

autonomic, 51, 57, 58, 60

basal ganglia, 35, 36, 82, 93, 116

beta oscillation, 8, 9, 24, 25, 27, 52, 68, 82, 112

biofeedback, 95

BOLD (blood oxygen level dependent), 25, 26, 53, 54, 60, 65, 66, 68-75, 87, 88, 90, 92, 94, 95, 108, 111

brain tumor, 8, 9, 88,

brainstem, 56, 57

C. *elegans*, 13, 16, 18, 33, 34, 37, 38, 40, 44, 45

cat, 38, 44, 45, 82, 102

cerebral blood flow (CBF), 52, 53, 108, 116

cholinergic, see acetylcholine

circadian, 7, 51, 56, 58-60

clustering coefficient, 4, 5, 10, 15, 16-19, 27, 32, 33-36, 38, 40, 42, 43, 46-48, 55

coherence (coherent), 5-10, 14, 15, 25-27, 35, 36, 39, 48, 52, 54, 67, 69, 81, 84, 89-91, 93,109, 112, 113

cognitive impairment, 28, 59, 74, 94

  mild, 8, 92

consciousness, 51, 70, 73, 74, 82, 88, 113, 114

corpus callosum, 23, 28, 84, 91, 103,

cortical thickness, 37-46

coupling, 4, 5, 7, 9, 10, 13-15, 19, 55, 57, 58, 60, 73, 75, 85, 89, 90, 92, 94, 118

cross correlation, 13-15

current source, 111, 114

default network, 4, 7-9, 26, 28, 39, 53, 54, 67, 68, 70, 73, 74

degree (graph metric), 15-19, 27, 34, 35, 39, 40, 42-44, 47, 48

delta oscillation, 24, 25, 55, 68, 70, 84

depression, 7, 10, 92, 100, 103, 104, 107, 114-118

detrended fluctuation analysis, 58

development, neural (developmental), 10, 21-29, 84, 90, 91, 94

diffusion spectrum imaging (DSI), 4, 5, 38-41, 44, 45

diffusion tensor imaging (DTI), 4, 5, 7, 9, 19, 22, 23, 28, 38, 43-46, 65, 72, 87, 89, 92

edge (graph metric), 13-19, 32-35, 38, 42-48

electrocardiogram (ECG, or EKG), 7, 57, 58, 67

electroencephalogram (EEG), 3-10, 13-15, 24, 25, 27, 28, 43, 51-60, 64-75, 83-85, 88-93, 95, 100, 104, 107-115, 118

encephalopathy, 9

endophenotype, 87

epilepsy, temporal lobe (TLE), 71, 72, 74, 89

epilepsy, generalized, 71-74, 89

evoked potentials, 85, 103, 113-15

exponential, 35, 39, 40, 44, 45, 47, 56, 57

facilitation (TMS), 103, 104, 117,

frontal cortex, 24-28, 39, 43, 44, 53, 68, 70, 73, 85-87, 90, 91

functional connectivity, 6-10, 19, 21, 23, 25, 26-28, 36, 46, 54, 55, 67, 70, 84, 89, 90-92, 94, 95, 100, 107-111, 118

functional magnetic resonance imaging (fMRI), 4-10, 25-28, 39, 40, 51, 53, 54, 60, 64-75, 84, 90-92, 100, 107, 108, 111, 112, 118

GABA (GABAergic), 56, 82, 88-90, 94, 95, 103, 104

gamma oscillation, 6, 8, 9, 25, 52, 82, 112

gap junction, 13, 85, 90

glutamate (glutamatergic), 82, 88, 90-92, 94, 104

graph theory, 4, 5, 6, 10, 25, 27, 33, 34, 46, 54, 55

hallucinations, 9, 85, 87-89

heart rate variability (HRV), 7, 57, 58

hippocampus (hippocampal), 9, 74, 82, 91, 92, 116

hypothalamus (hypothalamic), 53, 56, 57

hub, 16, 35, 38-40, 42, 44, 47, 54

insomnia, 7, 52, 54, 59,

inter-ictal activity (or discharges; IEA), 64, 71-75

intracranial recording, 54, 64, 72, 73, 75, 89

intelligence, 28, 35

Kevin Bacon, 33

language, 26, 28, 40, 41, 89, 90, 100, 107

local field potential (LFP), 66, 83, 93

localization (lesion), 3, 6, 7, 10, 72, 73

long term potentiation, 103, 104

long term depression, 103, 104

magnetoencephalography (MEG), 3-10, 51, 83, 84, 89, 91, 93, 95,

markov model, 56

maturation (brain), 22, 24-28

migraine, 8, 9

memory, 6, 53, 54, 70, 81-83, 85, 89, 91, 92, 94, 95, 107, 113, 115

modularity, 38, 40, 41, 48

monkey (or macaque), 37, 38, 44-47, 82,

motor evoked potential (MEP), 103, 104, 106, 113-115, 117

movement disorder, 3, 8, 93

multiple sclerosis, 7, 10, 40, 41, 65, 95,

near infrared spectroscopy (NIRS), 26

non-invasive, 3, 4, 6, 7, 59, 65, 71, 72, 75

nonlinear (or nonlinearity), 14, 15, 35, 92

non-REM sleep (NREM), 52-55, 57, 58, 60, 70, 113-115

occipital cortex, 5, 23-27, 35, 38, 39, 41, 44, 53, 68-70, 72, 82, 87, 102, 107, 108, 111-113, 117